Functional Illness of the Head and Neck

AF794026

Brian W. Blakley • Joan E. Blakley
Editors

Functional Illness of the Head and Neck

Springer

Editors
Brian W. Blakley
Otolaryngology
University of Manitoba
Winnipeg, MB, Canada

Joan E. Blakley
Winnipeg, MB, Canada

ISBN 978-3-031-12997-1 ISBN 978-3-031-12998-8 (eBook)
https://doi.org/10.1007/978-3-031-12998-8

© Editors 2023
This work is subject to copyright. All rights are reserved by the Publisher, whether the whole or part of the material is concerned, specifically the rights of translation, reprinting, reuse of illustrations, recitation, broadcasting, reproduction on microfilms or in any other physical way, and transmission or information storage and retrieval, electronic adaptation, computer software, or by similar or dissimilar methodology now known or hereafter developed.
The use of general descriptive names, registered names, trademarks, service marks, etc. in this publication does not imply, even in the absence of a specific statement, that such names are exempt from the relevant protective laws and regulations and therefore free for general use.
The publisher, the authors and the editors are safe to assume that the advice and information in this book are believed to be true and accurate at the date of publication. Neither the publisher nor the authors or the editors give a warranty, expressed or implied, with respect to the material contained herein or for any errors or omissions that may have been made. The publisher remains neutral with regard to jurisdictional claims in published maps and institutional affiliations.

This Springer imprint is published by the registered company Springer Nature Switzerland AG
The registered company address is: Gewerbestrasse 11, 6330 Cham, Switzerland

Preface

Functional disorders are the most common disorders encountered in clinical practice. This book is intended to help clinicians who deal with patients with functional disorders of the head and neck. Functional illness has been a fascination for me for years, but I don't think anyone truly masters the field. Although the book is focused on Otolaryngology, the lessons apply to all clinicians who treat patients with head and neck disorders, which includes essentially all clinicians. We have tried to keep the writing simple. The book is meant to outline some practical approaches to this challenging group of problems.

Approaches vary and this variation is welcome. The information contained is the responsibility of the authors of the applicable chapters. Notice that from many different angles there seems to be a convergence for some functional disorders toward the use of medications that affect serotoninergic signaling.

I hope you enjoy this book!

Winnipeg, Canada

Brian W. Blakley

Contents

Introduction What Is Functional Illness? 1

Brian W. Blakley

This chapter discusses what functional illness is generally and how it differs from other illness. Other chapters discuss specific problems.

Physicians love to think that we are in control, but we are not. Cognitive dissonance of the expert arises when the expert expects that they should "know" but find that they do not. This book is about coping with things that we do not know enough about. Some of us are uncomfortable with ambiguity and deny it. For linear thinkers, an admission that we "just don't know" is a failure or a sign of weakness. Actually, the opposite is true. Dealing with uncertainty requires strength. No one is just one thing though. We are all linear thinkers at times, and we are all non-linear thinkers at times. We just need to know when we cross from one to the other because each needs a different approach.

In this book, the term "functional illness" refers to symptoms and illness without adequate medical explanation after proper evaluation. "Functional illness" does not just mean "I don't know the cause." There must be an appropriate investigation. The word "idiopathic" has a similar meaning but is more often applied as a disease such as idiopathic pulmonary fibrosis. Of course, the word "disease" implies a known pathological process is ongoing so the term "idiopathic disease" may be an oxymoron. "Medically unexplained symptoms" is another term used. The opposite is often called "organic disease" to suggest that some organ function is deranged. "Linear medicine" is a similar term, referring to a logical sequence of cause-and-effect events that sometimes happens.

In the past, some clinicians used the term "functional illness" as a synonym for "psychogenic" or "imaginary," which is not the meaning herein or that used by modern thinkers [1]. The underlying assumption of those meanings is that anything that we do not understand must be imaginary but, we do not understand everything. This assumption is either cynical or naïve and has obstructed progress for decades.

B. W. Blakley (✉)
Department of Otolaryngology, University of Manitoba, Winnipeg, MB, Canada

© The Author(s), under exclusive license to Springer Nature Switzerland AG 2023

B. W. Blakley, J. E. Blakley (eds.), *Functional Illness of the Head and Neck*,
https://doi.org/10.1007/978-3-031-12998-8_1

Even if psychological factors underlie some symptoms, the assumption that psychological treatments are required does not have strong supportive evidence [2]. Symptoms can certainly be psychogenic [3] but organic causes must be ruled out. The Diagnostic and Statistical Manual of Mental Disorders version 5 (DSM-5) defines a more severe somatic symptom disorder as one "characterized by one or more somatic symptoms that are accompanied by excessive thoughts, feelings, and/or behaviors related to the somatic symptoms" [4]. Most functional disorders are not associated with particular behaviors or excessive thoughts. Some symptoms that are considered psychogenic by the best investigations available today may turn out to have some organic basis in the future. The first step is understanding so it would seem essential that we recognize what shortcomings we have so that we can then work toward their understanding.

There is lots of functional illness. Estimates for the incidence of functional disorders presenting to primary care physicians have been estimated at 15–30% in a Canadian study [5] and 33% in a British study [6]. These numbers are greater than for any of the single system (neoplastic, circulatory, respiratory, digestive systems) reported by the National Ambulatory Medical Care Survey in 2016 [7]. Fink et al. [8] report that estimates of patients with medically unexplained symptom from seven studies of secondary clinics range from 35% to 53%. The incidence may be lower in primary care clinics as Fink indicates that 7–33% of primary care patients across six studies had medically unexplained symptoms. Functional disorders are common in young people. For example, In the US military which should have a preponderance of the young and healthy, Garrett et al. reported that the incidence of functional neuropsychiatric disorders only was 37.5 per 100,000 [9].

Of course, we should take advantage of knowledge and evidence as far as it goes, but when we reach the end of "the known" we must embrace a different thought process. The approach to functional illness should differ from the approach to disorders with evidence base in four main ways.

First, there should be equipoise and individual thinking. Clinicians should acknowledge uncertainty to themselves and their patients. If treatments are non-standard or "off-label," patients must understand and agree. We should speak in terms of probability or "possibly" rather than "best treatment" as much as possible. Many treatments for non-functional diseases are only partially successful. Linear thinkers may provide a more confident but less honest prognosis that applies to groups. Concrete thinkers must learn psychological approaches.

Second, the clinician should pay close attention to treatments that patients think will work. While there are some thoughts that we should reject placebos or treatments that we think should not work, functional illness treatment tolerates placebos. Patients may even realize that the treatment that makes them feel better is a placebo. We should keep an open mind toward possible treatments or things that patients tell us but not support risky or expensive options. If a patient has a strong belief that a particular treatment will work, it is generally worth a try if it is inexpensive, safe, does not preclude other treatments and there is no conflict of interest. On the other hand, physicians sometimes see patients with malignancies or other serious disorders who refuse traditional treatment, deferring to "natural" methods. This is their right but should not be supported by ethical physicians. The physician is often blamed for a bad outcome so it is important to document patient attitudes and decisions and not support a dangerous course of action that may preclude other treatment.

Third, the functional illness approach is more trial-and-error than the linear medicine approach. Somehow this should be communicated when a functional disorder is encountered. Many patients will not cooperate with multiple visits particularly if their symptoms are mild. Reluctance to continue is acceptable if serious disease has been ruled out. Treating functional illness is difficult. The clinician is rarely a hero! Many (most?) patients with functional illnesses believe, or at least hope, that they have a simple treatable disorder, and are impatient with slow progress. Tinnitus is a good example of a disorder which many patients believe should be easily treatable, allowing them to be exploited by claims for cure on the Internet and public media.

Fourth, the functional thought process differs from the traditional, linear sequence of medical evaluation for organic disorders. Clinicians must not focus only on the presenting symptom but include an approach involving consideration of general well-being. For example, when prescribing an antidepressant for chronic pain, we should also ask how patients feel generally. Are they happier? Less stressed? Coping better? Functional illness involves data collected in quantal packages that may seem unrelated. Functional illness does not follow a linear pattern as in Fig. 1.1.

How many times have you seen treatment recommendations based on associated features? In treating functional illness particularly, we should be cautious about treating "correlations," even if they are strong. For example, does lipstick use cause pregnancy? Certainly, there would be a correlation among 1000 randomly selected people. Fortunately, we have other information about the cause of pregnancy, but causes may not be apparent in other situations. Ageing causes many symptoms, but we cannot reverse the aging process. Treating co-existing disorders is often useful but in general we want to treat causes not correlations. Correlations are inserted as proxies for causes. The point is that we should acknowledge whether we think we are treating a cause or an association.

Compliance with therapy is assumed but often absent. Most patients do not take medications as prescribed even if they say they do. If you suspect noncompliance with taking medications but it is being denied, a simple way of detecting false reports is to ask how many times per day they take the drug. If the response is something like, "Whatever it says on the bottle" you know that they have not taken the drug with any regularity.

The interplay between resiliency and burnout is a serious consideration for functional illness. Late signs of burnout include increases in interpersonal problems, physical illness, negative feelings, exhaustion, fatigue, and bad habits such as drugs, smoking, and anger. We all need to detect burnout early and take corrective action. Burnout is best avoided by changing lifestyle when first suspected and not taking on too many commitments. Burnout needs to be considered in functional illness. Burnout affects everyone and is increasing at a rapid rate in modern times. Remember the promises that we would have more leisure time with computers and technology? Somehow the high-tech world we live in has just created more pressure.

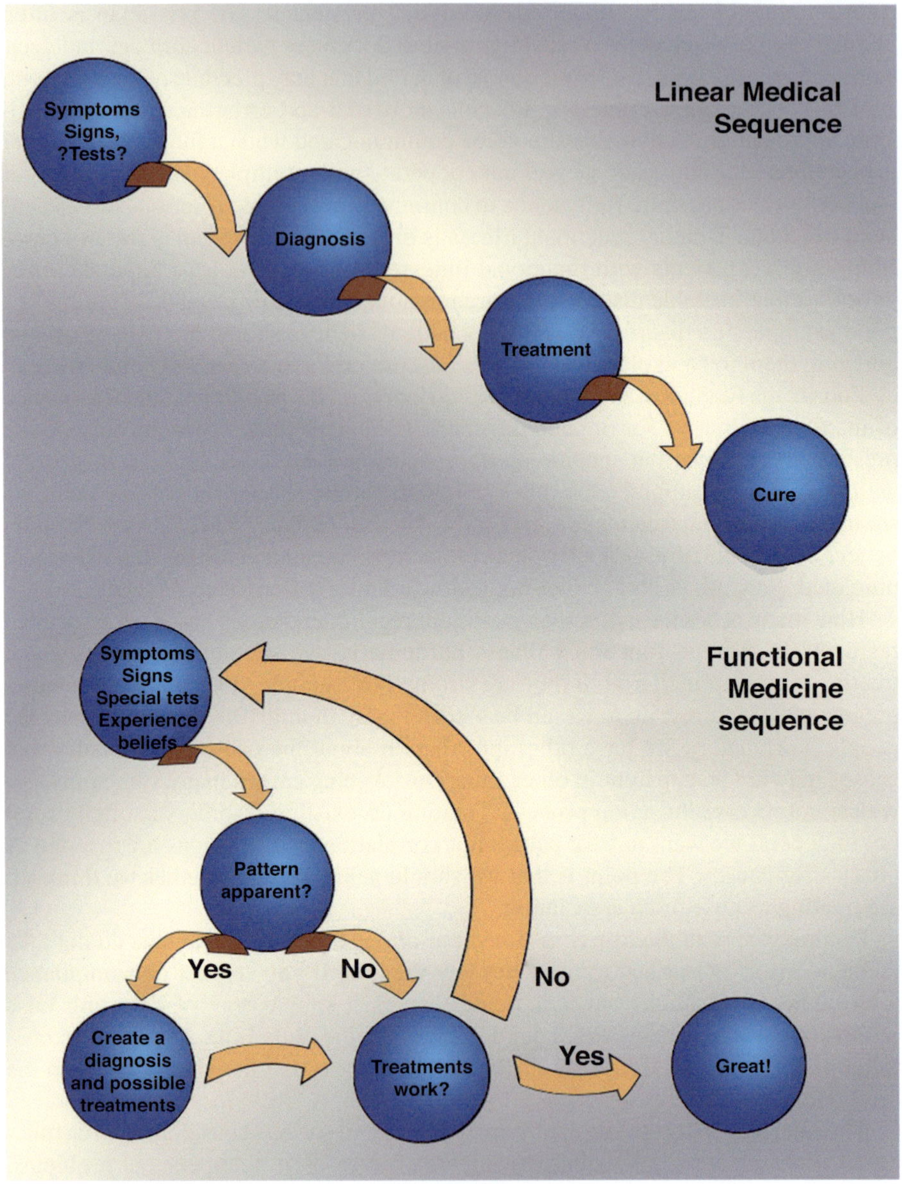

Fig. 1.1 Thought process for Linear versus functional illness contrasted

Reliable outcome percentages are rarely available for functional illness. Functional symptoms are difficult to standardize so there are few valid, randomized, controlled trials for functional illness. The evidence that does exist is fraught with opinion and uncertainty. There are opinions about evidence and evidence about opinions. We know that. Clinical judgement about each individual situation is required. There are no "cook-book" approaches to functional symptoms, but patience and persistence often pay off.

At this point, some rigid enthusiasts of systematic reviews and evidence-based medicine (EBM) will feel their upper lip rising into a sneer, asking, "How can we consider treatment without 'solid' evidence?" The answer is that we must because very few clinical decisions are backed by sufficient, objective, consistent evidence. Clinicians must use judgement, training, and experience. They need not apologize if evidence is lacking.

Evidence is important when available and is not just for bad clinicians anymore. The pinnacle of medical evidence is currently the Cochrane Review project, which is a great achievement. Cochrane methods demand rigor and standards, but most reviews do not reach a conclusion. Systematic reviews are good when the topic is discrete and objective but not for functional problems. We need evidence, but we should recognize that formal EBM and systematic reviews have serious shortcomings. They:

1. *Are not original work,* and have not, and cannot generate original discoveries.
2. *Assume a linear, deterministic world in which the same outcomes follow the same interventions usually under a "normal" or other parametric distribution,* but real life is highly non-linear. Big data findings apply to aggregate populations. Individuals have "contingencies" or circumstances that may become more important in decision making than small differences in mean values. Statistical methods that "control" for contingencies removes them even though they often carry more influence than the entity under study.
3. *Equate size with quality*. The opposite is often correct. Large size is good for aggregate statistics but problematic for individual cases. Large studies of symptoms or specific diseases cannot contain verifiable, quality, individual, clinical evaluations. Some studies involve billing data or other indirect proxies for individualized, quality clinical assessments by experts. Although it is commonly assumed that large sample sizes reduce error rates this is not true for type 1 errors (false positive conclusion) according to Sedgwick, who pointed out that the maximum probability of a type 1 error is always the alpha level involved [10].
4. *May not add up*. Have you ever wondered how an author found a thousand patients with a disorder to study that you, as a specialist in that area, see only four or five per year? In the United States, the Rare Diseases Act of 2002 [11] defines a rare disease as one that affects fewer than 200,000 people in the United States or a prevalence of about 1 in 1500 people. This definition implies that in order to study 1000 subjects, an author would have to personally see all cases of that disorder in a population of 1,500,000.
5. *Raise suspicion* of a finding that requires a thousand subjects to detect a small difference between two treatment means. If a meta-analysis is "needed," the effect is likely small. We should not be ashamed of small, quality studies.
6. *Select out clinically significant differences that become evident to competent clinicians in small studies*. Selecting out smaller, carefully done studies from the literature, favoring fewer, large "n" studies introduces bias. Most clinical

research questions cannot be standardized in homogeneous groups as required for large sample sizes. "One-time-only," "big money" projects may not be reproducible and often come to different conclusions if repeated. Even in areas that we might consider thoroughly researched and "well founded," recommendations may not be as objective as some might think. A review of the levels of evidence for the guidelines of the American College of Cardiology found that only 8.9% had level A evidence, 46.7% were of level B evidence, 44.5% were of level C evidence with large variability on the same topics [12]. Modern administrative roadblocks make it exceedingly difficult to conduct research without a large budget, staff and a pre-formed conclusion based on "pilot data." Small, well-done studies often have more than adequate power to show clinically significant differences. Small differences require large numbers to show statistical significance may not be clinically significant.

7. *Require that all topics of interest have adequate, comparable randomized trials.* Of course, investigators would not embark on a randomized trial of either a well-accepted treatment or highly disregarded treatment, so this assumption is commonly violated. The scope of clinical questions that can be answered with available EBM is limited. Ethical problems arise when randomizing patients to surgical treatments or to those that are known to work or not work.
8. *Suggest that the mean of large numbers*, usually with p-values, is the important parameter, whereas when treating an individual patient, the variability of outcomes is often more important. There is growing appreciation of this concept as evidenced by the increasing requirement for inclusion of effect size in many journals. Clinicians should consider effect size with clinical knowledge of the topic as well as the control group in a study. For example, if we know from clinical experience that half of the patients with a disorder improve spontaneously, we should be suspicious of a study reporting that 60% of the treatment group improves but only 10% of controls. The "number needed to treat" (NNT) can be a useful statistic. A useful exercise might be to add up all the incidences of all the disorders that you read about in a year then ask yourself how it is possible that there are any healthy people alive. Remember that 80% of statistics are made up [13].

We should pay attention to evidence when it makes sense, but how do we deal with functional problems when reliable evidence is not available? How do we proceed when we do not know what is best? For functional illness, we need to be empiric, not theoretical. We should simply do what works. There may be theories and basic science to support them, but these often change with time. Outcomes, regardless of pathophysiology do not change though. Empiricism is king in functional illness. Establishing and updating consensus about treatment outcomes across many centers should be the priority of guideline committees.

Down-sides to treatment options such as safety and cost must be considered. We should have more confidence in treatments for functional illnesses for which more unbiased consensus is evident. Understanding treatments and their limitations is the basis for medical training. Functional treatments come to be accepted by consensus established by formal communications such as meetings, books and published papers. The nature of functional illnesses dictates that some of the methods in such papers will be considered "flawed" and will require clinical knowledge and experience for interpretation, rather than blind reliance on statistics. Things can change though. As with evidence-based medicine, consensus should be under constant review and discussion, most of which will not be found in research papers—yet. There are degrees of consensus and uncertainty to weigh when considering a therapy.

Treatments for functional disorders should involve patient understanding, and be of low cost, low risk, and not preclude other proven treatments. Finally, the provider should not be in a conflict-of-interest situation. We propose consideration of the guidelines presented in Table 1.1 when recommending treatments for functional illness.

What is a cause anyway? We prefer to see an orderly linear progression of circumstances that follow one another and lead to some result as in Fig. 1.1. We assign the term "cause" to that progression, but It must be acknowledged that there are different levels of causation and they do not always follow a linear sequence. Alwyn Scott discusses these issues very well in his book The Nonlinear Universe: Chaos, Emergence Life [14]. Scott examines the thoughts of Aristotle who identified four levels of cause. The first is a "Material Cause" which refers to some physical substance that is necessary for an outcome. Obesity is caused by food, for example. The second level of cause is the "Formal cause" which refers to the need for certain materials to be present in a particular form. Food should be available after certain preparations have been made. The Material and Formal causes have been lumped together as *distal* causes according to Scott. The third level of cause is "Efficient Cause" which refers to the need for a particular agent that starts the process on its way. Someone must eat food for obesity to occur. The "efficient cause" is what science might think of as a *stimulus-response* relationship. For the mathematically inclined, Scott cites the use of a differential equation with a forcing term as an example of the Efficient cause of the dependent variable. Scott indicates that the Efficient cause can be thought of as the *proximate* cause which is used in the legal world to mean the act or action that caused a person's injury. Proximate cause is usually what we commonly think of as "the cause." The fourth level of cause is the "Final cause" which refers to the events that come about by the desire of an

Table 1.1 Guidelines for treatment of functional illness

Item	Discussion
Patient understands that treatment may not be "standard"	Some patients do not understand the subtleties of the issues involved
Low cost to the patient	Willingness to absorb costs varies across patients
Low risk to the patient	Risks vary across patients
Does not preclude other treatment	Time constraints or interactions may not allow or complicate some forms of treatment
No conflict of interest of the provider	Some providers have difficulty separating their interests from patient's interests

organism. Food digestion and metabolism must occur for obesity. The final cause is often thought to be teleological and disregarded, which is unfortunate. For functional illness we want to mitigate any cause that we can with a realistic intervention.

Even if there is a linear series of events leading to an outcome, there are always levels of understanding. For example, bacterial infection would seem to have a known cause and yet there are many aspects of infections that we do not understand. For example, why did this peritonsillar abscess happen now to this person and why in this location? It seems clear that better treatment results happen in disorders that we understand and that functional disorders have lower "cure" rates in general [15–17].

How do we cope when we do not understand something that we care about? First, we try to understand it. We think about it. We might read about it. We ask others about it. We develop theories and perform thought experiments to test the conclusions. Sometimes this works but often not. What do we do if we still cannot understand? At this point, actions vary, and these variations are important to recognize in ourselves, but more importantly in others. Some of us just adopt the best theory available as the truth. Some give up. Others just make up a new belief system and insist it is correct. Many of the key questions in life and death do not have provable answers yet many people have unshakeable beliefs about these issues. The noble action is to acknowledge ignorance and deliberately try to create knowledge. First, we must recognize the extent of our knowledge.

Medical specialty committees are fond of creating and revising guidelines and diagnostic criteria for functional disorders. Usually, these are sincere attempts to improve the lives of sufferers, but some are just guesswork. Some committees will conclude that different presentations and different constellations of symptoms are different diseases, but are they? If the treatment, prognosis and outcomes are similar perhaps they are the same thing with different presentations. How many times have the criteria for Meniere's disease changed without any new treatments or knowledge about the pathophysiology? Headache classifications identify different outcomes among different entities, but there is a lot of commonality too. Placing a name on something often makes us feel like we understand it and are in control, but we need to realize when this fallacy of control creates a false sense of security.

Committees are fond of "feel-good" recommendations such as a "multidisciplinary approach" but members rarely follow this advice themselves. True multidisciplinary clinics for functional illnesses are rare. Actual evidence that a committee effort is better than a coherent plan by an enlightened clinician is generally absent. "Multidisciplinary" often means "refer to many other specialists" but this may be just shifting responsibility and leaves the patient or even their primary care physician with nothing but a list of contradictory suggestions. Referral is certainly indicated if there is a valid indication but should not create a therapeutic merry-go-round that leads nowhere. Another "feel-good" suggestion that we should question is the implication that functional illness is always treatable if the patient just follows all the advice. In fact, we do not have all the answers and blaming the patient for failures is inappropriate.

Clinicians must also be aware that uncertainty opens the door to scams. Any medically bothersome disorder without a simple cure is an opportunity for scammers. Greater uncertainty begats more scams. The Internet is the largest source of misinformation on the planet and is hyped by the media, and conspiracy theorists creating doubt and a lack of trust for professionals. Arthritis, tinnitus, and mental health disorders are examples but there are many others. While we need to be open-minded about novel treatments, ethical clinicians have a duty to speak up when fraud arises.

Functional disorders frequently have certain characteristics. They are often vague, and their description varies if the patient is asked to describe the symptoms again. Functional symptoms may be present in patients who present with many unrelated symptoms [6]. Functional symptoms often have an identifiable trigger or inciting event [18] such as minor trauma, infection or stress. Viral illness is a common trigger. Interestingly, the trauma or viral illness that triggers is typically not severe itself.

Organic disorders are typically recognized with a single symptom or pattern of symptoms, but functional disorders tend to occur with multiple, variable symptoms. Escobar et al. defined somatization as four or more unexplained physical symptoms in men and six or more unexplained physical symptoms in women. Escobar et al. reported that the lifetime prevalence of somatization in was 4.4% [19]. Another study did not find that female gender was associated with functional disorders [20].

There is hope though. More clinicians are trying to cope with functional illness, trying treatments such as medications, psychological therapy, discussing personal issues (counselling) or sometimes just explanation. Attitudes are changing and there is more empathy for functional illness sufferers. The specifics are discussed in other chapters in this book, but as you look at the various chapters in this book, note for example, how many symptoms are now starting to be treated with antidepressants such as tricyclics, selective serotonin reuptake inhibitors (SSRIs), selective serotonin norepinephrine reuptake inhibitors (SNRIs). Up to 75% of patients with chronic dizziness improved with an SSRI [21].

References

1. Bransfield RC, Friedman KJ. Differentiating psychosomatic, somatopsychic, multisystem illnesses, and medical uncertainty. Healthcare (Basel). 2019;7:4.
2. Wilshire CE, Ward T. Psychogenic explanations of physical illness: time to examine the evidence. Perspect Psychol Sci. 2016;11(5):606–31.
3. Galli S, Tatu L, Bogousslavsky J, Aybek S. Conversion, factitious disorder and malingering: a distinct pattern or a continuum? Front Neurol Neurosci. 2018;42:72–80.
4. American Psychiatric Association. Diagnostic and statistical manual of mental disorders, fifth edition (DSM-5). 5th ed. Arlington: American Psychiatric Association; 2013.
5. Kirmayer LJ, Groleau D, Looper KJ, Dao MD. Explaining medically unexplained symptoms. Can J Psychiatr. 2004;49(10):663–72.
6. Duddu V, Husain N, Dickens C. Medically unexplained presentations and quality of life: a study of a predominantly south Asian primary care population in England. J Psychosom Res. 2008;65(4):311–7.

7. Rui POT. National Ambulatory Medical Care Survey: 2016 National Summary Tables 2016 [Table 14]. https://www.cdc.gov/nchs/data/ahcd/namcs_summary/2016_namcs_web_tables.pdf.
8. Fink PFK, Söllner W. Medically unexplained symptoms, somatisation and bodily distress: developing better clinical services. Cambridge: Cambridge University Press; 2011. p. 217–35.
9. Garrett A, Hodges S, Stalman S. Epidemiology of functional neurological disorder, Active Component, U.S. Armed Forces, 2000–2018 2020 [The Official Website of the Military Health System].
10. Sedgwick P. Pitfalls of statistical hypothesis testing: type I and type II errors. BMJ. 2014;349:g4287.
11. Rare Diseases Act, United States Congress, 107th session Sess. 2002.
12. Bevan GH, Kalra A, Josephson RA, Al-Kindi SG. Level of scientific evidence underlying the Current American College of Cardiology/American Heart Association clinical practice guidelines. Circ Cardiovasc Qual Outcomes. 2019;12(2):e005293.
13. BW B. OK. I made that statistic up. Had you thinking though didn't it? 2021.
14. Scott AC. The nonlinear universe: chaos, emergence, life. Springer; 2007. p. 371.
15. Häuser W, Fitzcharles MA. Facts and myths pertaining to fibromyalgia. Dialogues Clin Neurosci. 2018;20(1):53–62.
16. Kisely S, Forbes M, Sawyer E, Black E, Lalloo R. A systematic review of randomized trials for the treatment of burning mouth syndrome. J Psychosom Res. 2016;86:39–46.
17. Larun L, Brurberg KG, Odgaard-Jensen J, Price JR. Exercise therapy for chronic fatigue syndrome. Cochrane Database Syst Rev. 2016;12(12):Cd003200.
18. Albrecht PJ, Rice FL. Fibromyalgia syndrome pathology and environmental influences on afflictions with medically unexplained symptoms. Rev Environ Health. 2016;31(2):281–94.
19. Escobar JI, Burnam MA, Karno M, Forsythe A, Golding JM. Somatization in the community. Arch Gen Psychiatry. 1987;44(8):713–8.
20. Creed F, Barsky A. A systematic review of the epidemiology of somatisation disorder and hypochondriasis. J Psychosom Res. 2004;56(4):391–408.
21. Staab JP, Ruckenstein MJ, Amsterdam JD. A prospective trial of sertraline for chronic subjective dizziness. Laryngoscope. 2004;114(9):1637–41.

Some Basic Science and Functional Illness

2

Brian W. Blakley and Cory Bosecke

Psychological factors are critical in functional illness. Some basic science of anxiety is discussed in this chapter, and depression is considered in other chapters.

The Immune System and Inflammation

The immune system and the inflammatory response are not what they used to be, and it is not clear what they are anymore. The classic description of inflammation was proposed in the first century by Aulus Cornelius Celsus (in Latin) as redness (rubor), warmth (calor), swelling (tumor), and pain (dolor). In the nineteenth century, Virchow added loss of function to the list. He did not include leukocytosis, another classic feature. These classic concepts have served clinical practice well. Over time, though they have been abrogated by collections of cytokines and biomarkers, even in the absence of "classic signs" of inflammation as in Table 2.1.

Confusion about the nature of inflammation fosters promises that a product will "boost your immune system." These claims abound even though many functional disorders have hyperactive or autoimmune aspects. The logic of "boosting" a system that is already pathologically overactive seems perverse. Anti-inflammatory drugs often do not treat "inflammatory" disorders. Many "inflammatory" disorders have none of the classic signs of inflammation.

Part of the confusion results from the complexity of the immune system. The "immune system" is actually many systems and sub-systems. Even if one part is enhanced, others may not be. Medications may affect one part but not others.

B. W. Blakley (✉)
Department of Otolaryngology, University of Manitoba, Winnipeg, MB, Canada

C. Bosecke (✉)
Biomedical Engineering Program, University of Manitoba, Winnipeg, MB, Canada

© The Author(s), under exclusive license to Springer Nature Switzerland AG 2023

B. W. Blakley, J. E. Blakley (eds.), *Functional Illness of the Head and Neck*,
https://doi.org/10.1007/978-3-031-12998-8_2

Table 2.1 Classic features of inflammation

Localized	Systemic
Local wound redness	Fever
Local edema	Organ edema
Pain/tenderness	Generalized pain
Muscle, joint dysfunction	Organ failure
Histologic: Leukocyte response	Elevated WBC

Readers interested in more detail may consult a standard book in the field, such as the one by Roitt [1]. Briefly, there are two main immune systems to review and consider in patients with functional illness—the innate immune system and the adaptive immune system.

The *innate immune system* is present at birth and is inherited genetically. It has been thought to be minimally modifiable, but modern medicine has shown that parts of it can be "trained." The innate immune system is responsible for the "classic signs" of inflammation. It includes cellular barrier functions, the microbiome (population of bacteria in the GI tract principally), the inflammasome (which is a central immune regulator), pattern recognition receptors (PRRs) that are sensors of foreign peptides present on cell surfaces, pattern-associated molecular patterns (PAMPS), which are present on microbial cell surfaces, various intracellular enzymes, antimicrobial peptides, such as defensins and cathelicidins, cell sensors for bacteria, such as toll-like receptors (TLRs), cytokines, chemokines, and a variety of leucocytes and other cells. The innate system recognizes PRRs that are specific to microorganisms but not the host, such as lipopolysaccharide, a prototypical PAMP, which is common to a wide range of pathogens [2]. Vitamin D is important in innate immunity (see Chaps. 18 and 19).

Although often ignored, the innate immune system is critical for survival as a defense against microorganisms. The innate system is the first-line, rapid responder defense against microbes. Remember that it takes days or weeks to develop antibodies and mount defenses from the adaptive immune system, whereas bacterial counts can double in 30 min in the right environment if unchecked.

The other major immune system is the adaptive or acquired immune system. The major cellular components of the adaptive immune system are the B and T cells. B cells respond to antigens by producing antibodies which circulate in the blood and bind to specific antigens. If microorganisms enter the cell, T cells become critical. The T cells of most importance are helper T cells (TH cells or CD-4+ T cells) and cytotoxic T cells (CD8+ T cells). The two most important types of helper T cells (TH cells) are TH-1 and TH-2 cells. TH-1 cells produce interferon-gamma, interleukin (IL)-2, and tumor necrosis factor-beta(TNFβ)-, and are triggered by intracellular bacterial infections. TH-1 cells are thought to arise from the influence of microbiotia. TH-1 cells are associated with autoimmune disease of specific organs and skin disorders, among others. TH-1 inflammation is associated with IL-2, IL-12, interferon gamma (INF-γ), tumor necrosis factor alpha (TNF-α), and may be a consideration in treating functional illness. TH-2 cells produce IL-4, IL-5, IL-10, and IL-13 and are related to allergy and helminth infections [3]. Imbalance of TH-1 and TH-2 systems seems to contribute to recurrent infections and autoimmune disorder such as lupus.

Immune physiology is highly relevant when treating various functional disorders that may be inflammatory or allergic. NSAIDs inhibit cyclooxygenase enzymes (COX-1 and COX-2) that produce prostaglandins and prostacyclins, which are commonly used to treat some inflammatory conditions. See Fig. 2.1. On the other hand, many disorders caused by "inflammation" do not respond to NSAIDs, suggesting that the term "inflammation" may not apply there. Do biomarkers and cytokines trump classic signs and now define "inflammation"? There are clinical differences between presentations with classic inflammation and modern or "cytokine" inflammation. The disorders that respond best to NSAIDs are those with classic signs of inflammation, but the distinction is incomplete. Functional disorders without classic signs are less likely to find relief with NSAIDs or glucocorticoids.

"Neuroinflammation" has been implicated in many functional disorders, but what is it? Some authors paradoxically equate chronic pain without classic signs of inflammation as neuroinflammation. A recent review of neuroinflammation [4] discussed the cytokines involved in neuroinflammation, but classic signs of inflammation are notably absent. "Neuromodulation" refers to compounds that affect nerve function by modulating neurotransmitters and might be a more accurate term for some disorders caused by neuroinflammation.

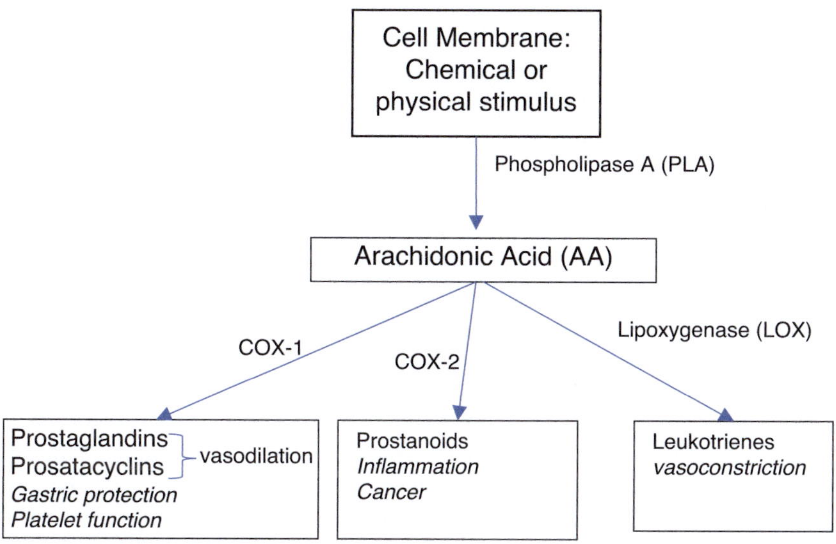

Fig. 2.1 Arachidonic acid (AA) and cyclooxygenase (COX) summary. Chemical or physical stimuli phospholipase A generates AA from cell membranes. Two of the metabolic pathways of AA metabolism are via COX and LOX. NSAIDS that are "specific" for COX-2 (celecoxib, rofecoxib and to a lesser extent, meloxicam and etodolac) should inhibit mediators of inflammation but tend to leave gastric protection and platelet function intact. LOX is not affected by COX-inhibitors

The question of autoimmunity arises frequently in functional illness. There are currently over 90 forms of autoimmunity, so the field is complex with a wide variety of mechanisms and levels of understanding. NSAIDs and glucocorticoids are appropriate for some disorders but not others, suggesting that the general implication of the immune system is open to question or at least re-definition. Obesity and diabetes mellitus are two common examples of "autoimmune" disorders without pain, fever, or leukocytosis, although loss of function is present. Additionally, simply finding an immune response in a disease state is not adequate to assume that autoimmune disease is present. Direct evidence of autoimmunity may involve the observation that transferring the antibody from diseased to healthy subjects induces the disease in question. There is no universal mechanism for autoimmunity.

Antioxidants

How often do you hear of someone advocating antioxidants? Daily someone insists that we should consume more antioxidants in our food, vitamins, supplements, or drugs. Are antioxidants even relevant? Actually, they are. Antioxidants relate to oxidation–reduction (REDOX) reactions. REDOX reactions involve loss or gain of electrons, which is a central consideration for biochemical antioxidant activity. REDOX considerations determine which chemical reactions will occur. Oxygen-free radicals are highly reactive REDOX chemical species with an unpaired electron in their outer shell, so they have the potential to cause great damage even though they typically last only a few milliseconds. Free radicals and REDOX considerations are known to be important in a wide range of diseases. These facts make antioxidant and REDOX considerations extremely important in physiology.

Simple REDOX reactions involve two chemical species—one loses electron(s) and is oxidized while another gains the electron(s) and is reduced. The species that is oxidized has reduced the other, so it can be called the reductant. Similarly, the other species is an oxidant. If you peruse topics at your local bookstore, you will come across a wide range of books that purport antioxidants for treatment of all sorts of medical problems, including cancer, infections, inflammation, diabetes, hypertension, etc. the list goes on. One could conclude from this that oxidation is the major cause of disease and should be stopped, but oxidation is not always undesirable. Many of the assertions in such books are based on unfounded beliefs. Not all antioxidants are good or bad. A complete discussion of REDOX issues is beyond the scope of this book. Readers who desire more in-depth biological REDOX information than contained in this very brief review may wish to consult a standard book on the topic such as the one by Halliwell and Gutteridge [5].

Many important intracellular REDOX events occur in the inner membrane of mitochondria where the electron transport chain is found. It is estimated that 80–90% of O_2 taken into our bodies is used in mitochondria to produce adenosine triphosphate (ATP). Biochemically, the process of conversion of food sources into energy results from the oxidation of sugars and fats. They are oxidized (lose electrons) to electron carriers such as nicotinamide adenine dinucleotide or flavins or other electron carriers, which are then metabolized to produce ATP. We need to seriously consider which processes should be stopped.

There are many REDOX paradoxes. For example, exercise is generally regarded as a very safe way to improve health in many aspects, but aerobic exercise is one of the most potent generators of oxygen-free radicals. Clinicians often supply oxygen to patients and consider reduced oxygen as bad, yet oxygen is toxic in high concentrations. In high, prolonged concentrations, oxygen damages lungs, causes retinopathy of prematurity, and enhances the toxicity of radiation on cells. Millions of years ago the atmosphere contained much less oxygen than in the present day so anaerobic organisms flourished. This changed so that about 300 million years ago the atmosphere contained about 35% O_2 and only those species that developed antioxidant defenses survived [5].

No chemical species is always an oxidant or a reductant by itself. Each species has a certain tendency to gain or lose electrons, but the direction of electron flow depends on the relative tendencies of the species involved. One is oxidized. The other is reduced, which is why they are called REDOX reactions. Each species operates as a half cell. Chemists use the standard hydrogen electrode (SHE) as a comparator to measure the tendency to gain or lose electrons against. The range of highly oxidizing to highly reducing biologically active half cells ranges from 2.31 to −2.84 V according to Table 2.3 from Halliwell and Gutteridge [5]. Although vitamins are often touted as powerful antioxidants, their half-cell potentials are usually in the midrange of that table and not particularly impressive. Ascorbic acid (vitamin C), for example, is 0.28 V and α-tocopherol (vitamin D) is 0.5 V referenced to SHE. These vitamins are not strong antioxidants, and this may be why these vitamins do not live up to the antioxidant hype.

Several questions arise for clinicians. Is there a benefit to changing the REDOX potential? If so, should we raise or lower it? How should we do it? While many diseases are thought to result from oxidative processes, we may upset an optimal equilibrium if we tamper inappropriately. The honest answer is that we don't know.

There is considerable room for suspicion of the health-related claims of antioxidants. Essentially, all compounds are antioxidants when compared to certain others. Even if they function as antioxidants in one chemical milieu, so what? What do they do for the rest of metabolism? For clinicians dealing with functional illness, it seems we should not worry too much about whether any drug or food is an antioxidant or not. We should rely on empirical, quality research if there is any, and then consensus if there is any, considering cost and safety before recommending any product.

Physiology of Pain

Pain is a major feature in many forms of functional illness. Acute pain is useful and important. It helps us avoid injury and alerts us when something is not right in our bodies. Chronic pain, typically defined as pain lasting longer than 3 months, can be a problem. Pain is complex. Complete discussion of pain is beyond the scope of this book, although some chapters discuss pain in their specific areas. Readers interested in richer information may wish to consult a book such as one by Cheng and Rosenquist [6]. Some key summary points to consider about pain are:

1. Chronic pain is often present without tissue damage or inflammation; however, inflammation is defined. Pains in the neck and low back and other areas are common and we often blame "arthritis" of the spine, but the degree of discomfort correlates poorly with radiologic and neurologic findings.
2. Peripheral and central sensitization commonly cause chronic pain. Neuropathies and neuralgias are examples of peripheral sensitization, and migraine and fibromyalgia are examples of central sensitization.
3. Nociceptors are sensory organs in the skin, muscles, joints, bone, viscera, and dura. Nociceptors sense pain caused by physical, thermal, or inflammatory tissue damage, called nociceptive pain, but they also sense touch and deep pressure. Nociceptive pain may respond to treatment with steroidal or non-steroidal anti-inflammatory (NSAID) medications, opioids, and other analgesics. Nociceptive pain occurs when the system is responding appropriately to some painful stimulus and may relate to classic inflammation. Many medications are reported to reduce markers of inflammation such as C-reactive protein (CRP), but lack evidence that they reduce pain. One example is the statins [7], but these are known to cause muscle pain.
4. Neuropathic pain occurs when the nervous system itself is faulty but is structurally intact. Neuropathic pain is common in functional illness. Post-herpetic neuralgia, peripheral neuropathy, migraine, and fibromyalgia are examples. Treatment of neuropathic pain with NSAIDs, and aspirin is thought to be ineffective. In clinical practice, this notion has merit and should be kept in mind when treating functional illness.

Neural Pain Pathways

Many textbooks discuss the spinal pathways from peripheral to sacral, lumbar, and thoracic regions to dorsal root ganglia, lateral spinothalamic tract, thalamus, and cortex. This information is helpful for neck and "infraclavicular" pain, but not for facial pain. In the head, the sensory information is carried by cranial nerve V, as well as VII, IX, and X, and reaches the trigeminal nucleus before entering the thalamus then the cortex. The default assumption is that physiology in the trigeminal nucleus is similar to that in the dorsal horn, but the histology in the two areas differs. This difference may underlie some clinical differences. For example, there is no migraine outside the head.

It appears that the perception that a stimulus is unpleasant occurs at the level of the thalamus. This consideration is of great importance when treating functional illness with chronic pain. Medications such as NSAIDS, and aspirin that act peripherally may be less effective for chronic functional head and neck pain. Medications that act centrally such as selective serotonin reuptake inhibitors (SSRIs), serotonin norepinephrine reuptake inhibitors (SNRIs) or "gabaergic" medications such as

Gabapentin, and Pregabalin are more likely to work but they take time. Remember that benzodiazepines are also gabaergic. These issues are discussed in more depth in other chapters.

Can massage help? Many patients report that simple massage helps their neck pain or headache. Children who fall or bump something often feel better if their parent rubs the overlying skin. Is this all placebo? Psychological factors account for some of the effect but a well-described physiological phenomenon is also involved. In 1965, Melzak and Wall were awarded the Nobel prize for reporting the "gate control" theory of pain control, which seems to be an explanation. To explain the gate control theory, we need a little neurophysiology of pain … not too much though. More might be painful.

Nociceptive fibers that conduct pain to the dorsal horns of the spine include "C" fibers, Aδ and Aβ fibers. Aβ fibers are myelinated, low-threshold fibers in the skin and joints that sense touch, movement, and vibration. Aδ fibers are thinly myelinated, high-threshold fibers that sense the acute, first wave of pain. "C" fibers are unmyelinated, high-threshold fibers that act of long duration and cause the sensation of pain to persist. For ongoing pain, it is the "C" fibers that we should shut down. Melzak and Wall showed that activation of the Aβ fibers can stimulate an interneuron that inhibits "C" fibers, so touch (Aβ sensation) can inhibit the response of "C" fibers through an interneuron, reducing pain (see Fig. 2.2). Discovery of the gate control mechanism led to the acceptance of the transcutaneous electrical nerve stimulation (TENS) devices. The same mechanism would explain some of the therapeutic benefits of topical gels, massage, and acupuncture, all of which should be considered when treating functional illness. Note that the Aβ fibers have low thresholds and are therefore activated by lesser degrees of stimulation than the "C" fibers. Aβ have some pain sensation as well, so do not press too hard.

Pain pathways are bidirectional, meaning that cortical activation and psychological factors can modify (either increase or reduce) the pain experience. During wars

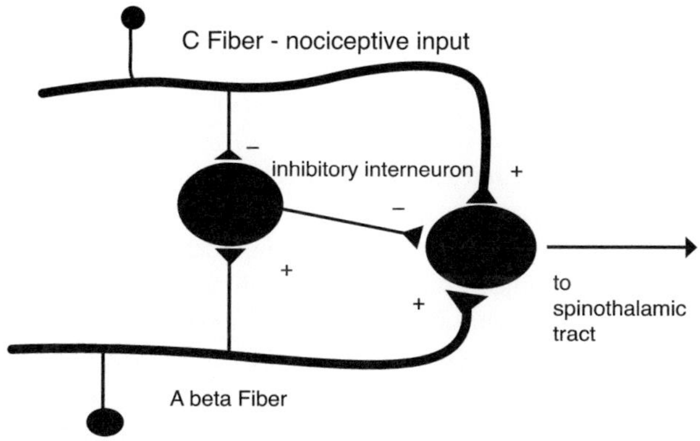

Fig. 2.2 Gate control theory of pain. Painful, nociceptive fibers conduct pain sensation to the thalamus via the spinothalamic tract. Activation of the touch receptor in A beta fibers can stimulate an interneuron that is inhibitory to the C fiber activity, reducing the pain sensation

or even major sporting events, participants may not realize that they have been injured until a time of relaxation occurs. Anxiety, depression, and other psychological factors can have a profound effect on pain perception.

One practical clinical application of Aβ physiology can be applied to patients who present with ear pressure but not pain, and do not have hearing loss, eustachian tube dysfunction, or middle ear fluid. In the absence of other findings, it is likely that idiopathic ear pressure is a variation of the sensation of pain/pressure mediated by Aβ fibers. Treatment for bothersome chronic functional ear pressure without pain should be considered with centrally acting agents such as SSRIs and SNRIs instead of NSAIDs or steroids.

Is there a Convergence of Treatment of Functional Symptoms?

There appears to be an evolving convergence that serotonergic medications such as SSRIs and SNRIs are useful in the treatment of some functional disorders but not others, suggesting that there could be some common causes. This convergence becomes apparent when considering other chapters in this book. The afferent and efferent neurotransmitters in the peripheral vestibular system are glutamine and acetylcholine, respectively, but glutaminergic anticholinergic medications do not seem to be as helpful for functional dizziness as the serotonergic group. The thalamus may be the site where sensations from the periphery are interpreted as unpleasant or not, suggesting a common site of dysfunction for some functional disorders such as chronic dizziness or pain. Neural pathways for anxiety involve the thalamus via the hippocampus. Inflammatory/autoimmune disorders such as Sjogren's disease, HIV, and sarcoidosis are associated with small fiber neuropathy, which is also implicated in fibromyalgia, metabolic syndrome, and neurotoxicity [8]. Perhaps there are some common causes.

There are efforts to identify neurological biomarkers for anxiety, which we explore next.

Anxiety by Cory Bosecke

The National Institute of Mental Health reports that anxiety disorders are the most common mental illnesses, as they affect 19.1% of Americans every year, with a lifetime prevalence of 31.1% [9]. Currently, diagnoses are based on psychiatric assessments that rely on subjective measures, such as self-reported symptoms and retrospective accounts of patient histories [10]. Patients are often misdiagnosed and many do not receive adequate treatment [10]. New technologies are needed to provide objective data that facilitate more accurate diagnoses, as the fields of neuroimaging and genetics have yet to uncover biomarkers that are sufficiently robust to be used in the clinic [11]. Meanwhile, only a few classes of drugs exist for treating anxiety disorders, but these drugs are not always effective and can produce intolerable side effects, suggesting research should identify new targets for therapeutic development [12]. Critically, articles dealing with anxiolytics seldom contain knowledge about the hippocampal theta rhythm (hTheta)—a potential biological marker for anxiety—the perturbance of which appears to be a common mechanism of action for drugs that treat anxiety [13]. A better understanding of the role hTheta plays in anxiety could lead to the development of new tools for diagnosing and treating patients with anxiety disorders [10, 13].

According to "The Diagnostic and Statistical Manual of Mental Disorders," fifth edition (DSM-5), the criteria for generalized anxiety disorder (GAD) begin with: "The presence of excessive anxiety and worry about a variety of topics, events, or activities [14]." GAD is interesting because drugs that treat it, namely "anxiolytics," lower the frequency of hTheta [15].

But what *is* anxiety—what is happening inside a brain that is in a state of anxiety—and how can it become pathological? Any attempt to uncover the neurological underpinnings of anxiety disorders should logically begin by identifying the mechanisms of anxiety proper. In this regard, MIT researchers developed an animal model for anxiety in which circuits that arise from networks of neurons, distributed among several *specific* brain regions, process stimuli to determine response [12]. The model describes four stages—"detection," "interpretation," "evaluation," and "response" circuits—that process stimuli and, if the environment is deemed sufficiently risky, drive an anxiety-like response [12]. Stimuli are *detected* in the thalamus, after which information travels forward and is *interpreted* by the amygdala, bed nucleus of the stria terminalis (BNST), ventral hippocampus (vHPC), and medial prefrontal cortex (mPFC), which then cause their downstream effectors that make up the *response* circuits (namely the hypothalamus, brainstem nuclei, and motor cortex), to trigger the observable effects of anxiety (e.g., increases in glucocorticoid circulation, heart rate, and risk avoidance, respectively) [12]. Information then travels backward, from the mPFC and vHPC to the BNST and amygdala, to *evaluate* interpretation and "prevent unchecked activation of proanxiety circuits [12]." See Fig. 2.3. Critically, *threat* is interpreted if more basolateral amygdala (BLA) neuronal populations are recruited by the projections of circuits pushing for defensive behavior than of those pushing for exploration [12].

It is important to note that anxiety is a normal, healthy function that is essential for survival [12], and is only pathological if it is persistent and there is significant difficulty controlling it [9, 16].

Calhoon and Tye (2015) suggest that *hTheta* could synchronize the local field potentials (LFPs) of regions in their model to time activity and facilitate "well-defined behavioural responses" [12]. This 1–2 mV, ~5–12 Hz nearly sinusoidal rhythm is the largest normal extracellular synchronous signal in the brains of mammals [17]. Elicited by brainstem nuclei, it originates in the HPC [17], and is believed to facilitate coordinated activity between distant regions [18]. It is thought to play an important role in several processes—including anxiety [19]—however, intracranial electrodes are required to record it directly [17]. Because of this, it has been recorded and studied extensively in animals, but very seldom in humans [20]. Despite this, much has been accomplished by the limited number of these intracranial electroencephalography (iEEG) studies that have been performed, as Ruzich

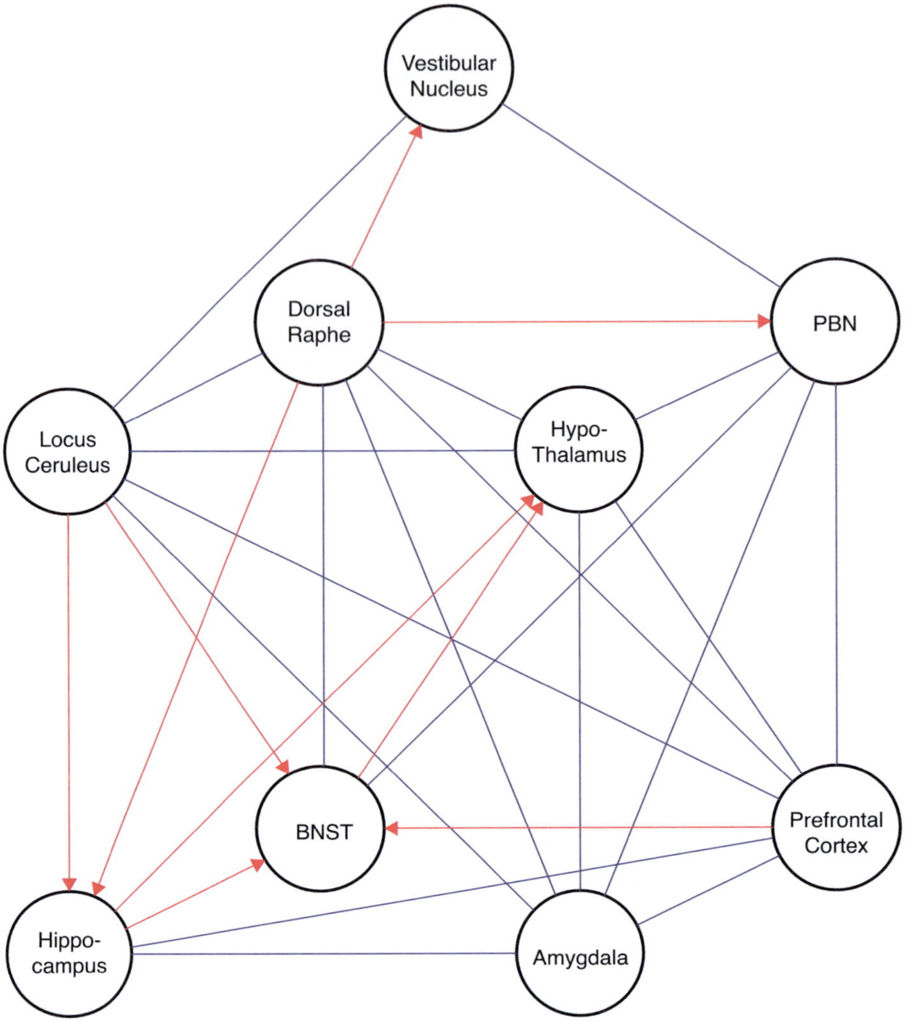

Fig. 2.3 Anatomical connections between the VN and main regions implicated in anxiety disorders. The blue lines represent bidirectional connections, and the red arrows are unidirectional projections

et al. (2018) point out [20], including the discovery of rhythmicity in the HPC that covers the same frequency range as hTheta in rodents, and that is similarly modified by behavior [21].

Lesion and inactivation studies have shown that the ventral hippocampus (vHPC) is necessary for mice to exhibit anxiety-like behavior (in free-roaming assays that model anxiety) [18, 22, 23].

EEG recording of hippocampal activity has been performed via intracranial electrodes, on a few occasions, in epilepsy patients undergoing seizure monitoring. In a 2005 study [21], Ekstrom et al. recorded signals from the hippocampus proper while patients navigated a virtual environment on a computer screen [21]. Interestingly, power spectra from the EEG data revealed prominent activity in the same (4–12 Hz) range that is seen in rodents [18, 21]. Signals increased in power and frequency with movement speed, which was virtual [21]. The authors declared that this was the first demonstration of behavior-modulated 4–7 Hz oscillations in the human HPC. They studied 4–7 Hz but pointed out *broadening the theta band to include frequencies classically analyzed in the rat does not affect our overall findings*, see Fig. 2.4 [21]. This study shows that there is theta range rhythmic activity in the human HPC that is modulated by behavior.

One of the difficulties in identifying biomarkers for anxiety disorders is that the deepest regions of the brain are implicated [20]. While functional magnetic resonance imaging (fMRI) can provide superior spatial resolution of neural activity among the anxiety-implicated hippocampus, amygdala, and prefrontal cortex (collectively, the "emotional triad"), activity is measured indirectly, via changes in blood flow, producing temporal resolution that is inadequate for monitoring the phasic interactions that putatively underlie anxiety communications [20]. Conversely, electroencephalography (EEG) and magnetoencephalography (MEG) directly estimate activity in these regions from electrophysiological data recorded at the skin's surface [20]; however, estimating the activity from these data requires source localization [20] which, for small, deep brain regions, is a complex process that has only been demonstrated in a few studies [20].

Fig. 2.4 Anxiolytics eliminate conflict-specific theta [10]. Placebo curve is expected effect in controls

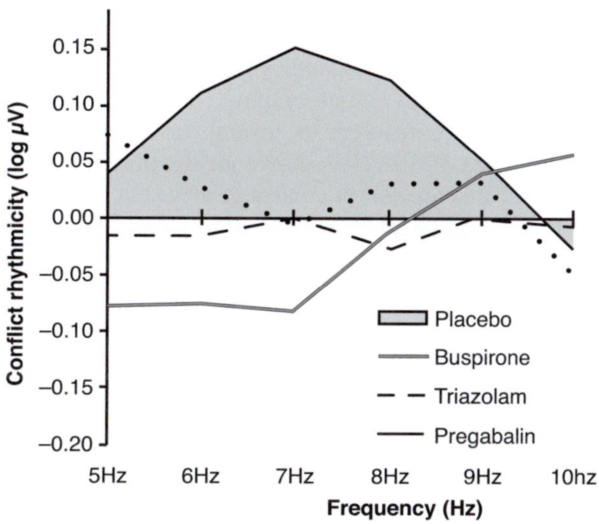

Anxiolytic Drugs and Theta

In 2013, McNaughton et al. [3, 24] documented "the first evidence for a human homologue of the 4–12 Hz rhythmicity," which they identified at the medial right frontal F8 EEG site [24]. In a previous study [25], they had detected 9–10 Hz conflict power at F8 that correlated with measures of trait anxiety and neuroticism [24]. Earlier [15], they demonstrated in mice that theta elicited by electrical stimulation of the reticular formation (RF) is reduced by systemic administration of drugs that lower anxiety (anxiolytics) [15]. This led them to accurately predict (in their 2013 paper) [24], that the 4–12 Hz conflict-specific rhythm they detected at F8 would be eliminated by triazolam, buspirone, and pregabalin—drugs which have only anxiolysis in common [24]. They concluded that: "there is a distinct rhythmic system in humans that is sensitive to both classical/GABAergic and novel/serotonergic anxiolytics; and this conflict-specific rhythmicity should provide a biomarker, with a strong pre-clinical neuropsychology, for a novel approach to classifying anxiety disorders [24]." They also suggested that: "a reduction in electrically-elicited theta predicts anxiolytic action with, after 30 years of testing, no false positives (even with sedatives) or negatives (even with drugs ineffective in panic or depression) [15, 24]."

McNaughton et al. [3] showed that the drugs used to treat GAD can modulate theta in humans. So, they provide a simple but powerful means of detection. Their results also confirm the existence of a functional homologue of rodent theta in the human mPFC.

Role of the Vestibular Nucleus

Evidence from previous studies suggests that the experimental diagnostic technique known as "Electrovestibulography" (EVestG) facilitated the identification of numerous possible biomarkers of several neurological disorders and diseases [11]. In some studies, EVestG has shown greater than 85% accuracy in discriminating individuals from case versus control groups [11].

The technique involves recording signals from electrodes placed in the outer ear canals of participants who are tilted in a hydraulic chair that elicits a response from the vestibular system (the brain's primary balance mechanism) [11]. The proximity of the ear drums to the vestibular peripheries allows measurement of peripheral afferent signals, which are shaped, in part, by the spontaneously active efferent vestibular system (EVS) that is, in turn, modulated by the vestibular nuclei (Fig. A in Appendix) [11]. The brainstem vestibular nucleus (VN) is connected to numerous regions of the brain, several of which are known to play a role in anxiety disorders [26]. Therefore, it is possible that inputs to the VN from these anxiety-implicated regions may alter VN efferent activity causing detectable perturbations in peripheral afferent signals.

Lithgow et al. reported that EVestG detected low-frequency modulation in vestibular afferents [11]. This might be explained by Tai et al. who found that vestibular stimulation elicits type 2 theta [27], and Sirota et al. who suggested that the HPC likely uses theta to phase-bias vestibular signals [28]. This suggests that type 2 theta is produced by vestibular stimulation and is detectable by EVestG.

Conclusion

There is a dire need for next-generation diagnostic and treatment technologies in the field of mental health, and anxiety disorders are the leading cause of disability. Generalized anxiety disorder is one of the most common forms, and it is an interesting condition for research.

There is a rhythm that represents a potential biomarker that has been identified in the prefrontal cortex and is believed to manifest elsewhere in locations that can only be accessed invasively.

This rhythm has been confirmed to manifest in humans as it does in animals. It is currently being developed as a part of a new diagnostic system that can separate individuals in fear- versus anxiety-like disorder groups. However, this technique has limitations that could be remedied by the discovery of another point from which to record this elusive rhythm.

The drugs that treat anxiety also treat balance disorders, and those same drugs reduce theta and have nothing else in common (largely opposing effects). This suggests that the underlying mechanism that explains comorbid anxiety and balance disorders is theta dysregulation.

References

1. Delves PJMS, Burton DR, Roitt IM. Roitt's essential immunology. 13th ed. Wiley Blackwell; 2017.
2. Guthrie LA, McPhail LC, Henson PM, Johnston RB Jr. Priming of neutrophils for enhanced release of oxygen metabolites by bacterial lipopolysaccharide. Evidence for increased activity of the superoxide-producing enzyme. J Exp Med. 1984;160(6):1656–71.
3. Moss RB, Moll T, El-Kalay M, Kohne C, Soo Hoo W, Encinas J, et al. Th1/Th2 cells in inflammatory disease states: therapeutic implications. Expert Opin Biol Ther. 2004;4(12):1887–96.
4. Mukhara D, Oh U, Neigh GN. Neuroinflammation. Handb Clin Neurol. 2020;175:235–59.
5. Halliwell BGJ. Free radicals in biology and medicine. 5th ed. Oxford University Press; 2015.
6. Cheng JRR, editor. Fundamentals of pain medicine. Springer; 2018.
7. Plenge JKHT, Weil KM, Poirier P, Grunwald GK, Marcovina SM, Eckel RH. Simvastatin lowers C-reactive protein within 14 days: an effect independent of low-density lipoprotein cholesterol reduction. Circulation. 2002;106(12):1447.
8. Bailly F. The challenge of differentiating fibromyalgia from small-fiber neuropathy in clinical practice. Joint Bone Spine. 2021:105232.
9. National Institute of Mental Health. Prevalence of any anxiety disorder among adults 2017. https://www.nimh.nih.gov/health/statistics/any-anxiety-disorder.shtml.
10. McNaughton N. What do you mean 'anxiety'? Developing the first anxiety syndrome biomarker. Taylor & Francis. 2017:1–14.
11. Lithgow BJ, Garrett AL, Moussavi ZM, Gurvich C, Kulkarni J, Maller JJ, et al. Major depression and electrovestibulography. World J Biol Psychiatry. 2015;16(5):334–50.

12. Calhoon GG, Tye KM. Resolving the neural circuits of anxiety. Nat Neurosci. 2015;18(10):1394.
13. Korotkova T, Ponomarenko A, Monaghan CK, Poulter SL, Cacucci F, Wills T, et al. Reconciling the different faces of hippocampal theta: the role of theta oscillations in cognitive, emotional and innate behaviors. Neurosci Biobehav Rev. 2018;85:65–80.
14. American Psychiatric Publishing. Diagnostic and statistical manual of mental disorders : DSM-5. 5th ed. Washington, D.C: American Psychiatric Publishing; 2013.
15. McNaughton N, Kocsis B, Hajós M. Elicited hippocampal theta rhythm: a screen for anxiolytic and procognitive drugs through changes in hippocampal function? Behav Pharmacol. 2007;18(5–6):329–46.
16. International Statistical Classification of Diseases and Related Health Problems 10th Revision (ICD-10) Version for 2010. Neurotic, stress-related and somatoform disorders (F40-F48) 2010 http://apps.who.int/classifications/icd10/browse/2010/en#/F41.1.
17. Vertes RP, Kocsis B. Brainstem- diencephalo-septohippocampal systems controlling the theta rhythm of the hippocampus. Neuroscience. 1997;81(4):893.
18. Adhikari A, Topiwala MA, Gordon JA. Synchronized activity between the ventral hippocampus and the medial prefrontal cortex during anxiety. Neuron. 2010;65(2):257–69.
19. Lee AT, Cunniff MM, See JZ, Wilke SA, Luongo FJ, Ellwood IT, et al. VIP interneurons contribute to avoidance behavior by regulating information flow across hippocampal-prefrontal networks. Neuron (Cambridge, Mass). 2019;102(6):1223–34.e4.
20. Ruzich E, Crespo-García M, Dalal SS, Schneiderman JF. Characterizing hippocampal dynamics with MEG: a systematic review and evidence-based guidelines. Hum Brain Mapp. 2019;40(4):1353–75.
21. Ekstrom AD, Caplan JB, Ho E, Shattuck K, Fried I, Kahana MJ. Human hippocampal theta activity during virtual navigation. Hippocampus. 2005;15(7):881–9.
22. File SE, Gonzalez LE, Andrews N. Comparative study of pre- and postsynaptic 5-HT1A receptor modulation of anxiety in two ethological animal tests. J Neurosci. 1996;16(15):4810.
23. Deacon RMJ, Bannerman DM, Rawlins JNP. Anxiolytic effects of cytotoxic hippocampal lesions in rats.(abstract). Behav Neurosci. 2002;116(3):494.
24. McNaughton N, Swart C, Neo P, Bates V, Glue P. Anti-anxiety drugs reduce conflict-specific "theta"—A possible human anxiety-specific biomarker. J Affect Disord. 2013;148(1):104–11.
25. Neo P, Thurlow J, McNaughton N. Stopping, goal- conflict, trait anxiety and frontal rhythmic power in the stop-signal task. Cognitive, Affective, & Behavioral Neuroscience. 2011;11(4):485–93.
26. Balaban CD, Jacob RG, Furman JM. Neurologic bases for comorbidity of balance disorders, anxiety disorders and migraine: neurotherapeutic implications. Expert Rev Neurother. 2011;11(3):379–94.
27. Tai SK, Ma J, Ossenkopp KP, Leung LS. Activation of immobility-related hippocampal theta by cholinergic septohippocampal neurons during vestibular stimulation. Hippocampus. 2012;22(4):914–25.
28. Sirota A, Montgomery S, Fujisawa S, Isomura Y, Zugaro M, Buzsáki G. Entrainment of neocortical neurons and gamma oscillations by the hippocampal theta rhythm. Neuron. 2008;60(4):683–97.

Altered Sensation

3

Brian W. Blakley

Introduction

A 54-year-old man presents with chronic, non-pulsatile ringing tinnitus and mild sensorineural hearing loss in both ears. He also indicates that he is upset by a marked sensation of tingling on the tip of the pinna on the right. Tactile sensation is normal but when the pinna is examined, the patient reports worsening of the tingling, questionably to the point of pain. We do not really understand tinnitus, but it is common, and we can deal with it, but what do we make of the tingling sensation? It doesn't seem to fit. Is he malingering? What do we think of symptoms that we have no explanation for? We will come back to this patient at the end of this chapter.

We should not be surprised that nerves do not always function optimally. The traditional concept of named, sensory nerves conducting impulses along anatomic pathways to the brain holds, but nerves are not just one-way wires. Recent evidence suggests that nerves have two-way communication as well as inter- and intra-neuronal communication. Nerves are really glands, secreting a variety of substances. We can understand reduced function such as numbness if a sensory nerve is cut or damaged, but for some reason, we have trouble considering that nerves can hyper-function or function abnormally but still be physically intact. It is curious that we expect that the 90 billion or so nerve cells in our body should all function optimally all the time.

Neuropathy refers to damage or pathology of nerves with resulting dysfunction. Typically, the term "neuropathy" refers to peripheral neuropathy with symptoms of tingling, pain that is shooting or burning, numbness or other odd sensations. "Peripheral neuropathy", often due to diabetes and some chemotherapeutic medications is well accepted but not well understood. "Central neuropathy" also exists. Central neuropathy causing pain is often called neuropathic pain. The term

B. W. Blakley (✉)
Department of Otolaryngology, University of Manitoba, Winnipeg, MB, Canada

© The Author(s), under exclusive license to Springer Nature Switzerland AG 2023

B. W. Blakley, J. E. Blakley (eds.), *Functional Illness of the Head and Neck*,
https://doi.org/10.1007/978-3-031-12998-8_3

"neuropathy" in general, could include allodynia, hyperalgesia and hypersensitivity. The distinction between peripheral and central neuropathy may be indistinct. For example, atypical facial pain, tinnitus, TMJ disorders or pain in distant sites of the body commonly co-exist. This widespread dysfunction should be mediated centrally or by similar pathology developing simultaneously at random in multiple peripheral nerves. The notion of discrete all-or-none "labelled lines" does not make sense for neuropathy.

The "gate theory" as discussed in Chap. 2 of this book illustrates an important interaction between neurons indicating that activation of one neuron can deactivate another. Expansion of the gate theory across groups of neurons should lead us to anticipate complex interactions and altered sensation.

Allodynia

Allodynia is defined as pain elicited by a stimulus that should not cause pain. In the past, tenderness over the maxillary sinus was thought to indicate acute sinusitis. This never made sense under traditional linear thinking. The inflammation is inside the sinus. Unless the bone has been eroded, the outside bone should not be tender. Improved imaging and revised thinking would suggest that atypical facial pain without sinusitis is more likely.

Allodynia can often cause referred pain to nearby locations. The referral patterns do not always follow dermatome patterns, indicating that aberrant central processing must be involved.

Hyperalgesia

Hyperalgesia is defined as a pain response that is out of proportion to the stimulus. One example is extreme pain reported when removing cerumen peripherally from a normal ear canal, as in our patient above. Ear canals are sensitive, but gentle manipulation, at least of the periphery, should be well tolerated in the absence of infection. Of course, anxiety will amplify hyperalgesia. Often, over repeated visits with gentle technique, the anxiety can fade, allowing more complete procedures in normal adults.

Hypersensitivity

Hypersensitivity is an exaggerated response to a stimulus. The term applies to immunologic, sensory, psychological or many other systems. Hyperacusis is an example. Spontaneous tinnitus, without a stimulus, is often lumped with hyperacusis, but the two disorders seem to be different. Anxiety, hyperalgesia and allodynia may also be examples of hypersensitivity. Migraine and fibromyalgia are probably the most well-recognized forms of central hypersensitivity. Central and peripheral hypersensitization have been studied, and a large literature base has resulted.

Peripheral Sensitization

NSAIDS may prevent nociceptor sensitization of receptors by modulating cyclo-oxygenase products, and opioids may act by direct action on nitric oxide (NO) [1]. "Neuroinflammation" [2], inflammatory mediators [3] and calcitonin gene-related peptide (CGRP) may be active in up-regulating receptors in peripheral and central sensitization [4]. Nerve growth factors are thought to be involved in facial sensitization [5].

Central sensitization is characterized by migraine and fibromyalgia, but there are many other examples. Hyperexcitable neurons in the spinal cord and brain amplify sensation from peripheral inputs and may spread responses from nearby sites. Shaible (2004) gives an example of infection in the thigh with a tenderness that spreads to normal surrounding tissues, even crossing dermatome barriers. The site of cross-over appears to be the medial thalamocortical system, consisting of the medial thalamus, anterior cingulate cortex, insula and prefrontal cortex [6]. Other authors report that synaptic plasticity caused by neuroinflammation and various cytokines is sensitizing [7].

Mechanisms of central sensitization may include up-regulation of glutamate receptors, activating protein kinase C, leading to phosphorylation of one or more members of the transient receptor potential (TRP), typically transient receptor potential vanilloid 1 (TRPV1), by inflammatory mediators [8–10]. TRPs are the target of drug research in the hopes of blocking pain sensitization [11, 12]. Calcitonin gene-related peptide (CGRP) appears to be involved in migraine, particularly [13].

There is no particular reason that pain should be the only symptom of sensitization. The most well-accepted examples of central hypersensitivity are fibromyalgia and migraine, both of which cause more than pain alone. There are strong indications that central sensitization results in many symptoms in addition to pain [14, 15], which seems reasonable and would explain why some patients report multiple symptoms that would appear to be unrelated according to the linear thinking model. In addition to allodynia and hyperalgesia, it is likely that dysosmia, dysgeusia, hyperacusis, dizziness and a variety of other symptoms relate to nerve dysfunction without structural abnormalities. The mechanisms are basically not known. At our present level of understanding, it seems appropriate to consider them as "neuropathy".

At this point, we cannot identify any unified mechanism that sensitizes nerves, but sensitization certainly happens and causes many symptoms. Whatever the mechanism(s) may be, there are indications that dopamine, serotonin and/or norepinephrine metabolism are often involved [16]. This observation implies that treatment for some of these symptoms with medications that affect serotonin, dopamine or norepinephrine may be worthwhile. Central and peripheral sensitization overlap so that allodynia and hyperalgesia commonly co-exist [17]. The patient at the beginning of this chapter is an example. Hypersensitivity of the ear canal exists in association with other nerve dysfunction—tinnitus and hearing loss. For him, it seems appropriate to remove the cerumen and rule out infection or other illnesses. If other disease is absent, discuss the severity of symptoms and his desires with him to see if a trial of a serotonergic medication might be reasonable for pain. There is little evidence that this treatment would alleviate the tingling or hearing loss though. He may be happy knowing that there is no serious pathology. After all, ear canal tenderness may be his worst symptom, and how often does one have to manipulate the ear canal?

Summary

The main point of this chapter is to point out that neuropathies exist, are common, and are not imaginary. These common occurrences should be given careful consideration in clinical medicine.

References

1. Gomes FIF, Cunha FQ, Cunha TM. Peripheral nitric oxide signaling directly blocks inflammatory pain. Biochem Pharmacol. 2020;176:113862.
2. Seifert O, Baerwald C. Interaction of pain and chronic inflammation. Z Rheumatol. 2021;80(3):205–13.
3. Oostinga D, Steverink JG, van Wijck AJM, Verlaan JJ. An understanding of bone pain: a narrative review. Bone. 2020;134:115272.
4. Iyengar S, Ossipov MH, Johnson KW. The role of calcitonin gene-related peptide in peripheral and central pain mechanisms including migraine. Pain. 2017;158(4):543–59.
5. Mai L, Huang F, Zhu X, He H, Fan W. Role of nerve growth factor in orofacial pain. J Pain Res. 2020;13:1875–82.
6. Schaible HG, Richter F. Pathophysiology of pain. Langenbeck's Arch Surg. 2004;389(4):237–43.
7. Ji RR, Nackley A, Huh Y, Terrando N, Maixner W. Neuroinflammation and central sensitization in chronic and widespread pain. Anesthesiology. 2018;129(2):343–66.
8. Chung MK, Ro JY. Peripheral glutamate receptor and transient receptor potential channel mechanisms of craniofacial muscle pain. Mol Pain. 2020;16:1744806920914204.
9. Matsuda M, Huh Y, Ji RR. Roles of inflammation, neurogenic inflammation, and neuroinflammation in pain. J Anesth. 2019;33(1):131–9.
10. So K. Roles of TRPA1 in painful dysesthesia. Yakugaku Zasshi. 2020;140(1):1–6.
11. Khan A, Khan S, Kim YS. Insight into pain modulation: nociceptors sensitization and therapeutic targets. Curr Drug Targets. 2019;20(7):775–88.
12. Kremer M, Salvat E, Muller A, Yalcin I, Barrot M. Antidepressants and gabapentinoids in neuropathic pain: mechanistic insights. Neuroscience. 2016;338:183–206.
13. Iyengar S, Johnson KW, Ossipov MH, Aurora SK. CGRP and the trigeminal system in migraine. Headache. 2019;59(5):659–81.
14. Littlejohn G, Guymer E. Neurogenic inflammation in fibromyalgia. Semin Immunopathol. 2018;40(3):291–300.
15. Reynolds WS, Dmochowski R, Wein A, Bruehl S. Does central sensitization help explain idiopathic overactive bladder? Nat Rev Urol. 2016;13(8):481–91.
16. Clauw DJ, Essex MN, Pitman V, Jones KD. Reframing chronic pain as a disease, not a symptom: rationale and implications for pain management. Postgrad Med. 2019;131(3):185–98.
17. Finnerup NB, Kuner R, Jensen TS. Neuropathic pain: from mechanisms to treatment. Physiol Rev. 2021;101(1):259–301.

Stress and Functional Illness

4

Avni A. Shah and Ashley D. Agan

In today's world, stress has become an ubiquitous part of life. Daily stressors repeatedly trigger our body's innate stress response system. In the short term, this stress response is vital to maintaining homeostasis but, over time, can become maladaptive with chronic activation, leading to myriad ill effects.

For the patients presenting with functional ear, nose, and throat ailments, it is important to consider the role stress may have in the pathophysiology of their illness. In this chapter, we will first refresh the basics of the stress response, including sympathetic activation, the hypothalamic–pituitary–adrenal (HPA) axis, and important neurotransmitters. Then, we will explore the relationships between stress and functional illness and how stress may precipitate, worsen, or prolong various ear, nose, and throat complaints.

The Physiology of Stress

The stress response begins in the amygdala, a small, almond-shaped region of the brain important in the fight-or-flight response, emotional learning, and emotional memory formation [1, 2]. Normally, the amygdala remains quiet under tonic GABAergic inhibition. However, conditioned and unconditioned stimuli can trigger the amygdala, removing this tonic inhibition. Input from several regions of the brain, including the prefrontal cortex, stria terminalis, hippocampus, and sensory regions, is received and processed by the lateral and basal nuclei of the amygdala.

A. A. Shah
University of Texas Southwestern Medical Center, Dallas, TX, USA

A. D. Agan (✉)
Department of Otolaryngology-Head and Neck Surgery, University of Texas Southwestern Medical Center, Dallas, TX, USA
e-mail: ashley.agan@utsouthwestern.edu

© The Author(s), under exclusive license to Springer Nature Switzerland AG 2023

B. W. Blakley, J. E. Blakley (eds.), *Functional Illness of the Head and Neck*,
https://doi.org/10.1007/978-3-031-12998-8_4

This information is then passed along to the central nuclei of the amygdala [3]. The amygdala then activates the hypothalamus. Once activated, the hypothalamus stimulates the sympathetic arm of the autonomic nervous system and the HPA axis. Interestingly, several studies have found chronic stress exposure may precipitate structural and functional changes in the amygdala that result in hyperreactivity, leading to an overactive response to fear and anxiety-inducing stimuli [4–6].

The peripheral nervous system is split into the somatic nervous system and the autonomic nervous system, which is further subdivided into the parasympathetic and sympathetic nervous systems.

The sympathetic nervous system classically controls the immediate fight-or-flight response to stressors [7]. Sympathetic stimulation activates epinephrine and, to a lesser degree, norepinephrine release from the adrenal medulla. These catecholamine neurotransmitters travel through the bloodstream, precipitating widespread effects, which prepare the body to take action [8]. The parasympathetic nervous system, colloquially known as the "rest and digest" system, demonstrates largely opposite effects to the sympathetic nervous system. These effects are summarized in Table 4.1.

Norepinephrine and epinephrine are catecholamine neurotransmitters derived from tyrosine. Norepinephrine is largely utilized for communication within the nervous system. Epinephrine is synthesized from norepinephrine in the adrenal medulla in a reaction catalyzed by phenylethanolamine-N-methyltransferase. While both epinephrine and norepinephrine are released from the adrenal medulla during times of stress, epinephrine is released at the four times greater rate. With chronic stimulation, tyrosine hydroxylase, an upstream, rate-limiting enzyme in catecholamine synthesis, is upregulated via transcriptional and post-transcriptional effects [9]. These catecholamines create rapid effects but are removed just as rapidly via reuptake, uptake into tissues, and inactivation in the liver via catechol-O-methyltransferase (COMT) and monoamine oxidase (MAO). They are excreted by the kidney as vanillylmandelic acid (VMA) or metanephrines [9].

While the sympathetic nervous system mediates our immediate response to stress, activation of the HPA axis follows close behind. The term "HPA axis" refers to the neuroendocrine relationship between the hypothalamus, pituitary, and adrenals.

The hypothalamus is located at the base of the brain and produces many stimulatory and inhibitory hormones destined for the pituitary, including corticotropin releasing hormone (CRH) [10]. The pituitary gland is composed of two parts: the anterior pituitary (adenohypophysis) and the posterior pituitary (neurohypophysis). The anterior pituitary receives stimulatory and inhibitory hormones from the

Table 4.1 Effects of sympathetic versus parasympathetic stimulation

Organ	Sympathetic NS	Parasympathetic NS
Pupil	Dilate	Constrict
Heart	Increases heart rate, cardiac output	Decreases heart rate, cardiac output
Lungs	Dilates airways	Constricts airways
GI tract	Reduced secretion, peristalsis	Increased secretion, peristalsis
Urinary system	Relax bladder	Contract bladder

hypothalamus via the hypophyseal portal system, and it releases several hormones, including adrenocorticotropic hormone (ACTH). In response to stressors, limbic structures stimulate the paraventricular nucleus of the hypothalamus, which releases corticotropin releasing hormone (CRH). CRH travels to the anterior pituitary via the hypophyseal portal system and triggers the release of adrenocorticotropic hormone (ACTH). ACTH then travels in the bloodstream to the adrenal cortex and stimulates the release of cortisol from the zona fasciculata [11].

Cortisol inhibits further ACTH release, forming a negative feedback loop [9]. Once ACTH and cortisol levels drop sufficiently, CRH release is triggered once more, and the cycle continues. In this manner, cortisol levels naturally rise and fall throughout the day in 7–15 episodic bursts. A major burst is noted in the morning around 8 AM, and this is often pointed to as the cause of increased rates of myocardial infarction and sudden cardiac death in the mornings [9, 12]. Chronic ACTH stimulation induces hypertrophy of the adrenal glands, and resultantly, cortisol secretion can rise to 200–250 mg/day—nearly 10–20 times the normal amount. In the short term, cortisol elevations are normal, healthy responses to daily circadian rhythms and stressors, but chronic elevation can be harmful [9].

Cortisol has many effects throughout the body. Cortisol stimulates protein catabolism in the skeletal muscles and connective tissue. However, cortisol excess results in muscle atrophy and weakness, skin thinning, and bone matrix/mass reduction. In the immune system, cortisol demonstrates anti-inflammatory effects by reducing cytokine release, but with chronic activation can result in immune suppression. Some studies have demonstrated links between fetal glucocorticoid exposure and development of hypertension, coronary artery disease, and obesity later in life [9, 13, 14]. Cortisol also stimulates synthesis of phenylethanolamine-N-methyltransferase, the very enzyme that converts norepinephrine to epinephrine in the adrenal medulla [9].

Chronic Stress

In the short term, the physiologic response described above can be vital in maintaining homeostasis in the face of stressors. However, repeated activation of these pathways due to chronic stress generates widespread, negative impacts to health. Long-term effects of chronic stress can include anxiety, depression, weight gain, immune suppression, difficulty concentrating, difficulty sleeping, changes in weight, digestive issues, and headache [15]. Stress also impairs memory. A study of mice demonstrated a significant reduction in long-term potentiation, a key neural process for memory and learning, in the CA3 pyramidal neurons and dentate nucleus of the hippocampus 48 hours after 21 days of chronic stress exposure [16].

Stress can also increase susceptibility to pathogens. Stress alters Type I and Type II cytokine levels, affecting the balance between adaptive and innate immune responses. Stress impairs the trafficking, function, and even quantity of immune cells [17]. Stress can even impact our response to vaccination. A meta-analysis of 13 studies, with a total of 1158 participants, demonstrated a statistically significant inverse association between psychologic stress and peak antibody response to influenza vaccination, which was determined by measuring antibody titers after vaccination in stressed individuals compared to unstressed individuals [18]. The clinical significance of this is unknown. There are a number of studies that have demonstrated associations between anxiety and depression and viral illnesses; however, causality has not been investigated [19]. It has also been shown that elevated cortisol levels can result in impaired wound healing [20].

Of note, the impact of stress on the immune system is often paradoxical. Immune suppression from stress can worsen the risk of infection or cancer, but it can also worsen asthma, autoimmune, and inflammatory conditions. We might expect improvements in these conditions in response to immunosuppression; however, that is not what is observed. Certainly, the effects of stress on the immune system are not linear or one-size-fits-all. They are highly dependent on the individual, their environment, exposure to stress early in life, the nature of the stressor, the timing of the stressor, and many other variables [21].

The Stress Experience

Now that we have thoroughly explored the physiologic effects of acute and chronic stress, it is important to understand the myriad ways stress can present in a patient. For example, stress-mediated sympathetic activation can lead to palpitations and the sensation of a pounding heart. Blood pressure may also spike. Anxious feelings might result in abdominal pain, a sensation of tingling or butterflies, nausea, diarrhea, or constipation [22]. Job stress is linked with muscle tension, especially in the neck, shoulders, and lower back. This can also generate tension and migraine headaches. Acute, severe stress can trigger asthma attacks [23]. Chronic stress hampers our body's immune system and can manifest as repeated colds and infections [24]. Immune system suppression in chronic stress has also been connected to the development of chronic fatigue and metabolic disorders. Chronic stress increases the risk of hypertension, heart attacks, and stroke [23].

The effects of stress on the body are not limited to those described above. Physical tension from stress can manifest as a wide range of symptoms, including but not limited to, muscle pain, muscle tension, chest pain, trouble sleeping, fatigue, headaches, gastrointestinal dysfunction, light-headedness, changes in urinary frequency, and sexual dysfunction [25]. More subtle manifestations include tremors, fidgeting, stuttering, jaw clenching, heartburn, flatulence, appetite changes, ringing/popping/buzzing sounds, dry mouth, and difficulty swallowing. Importantly, patients may also experience increased irritability, difficulty concentrating, racing thoughts, forgetfulness, social withdrawal, anxiety, depression, and panic attacks [24].

Stress affects brain–gut communication and can result in abdominal pain, bloating, and discomfort [23]. Stress may even impact the delicate balance of our gut bacteria [26]. In settings of stress, intestinal cells release catecholamines and other hormones that alter the growth of these bacteria. Reduced gut motility and gut perfusion in stress can alter intestinal epithelial permeability, leading to local gastrointestinal environmental changes [27]. One randomized controlled trial with 73 military recruits found that physical stress increased intestinal permeability, changing the gut microenvironment and decreased common gut bacterial species such as *Bacteroides* in favor of less common species [28].

Clearly, the widespread effects of stress on the body should not be underestimated. It is not unreasonable to imagine that stress, especially chronic stress, plays a role in the pathogenesis and/or prolongation of various functional disorders. In fact, several well-known relationships between stress and illness in other medical fields can attest to this. For example, inflammatory bowel disease relapse is associated with stress-induced changes in immune and inflammatory function [29, 30]. States of high psychological stress are associated with greater disease severity in interstitial cystitis/bladder pain syndrome and overactive bladder [31, 32]. When it comes to otolaryngologic symptoms for which no organic cause can be identified, it is important to consider and explore the role stress may have.

Functional ENT Illness and Stress

For many functional ENT illnesses, patients describe symptom exacerbation or even first-time symptom onset in the setting of stress. While unequivocal biochemical links have not yet been established, the relationship between stress and functional ENT illness is far from anecdotal.

Tinnitus is one of the most common otologic complaints and, in its subjective form, is often associated with stress. Tinnitus is characterized by the perception of sound in the absence of external stimuli and is extremely heterogeneous in its development and character. Tinnitus may be subjective (heard only by the patient) or objective (heard by the examiner as well, i.e., a bruit from vascular malformation). Tinnitus may be idiopathic (primary) or present secondary to a specific underlying cause (hearing loss, traumatic injury, otosclerosis, TMJ, ototoxic medications) [33, 34].

The patient experience of tinnitus ranges from a mild annoyance to a debilitative condition. Anxiety and depression are well-known comorbidities of tinnitus [33, 35, 36]. A study of 122 tinnitus patients in Germany during the COVID-19 lockdown found patients who experienced high levels of grief, frustration, stress, and nervousness had worsened tinnitus symptoms [37]. There is evidence that cognitive behavioral therapy (CBT) can help patients reframe their tinnitus (from “fighting it” to “allowing it”) in order to reduce associated stress and improve overall wellbeing [38]. Such interventions for severe tinnitus may help patients reduce stress caused by the disease itself, and thereby (1) reduce the negative impact of tinnitus on their daily life and (2) break the stress-illness cycle that may be perpetrating or worsening their symptoms. In fact, mindfulness-based cognitive therapy (MCBT) was able to reduce tinnitus-related distress in 50% of study participants and reduce psychological distress in 41.2% of participants [39]. It stands to reason, if such non-pharmacologic therapy can improve disease and psychological distress in these patients, non-organic tinnitus may have a strong association with mental state. CBT or MCBT should be considered as important options in multi-modal treatment of tinnitus [40]. In patients with comorbid depression, treatment of depression improved patient symptoms of both depression and tinnitus. One study of 30 chronic tinnitus patients with comorbid depression found SSRI treatment reduced major depression in 66% of patients, and many also noticed a significant decrease in tinnitus symptoms by the tinnitus severity index [41]. However, in patients without comorbid depression, anti-depressants may prove to be less effective [42].

Stress can also influence dizziness and balance conditions. For example, a longitudinal study which recorded Meniere's symptoms, stress levels, and unusual events in 1031 participants found a strong association between attacks and worsening of symptoms with stress or unusual events [43]. Meniere's disease, characterized by episodes of vertigo, tinnitus, and sensorineural hearing loss, is generally treated with anti-nausea medication, diuretics, low-salt diets, and/or vestibular rehabilitation [44]. However, the results of this study suggest that adding stress management counseling to the treatment plan might improve symptoms and give the patient strategies to cope with stress-related exacerbations. It is also important to factor in how patient stress about the disease itself can exacerbate symptoms. Stress can precipitate an attack, which can generate patient stress and fear of another attack, which might go on to generate another attack, and so on. By assisting the Meniere's disease patient with a range of interventions, including stress management counseling, providers can work toward reducing both the severity of Meniere's symptoms and the distress caused by the condition.

Another functional ENT illness with links to stress is globus sensation. Globus is a persistent feeling of a "lump" in the throat that arises from a variety of etiologies, such as GERD, esophageal sphincter abnormalities, esophageal motility disorders, tumors, or psychological factors and stress. Many globus sensation patients experience worsened symptoms during stress. Further, stressful life events are often noted before the precipitation of globus sensation [45]. If organic causes can be excluded, and the patient's symptoms do not respond to PPI therapy, cognitive behavioral therapy, anti-depressants, or gabapentin may be considered [46].

In summary, sympathoadrenal activation occurs when we are faced with a threat to homeostasis, be it real or imagined. Stress, in both acute and chronic forms, has a significant widespread impact on the body. For patients presenting with functional ENT illness, it is vital to consider the role stress may have in their illness. While addressing stressors may not eliminate the condition in its entirety, it can reduce symptom severity and mental stress regarding the condition itself, thereby improving the patients' day-to-day experience. Functional illnesses are challenging to understand, diagnose, and treat. However, by acknowledging the validity of the patient's experience and exploring multiple influencing factors, such as stress, providers can better treat these conditions.

References

1. Zhang X, Ge TT, Yin G, Cui R, Zhao G, Yang W. Stress-induced functional alterations in amygdala: implications for neuropsychiatric diseases. Front Neurosci. 2018;12:367.
2. LeDoux JE. Brain mechanisms of emotion and emotional learning. Curr Opin Neurobiol. 1992;2(2):191–7.
3. Ressler KJ. Amygdala activity, fear, and anxiety: modulation by stress. Biol Psychiatry. 2010;67(12):1117–9.
4. Joss D, Khan A, Lazar SW, Teicher MH. A pilot study on amygdala volumetric changes among young adults with childhood maltreatment histories after a mindfulness intervention. Behav Brain Res. 2021;399:113023.
5. Morey RA, Gold AL, LaBar KS, Beall SK, Brown VM, Haswell CC, et al. Amygdala volume changes in posttraumatic stress disorder in a large case-controlled veterans group. Arch Gen Psychiatry. 2012;69(11):1169–78.
6. Klaming R, Spadoni AD, Veltman DJ, Simmons AN. Expansion of hippocampal and amygdala shape in posttraumatic stress and early life stress. NeuroImage: Clinical. 2019;24:101982.
7. Cannon WB. Bodily changes in pain, hunger, fear, and rage. D. Appleton and company; 1915.
8. Robertson DW, Biaggioni I, Burnstock G, Low P, Paton JFR. Primer on the autonomic nervous system. Elsevier Inc.; 2012. p. 703.
9. Auchus RJ, Parker KL. The adrenal glands. Textbook of endocrine physiology. 6th ed. Oxford University Press; 2011.
10. Shahid Z, Asuka E, Singh G. Physiology, hypothalamus. Treasure Island (FL).: StatPearls Publishing. Copyright © 2021, StatPearls Publishing LLC.: StatPearls; 2021.
11. Ojeda SR. The anterior pituitary and hypothalamus. Textbook of endocrine physiology. 6th ed. Oxford University Press; 2011.
12. Willich SN, Klatt S, Arntz HR. Circadian variation and triggers of acute coronary syndromes. Eur Heart J. 1998;19(Suppl C):C12-23.
13. Benediktsson R, Lindsay RS, Noble J, Seckl JR, Edwards CR. Glucocorticoid exposure in utero: new model for adult hypertension. Lancet. 1993;341(8841):339–41.
14. Harris A, Seckl J. Glucocorticoids, prenatal stress and the programming of disease. Horm Behav. 2011;59(3):279–89.
15. Chronic stress puts your health at risk. Mayo Clinic; 2019. https://www.mayoclinic.org/healthy-lifestyle/stress-management/in-depth/stress/art-20046037.
16. Pavlides C, Nivón LG, McEwen BS. Effects of chronic stress on hippocampal long-term potentiation. Hippocampus. 2002;12(2):245–57.
17. Dhabhar FS. Effects of stress on immune function: the good, the bad, and the beautiful. Immunol Res. 2014;58(2–3):193–210.
18. Pedersen AF, Zachariae R, Bovbjerg DH. Psychological stress and antibody response to influenza vaccination: a meta-analysis. Brain Behav Immun. 2009;23(4):427–33.
19. Coughlin SS. Anxiety and depression: linkages with viral diseases. Public Health Rev. 2012;34(2):7.
20. Ebrecht M, Hextall J, Kirtley L-G, Taylor A, Dyson M, Weinman J. Perceived stress and cortisol levels predict speed of wound healing in healthy male adults. Psychoneuroendocrinology. 2004;29(6):798–809.
21. Dhabhar FS. Enhancing versus suppressive effects of stress on immune function: implications for immunoprotection and immunopathology. Neuroimmunomodulation. 2009;16(5):300–17.
22. Wirsching M, McDaniel SH, Fritzsche K. Psychosomatic medicine : an international guide for the primary care setting. 2nd ed. Springer; 2020.
23. Stress effects on the body: American Psychological Association; 2018 https://www.apa.org/topics/stress/body.

24. Stress Effects: The American Institute of Stress; 2020 https://www.stress.org/stress-effects.
25. Stress: Cleveland Clinic; 2021 https://my.clevelandclinic.org/health/articles/11874-stress
26. Madison A, Kiecolt-Glaser JK. Stress, depression, diet, and the gut microbiota: human-bacteria interactions at the core of psychoneuroimmunology and nutrition. Curr Opin Behav Sci. 2019;28:105–10.
27. Karl JP, Hatch AM, Arcidiacono SM, Pearce SC, Pantoja-Feliciano IG, Doherty LA, et al. Effects of psychological, environmental and physical stressors on the gut microbiota. Front Microbiol. 2018;9:2013.
28. Karl JP, Margolis LM, Madslien EH, Murphy NE, Castellani JW, Gundersen Y, et al. Changes in intestinal microbiota composition and metabolism coincide with increased intestinal permeability in young adults under prolonged physiological stress. Am J Physiol Gastrointest Liver Physiol. 2017;312(6):G559-g71.
29. Mawdsley JE, Rampton DS. Psychological stress in IBD: new insights into pathogenic and therapeutic implications. Gut. 2005;54(10):1481–91.
30. Brown CH. Acute emotional crises and ulcerative colitis. Am J Dig Dis. 1963;8(6):525–36.
31. Grundy L, Caldwell A, Brierley SM. Mechanisms underlying overactive bladder and interstitial cystitis/painful bladder syndrome. Front Neurosci. 2018;12:931.
32. Birder LA. Pathophysiology of interstitial cystitis. Int J Urol. 2019;26(Suppl 1):12–5.
33. Baguley D, McFerran D, Hall D. Tinnitus. Lancet. 2013;382(9904):1600–7.
34. Esmaili A, Renton J. Tinnitus. Aust J Gen Pract. 2018;47:205–8.
35. Bhatt JM, Bhattacharyya N, Lin HW. Relationships between tinnitus and the prevalence of anxiety and depression. Laryngoscope. 2017;127(2):466–9.
36. Durai M, Searchfield G. Anxiety and depression, personality traits relevant to tinnitus: a scoping review. Int J Audiol. 2016;55(11):605–15.
37. Schlee W, Hølleland S, Bulla J, Simoes J, Neff P, Schoisswohl S, et al. The effect of environmental stressors on tinnitus: a prospective longitudinal study on the impact of the COVID-19 pandemic. J Clin Med. 2020;9:9.
38. Marks E, Smith P, McKenna L. I Wasn't at war with the noise: how mindfulness based cognitive therapy changes Patients' experiences of tinnitus. Front Psychol. 2020;11:483.
39. McKenna L, Marks EM, Vogt F. Mindfulness-based cognitive therapy for chronic tinnitus: evaluation of benefits in a large sample of patients attending a tinnitus clinic. Ear Hear. 2018;39(2):359–66.
40. Nolan DR, Gupta R, Huber CG, Schneeberger AR. An effective treatment for tinnitus and hyperacusis based on cognitive behavioral therapy in an inpatient setting: a 10-year retrospective outcome analysis. Front Psych. 2020;11:25.
41. Folmer RL, Shi YB. SSRI use by tinnitus patients: interactions between depression and tinnitus severity. Ear Nose Throat J. 2004;83(2):107–8. 10, 12 passim
42. Baldo P, Doree C, Molin P, McFerran D, Cecco S. Antidepressants for patients with tinnitus. Cochrane Database Syst Rev. 2012;2012(9):Cd003853.
43. Yeo NL, White MP, Ronan N, Whinney DJ, Curnow A, Tyrrell J. Stress and unusual events exacerbate symptoms in Menière's disease: a longitudinal study. Otol Neurotol. 2018;39(1):73–81.
44. Basura GJ, Adams ME, Monfared A, Schwartz SR, Antonelli PJ, Burkard R, et al. Clinical Practice Guideline: Ménière's Disease. Otolaryngol Head Neck Surg. 2020;162(2_suppl):S1-s55.
45. Lee BE, Kim GH. Globus pharyngeus: a review of its etiology, diagnosis and treatment. World J Gastroenterol. 2012;18(20):2462–71.
46. Manabe N, Tsutsui H, Kusunoki H, Hata J, Haruma K. Pathophysiology and treatment of patients with globus sensation—from the viewpoint of esophageal motility dysfunction. J Smooth Muscle Res. 2014;50:66–77.

Allergy and Environmental Illness

5

Ilka C. Nauman

Allergy

Positive allergy testing either in vitro (blood draw) or in vivo (skin prick or intradermal) confirms the presence of allergic disease. Often, medical management is straight-forward and for many patients immunotherapy "cures" sinonasal allergies long term.

The challenge for clinicians are patients with negative test results, but symptoms that are classic of allergies such as nasal congestions, nasal drainage, dryness feeling and increased sensitivity, eye and skin itching, as well as cough. They are often classified as "idiopathic and nonallergic" and continue to be difficult to treat. For non-allergic nasal symptoms, conventional allergy treatments are often tried, and some patients have a positive response to topical glucocorticoid sprays. Those are considered to have very localized allergic disease called local atopy (entopy) of the nose and sinuses without measurable response in the blood and the skin, hence the negative test [1].

More often than not patients are told they "don't have allergies," which is based on an allergy test of 24 or may be 36 allergens, and patients continue to suffer with their symptoms. Uncommon or untested allergens, chemical sensitivity, or hyper-responsiveness may be the underlying trigger of the "allergy and sinus" symptoms.

In regard to non-allergic rhinitis, various underlying pathomechanisms have been described, among others, autonomic dysfunction but also dysfunction of nociceptive nerve sensor and ion channel proteins [1].

Nociceptive hyper-responsiveness is a response of the trigeminal nerve fibers innervating the nasal mucosa and modulating the tonicity and osmolarity of the nasal mucosal lining and secretions through activation of specific ion channels.

I. C. Nauman (✉)
Michigan Ear Institute, Michigan State University, East Lansing, MI, USA

Oakland University Beaumont Hospital, Farmington Hills, MI, USA

© The Author(s), under exclusive license to Springer Nature Switzerland AG 2023

B. W. Blakley, J. E. Blakley (eds.), *Functional Illness of the Head and Neck*,
https://doi.org/10.1007/978-3-031-12998-8_5

Those respond strongly to thermal changes of inhaled air. Cold, dry air is one of the most common triggers of nasal symptoms followed by changes in temperature, barometric pressure changes or humidity [2].

The cold air will stimulate the trigeminal nerve and trigger a strong cholinergic parasympathetic reflex response arc and augmented glandular response with increased nasal congestion and copious discharge. Other triggers of the same nerve fibers may be methacholine, nicotine/cigarette smoke, as well as capsaicin and nonspecific stimuli such as irritants (perfumes, cleaning fluids, gasoline), bright lights (photic sneeze reflex), and spicy foods (gustatory rhinitis).

The connection of runny nose (vasomotor rhinitis) and the dysfunction of the autonomic nervous system was established more than 50 years ago and represents an imbalance between the parasympathetic and sympathetic nervous systems with a strong vasodilatory response of the parasympathetic system [3]. A history of nasal trauma in itself may pose a great risk for developing vasomotor rhinitis [4] and should be asked about when obtaining the history. Autonomic dysfunction as the underlying cause of the nasal symptoms, facial pain, and headaches may not be found unless a comprehensive history about the multi-organ symptoms is taken, and treatment should be tailored to each patient in close collaboration with a neurologist, cardiologist, and even gastroenterologist (as patients can exhibit symptoms of gastroesophageal reflux disease) [2].

Anticholinergic treatments (e.g., ipratropium) and a last resort surgical treatments of intranasal cautery/cryotherapy of the turbinates but also posterior nasal and vidian nerve ablation could be considered for rhinorrhea complaints.

Congestion can be effectively treated with warm steam inhalation and irrigation with hypertonic saline solution. Aerosolizing essential oils (menthol, eucalyptus, and camphor oil) can greatly improve the perception of nasal patency and have been used for centuries. Menthol has no effect on objective measures of airflow in the nose but significantly increases the perception of nasal patency [5] by stimulating the trigeminal cold receptors of the nose [6]. This points to the significance of the perception and sensation of airflow inside the nose rather than the objectively measurable airflow itself.

Pollution in the Environment at Large

Pollution in our environment poses a great health risk and impacts our wellbeing. Numerous studies link environmental toxins and particulate matter inhalation in large cities as causes for premature death and sickness. Chemicals like black carbon, nitrogen dioxide, sulfur dioxide, ozone, and carbon monoxide, as well as particles with an aerodynamic diameter of less than 2.5 μm (also referred to as PM2.5) are often made responsible to induce systemic inflammation.

Those reactions far exceed the apparent exposure of the upper and lower airway (respiratory symptoms) and explain the connection to cardiovascular events and even neurologic effects. Cognitive decline in older patients [7] and lower cognitive and motor skills in kids and adolescence [8] have been described. In a more subtle way, a decrease in general brain productivity, which is often termed "brain fog" has been described with air pollution [9].

Urban air pollution has been studied and found to be associated with systemic inflammation/oxidative stress, impairment of the fibrinolytic system, activation of blood coagulation, and alterations in autonomic nervous system [10], explaining the well-studied connection between exposure and premature death from cardiovascular diseases especially in patients with systemic inflammation and obesity [11].

Pollution compounds cause breakdown of the blood–brain barrier, alveolar capillary, and intestinal barriers and can worsen the effect of other chemicals and heavy metals that enter the body.

On a lighter side, chocolate consumption seems to have a protective effect from pollution damage in the brain [12]. The antioxidant-rich polyphenols of the chocolate have been found to lead to the expression of neuroprotective and neuromodulatory proteins that promote neurogenesis, neuronal function, brain connectivity, and angiogenesis [13].

Pollution at Work Spaces—Occupational Exposure

Occupational exposure to (often highly toxic) fumes and gases carries its own often well-documented set of risks. Most often, the respiratory tract is at highest risk for exposure entering the body through inhalation. Silicosis of miners, byssinosis of cotton workers and sinonasal cancers in woodworkers are just a few examples of well-established devastating occupational diseases.

The damaging effects of occupational toxins may be carried through the body and reach every system, including the central nervous system. Complaints of numbness and tingling or weakness are early signs of peripheral neuropathy, and "segmental demyelination" has been associated with heavy metal toxicity such as lead (battery manufacturing), arsenic, or thallium (glass industry).

Trichloroethylene, for example, a potent neurotoxin (found in some household cleaners, paint removers, carpet cleaners, and spray adhesives) has a predilection for the trigeminal nerve leading to numbness. A thorough otolaryngological examination may expose the finding, but the connection to a chemical in the work environment may never be made [14]. Often laboratory toxicologic tests have limited application for the etiologic diagnosis of neurotoxic disorders as in most cases the chemical is no longer detectable [15].

Strict guidelines from the Occupational Health and Safety Administration (OSHA) are set for workers with risks of exposure, and standards should be enforced to ensure safe working conditions [16]. Inadequate use of resources or appropriate training in safety protocols, sometimes simply not following the guidelines and lack of concern can lead to unsafe exposures. Acute but more often chronic adverse health effects occur. Unless a vigilant clinician suspects exposure, when several patients present with similar symptoms and further history taking make the connection, the link of an exposure maybe completely missed, or the condition attributed to other chronic ailments.

Pollution at Work Spaces—Office Space

In contrast to factory work with known risks, it appears even harder to pinpoint exposure to chemicals and toxins in an office setting. Essentially every office, even academic institution, relies on laser printers and photocopiers for their daily operations. Toner-based printing equipment not only contains several engineered nanomaterials in the inks but also emits ozone, volatile organic compounds, and heavy metals such as cadmium, selenium, arsenic, zinc, and nickel [17].

Toxicity of those particles has only been studied in recent years, and large epidemiological studies have not been conducted. In vitro experiments show significant cytotoxicity resulting in gene regulation of cytokines responsible for leukocyte migration, cellular antioxidant status, and modulation of pro-inflammatory responses [18]. Several clinical studies confirm that exposure in humans leads to inflammation and oxidative stress persisting for days after the exposure [19]. In combination with poorly ventilated spaces, even with moderate use, effects have been demonstrated. A family study of sarcoidosis in African Americans found a positive association between sarcoidosis and occupations with exposure to photocopier toner dust of clerical workers [20].

Pollution at Work Spaces—Sick-Building Syndrome

The term sick-building syndrome applies to the development of reproducible symptoms that might be rather non-specific while in a building (work space or home). There is a distinctive temporal relation with visits or prolonged stay in a particular building. Symptoms occur within a few hours of entering the building and often improve rather quickly when exiting the building. Most often, the term sick-building syndrome is used for work space environments rather than a domestic dwelling, although problems with indoor air also occur in private homes. Dwellings with water damage where fungal spores are felt to be the culprit, or poorly ventilated attic and basement spaces with high airborne dust particles can set off symptoms repeatedly. Chemical outgassing from structural components (e.g., paints, formaldehyde) may play a role in the development of symptoms.

General symptoms of sick-building syndrome are dull headache and lethargy, dizzy symptoms, ENT membrane symptoms such as stuffy nose, occasionally sneezing, dry throat, and asthma. Symptoms can be uncomfortable and at times disabling but usually not chronic [21]. Treatment involves much less the patient rather the building itself and an assessment of the building should be considered high priority [22]. Frequently, ventilation plays a key role in improving air quality and decreasing symptoms. Low ventilation rates in air-conditioned buildings of less than 10 l/s/person are associated with increased symptoms [23]. Simple measures such as increasing the airflow of the air-conditioning units might help to improve symptoms.

Psychological factors, such as stress and work dissatisfaction, as well as environmental factors such as poor lighting, noise and ergonomic factors may contribute to worsening symptoms.

There is a strong association between lack of control of the office environment and symptoms [24]. Employees who are more stressed and feel they have no sense of control generally have more symptoms [25].

Air Filtration

Key to improved indoor air quality is ventilation and filtration. Ventilation becomes important when the indoor environment has a high concentration of toxic compounds. Increasing the airflow in the air-conditioning units or opening doors and windows can be an efficient way to improve the indoor air quality quickly. Filtration systems are necessary in buildings to improve the indoor air quality either because ventilation is inadequate, or the air quality remains poor.

Air purifiers usually use a multilayer filter system of a pre-filter, a carbon filter, an antibacterial filter, and a high-efficiency particle air filter (HEPA). Adding a potent HEPA filtration system will effectively decrease fine and ultrafine particles from closed spaces as it removes 99.97% of particles greater than 0.3 μm [26].

It has been shown to be an effective tool in asthma control from traffic-related airborne particles [27], for controlling sinonasal symptoms of environmental allergies and to reduce the ill effects of cigarette smoke [28].

The removal efficiencies generally increased with manufacturer-reported filter ratings and with filter thickness, but significant variability in effectiveness seems to be common [29]. The highest filter quality (MERV 16) seems to remove particles two to three times more efficiently than the lower quality ones [30]. Consumers are often overwhelmed by the number of available models and brands. Most valuable recommendation in the authors' practice has been made based on Consumer Report reviews as an independent, non-profit organization making direct comparison of features and performance. (https://www.consumerreports.org/cro/air-purifiers/buying-guide/index.htm).

Environmental Noise and Sound Pollution

Loud noise as a nonspecific stressor impairs physical and mental wellbeing. Excessive and prolonged noise exposure has been associated with multiple health-related problems, from stress, poor concentration, and loss of productivity to loss of sleep and cardiovascular disease [31]. Its mechanism has been postulated to activate the general oxidative stress pathway of nitric oxide and impair endothelial function. Besides the direct stimulation of noise affecting the hearing pathways, an indirect activation, leading to a cognitive and emotional response has been described [32]. Noise activates the autonomic nervous system as well as endocrine system [33]. Particularly road, railroad and aircraft noise in urban areas have been studied and clearly shown to increase the risk of ischemic heart disease, heart attacks as well risk of high blood pressure [34]. The discovery of loud noise effects on the cardiovascular system by secretions of catecholamines [35] and vasoconstriction [36] date back to studies in the 1960s. Even low-level noise exposure was found to have a similar effect on the autonomic nervous and cardiovascular system [37]. There is robust evidence for a negative effect of industrial noise exposure in school children's reading skills and memory, as well as on standardized academic test scores [38].

Noise in the environment disrupts sleep and causes repeated awakening. Changes in sleep architecture of REM sleep and also changes in Stages 3 and 4 have been documented [39]. Total sleep time can be reduced by both longer time to fall asleep and premature awakening [40]. The sleep may also become fragmented or deep sleep may shift to lighter sleep stages [41]. Daytime noise is suspected to have a sustained effect on nighttime sleep quality, specifically on slow wave sleep and sleep efficiency [42]. An older study links louder noise exposure to the preference for sweet taste [43] and with that potentially a risk to consume more calories. Greater rates of weight gain have been causally related to poor sleep, maybe from increased dietary intake itself or decreased physical activity [44]. Obesity then leads to many co-morbidities including sleep apnea, which disrupts the sleep at a physical level, a vicious cycle begins.

Work Stress

Worldwide, mental health illnesses, burnout, and other conditions related to stress are on the rise. Emotional depletion or loss of motivation are the first consequences of prolonged exposure to chronic emotional and interpersonal stressors on the job [45].

Work environmental stressors may include:

1. Organizational constraints.
   - problems with equipment, supplies, or soft or hardware,
   - work content such as unclear roles, work volumes.
2. Temporal factors such as shift work.
3. Interpersonal stressors.
   - Discrimination—bias, sexual harassment – Coworker interactions—lack of support from colleagues, interpersonal conflict, inequitable workload, and unsuitable partners—Supervision—criticism, lack of feedback, and unequal treatment [46].

Exposure to occupational stressors is related to the development and/or exacerbation of physical symptoms. For example work-related upper extremity shoulder and neck pain symptoms in office workers are strongly associated with the amount of job stress [47]. Of a cohort of "healthy people," almost 47% reported muscle pain in the head/neck region that interfered with their ability to work, which all reflected measurable in their work performance [48].

Decreased productivity and sick leave on a personal level, financial and social cost for the family and high economic burden for the company and society as a whole are the consequences of unaddressed work stress. Interventions by the employer that enhance individual protective factors may be most effective in reducing stress and illness among employees [49]. Resilience training, yoga, and mindfulness-based stress reduction have been validated as effective tools to reduce stress, improve well-being and emotional regulation. Individuals with greater positive self-perceptions lived longer and tended to practice more preventive health behaviors [50].

Burnout, as one symptom of work-related stress may affect as many as 10% of the working population and 44% of US physicians experience symptoms of burn-out [51].

In the times of the COVID-19 pandemic when this chapter was written, a state of fear and panic affects patient and treating health care professionals alike. With great fear, clinical outcomes can potentially worsen due to uncertainty and the Nocebo effect, in which negative expectations can lead to negative outcomes [52] for the patient and a significant increase in work stress amongst health care workers.

The link between physiology, pathophysiology, and psychology in any environment cannot be over-emphasized at any time, but especially in times of a disaster, the impact on mental health needs to be a primary concern. Therefore, it remains of upmost importance to actively engage in behaviors aiding in stress management, encouraging nurturing human interactions, fostering connectedness and healthy communities.

References

1. Baraniuk JN. Pathogenic mechanisms of idiopathic nonallergic rhinitis. World Allergy Organ J. 2009;2(6):106–14. Published 2009 Jun 15
2. Elsheikh MN, Badran HM. Dysautonomia rhinitis: associated otolaryngologic manifestations and characterization based on autonomic function tests. Acta Otolaryngol. 2006;126(11):1206–12.
3. Jaradeh SS, Smith TL, Torrico L, Prieto TE, Loehrl TA, Darling RJ, Toohill RJ. Autonomic nervous system evaluation of patients with vasomotor rhinitis. Laryngoscope. 2000;110(11):1828–31.
4. Segal S, Shlamkovitch N, Eviatar E, Berenholz L, Sarfaty S, Kessler A. Vasomotor rhinitis following trauma to the nose. Ann Otol Rhinol Laryngol. 1999;108:208–10.
5. Kenia P, Houghton T, Beardsmore C. Does inhaling menthol affect nasal patency or cough? Pediatr Pulmonol. 2008;43(6):532–7.
6. Burrow A, Eccles R, Jones AS. The effects of camphor, eucalyptus and menthol vapour on nasal resistance to airflow and nasal sensation. Acta Otolaryngol. 1983;96(1-2):157–61.
7. Weuve J, Puett RC, Schwartz J, Yanosky JD, Laden F, Grodstein F. Exposure to particulate air pollution and cognitive decline in older women. Arch Intern Med. 2012;172(3):219–27.
8. Lopuszanska U, Samardakiewicz M. The relationship between air pollution and cognitive functions in children and adolescents: a systematic review. Cogn Behav Neurol. 2020;33(3):157–78.
9. Patten KT, González EA, Valenzuela A, et al. Effects of early life exposure to traffic-related air pollution on brain development in juvenile Sprague-Dawley rats. Transl Psychiatry. 2020;10:166.
10. Chuang KJ, Chan CC, Su TC, Lee CT, Tang CS. The effect of urban air pollution on inflammation, oxidative stress, coagulation, and autonomic dysfunction in young adults. Am J Respir Crit Care Med. 2007;176(4):370–6.
11. Huang W, Zhu T, Pan X, et al. Air pollution and autonomic and vascular dysfunction in patients with cardiovascular disease: interactions of systemic inflammation, overweight, and gender. Am J Epidemiol. 2012;176(2):117–26.

12. Calderón-Garcidueñas L, San Juan Chávez V, Vacaseydel-Aceves NB, Calderón-Sánchez R, Macías-Escobedo E, Frías C, Giacometto M, Velasquez L, Félix-Villarreal R, Martin JD, Draheim C, Engle RW. Chocolate, air pollution and children's neuroprotection: what cognition tools should be at hand to evaluate interventions? Front Pharmacol. 2016;7:232.
13. Sokolov AN, Pavlova MA, Klosterhalfen S, Enck P. Chocolate and the brain: neurobiological impact of cocoa flavanols on cognition and behavior. Neurosci Biobehav Rev. 2013;37(10 Pt 2):2445–53.
14. Feldman RG. Occupational neurology. Yale J Biol Med. 1987;60(2):179–86.
15. Lotti M, Aminoff MJ. Evaluating suspected work-related neurologic disorders (clinical diagnosis). Handb Clin Neurol. 2015;131:9–21.
16. https://www.osha.gov/
17. Nandan A, Siddiqui NA, Kumar P. Assessment of environmental and ergonomic hazard associated to printing and photocopying: a review. Environ Geochem Health. 2019;41(3):1187–211.
18. Pirela SV, Martin J, Bello D, Demokritou P. Nanoparticle exposures from nano-enabled toner-based printing equipment and human health: state of science and future research needs. Crit Rev Toxicol. 2017;47(8):678–704.
19. Khatri M, Bello D, Gaines P, Martin J, Pal AK, Gore R, Woskie S. Nanoparticles from photocopiers induce oxidative stress and upper respiratory tract inflammation in healthy volunteers. Nanotoxicology. 2013;7:1014–27.
20. Rybicki BA, Amend KL, Maliarik MJ, Iannuzzi MC. Photocopier exposure and risk of sarcoidosis in African-American sibs. Sarcoidosis Vasc Diffuse Lung Dis. 2004;21(1):49–55.
21. Redlich CA, Sparer J, Cullen MR. Sick-building syndrome. Lancet. 1997;349(9057):1013–6. https://doi.org/10.1016/S0140-6736(96)07220-0.
22. Burge PS. Sick building syndrome. Occup Environ Med. 2004;61(2):185–90.
23. Mendell MJ, Smith AH. Consistent pattern of elevated symptoms in airconditioned office buildings: a reanalysis of epidemiologic studies. Am J Public Health. 1990;80(1193–9):43.
24. Burge PS, Hedge A, Wilson S, et al. Sick building syndrome; a study of 4373 office workers. Ann Occup Hyg. 1987;31:493–504.
25. Menzies D, Pasztor J, Nunes F, et al. Effects of new ventilation system on health and well-being of office workers. Arch Environ Health. 1997;52:360–7.
26. Vijayan VK, Paramesh H, Salvi SS, Dalal AA. Enhancing indoor air quality—the air filter advantage. Lung India. 2015;32(5):473–9.
27. James C, Bernstein DI, Cox J, Ryan P, Wolfe C, Jandarov R, Newman N, Indugula R, Reponen T. HEPA filtration improves asthma control in children exposed to traffic-related airborne particles. Indoor Air. 2020;30(2):235–43.
28. Sublett JL. Effectiveness of air filters and air cleaners in allergic respiratory diseases: a review of the recent literature. Curr Allergy Asthma Rep. 2011;11:395–402.
29. Fazli T, Zeng Y, Stephens B. Fine and ultrafine particle removal efficiency of new residential HVAC filters. Indoor Air. 2019;29(4):656–69.
30. Stephens B, Siegel JA. Ultrafine particle removal by residential heating, ventilating, and air-conditioning filters. Indoor Air. 2013;23(6):488–97.
31. Berglund B, Lindvall T, editors. Community noise. Archives of the Center for Sensory Research. 1995;2(1):1–195.
32. Münzel T, Sørensen M, Schmidt F, et al. The adverse effects of environmental noise exposure on oxidative stress and cardiovascular risk. Antioxid Redox Signal. 2018;28(9):873–908.
33. Babisch W. Stress hormones in the research on cardiovascular effects of noise. Noise Health. 2003;5(18):1–11.
34. https://www.who.int/quantifying_ehimpacts/publications/e94888.pdf?ua=1
35. Jansen G. Effects of noise on health. Ger Med Mon. 1968;13:446–8.
36. Jansen G. The effect of noise during physical work [in German]. Int Z Angew Physiol. 1964;20:233–9.
37. Ising H, Dienel D, Günther T, et al. Health effects of traffic noise. Int Arch Occup Environ Heath. 1980;47:179–90.
38. Stansfeld S, Clark C. Curr Environ. Health Rep. 2015;2(2):171–8.

39. Arnberg P, Eberhardt JL. Sleep disturbances caused by vibrations from heavy road traffic. J Acoust Soc Am. 1990;88(3):1486–93.
40. Muzet A. Environmental noise, sleep and health. Sleep Med Rev. 2007;11:135–42.
41. Hume KI, Brink M, Basner M. Effects of environmental noise on sleep. Noise Health. 2012;14(61):297–302.
42. Lin CY, Tsai PJ, Lin KY, Chen CY, Chung LH, Wu JL, Guo YL. Will daytime occupational noise exposures induce nighttime sleep disturbance? Sleep Med. 2018;50:87–96.
43. Ferber C, Cabanac M, Influence of noise on gustatory affective ratings and preference for sweet or salt Appetite, Volume 8, Issue 3, 1987, Pages 229-235, ISSN 0195-6663.
44. Ogilvie RP, Patel SR. The epidemiology of sleep and obesity. Sleep Health. 2017;3(5):383–8.
45. Alvarez E, Sutton A, Barton B, Vaidya S. Evaluating a group-based yoga of stress resilience programme: a pragmatic before-after interventional study protocol. BMJ Open. 2020;10(3):e035862. Published 2020 Mar 31
46. Morris A. Gender and ethnic differences in social constraints among a sample of New York City police officers. J Occup Health Psychol. 1996;1(2):224–35.
47. Haufler AJ, Feuerstein M, Huang GD. Job stress, upper extremity pain and functional limitations in symptomatic computer users. Am J Ind Med. 2000;38(5):507–15.
48. Suvinen TI, Ahlberg J, Rantala M, Nissinen M, Lindholm H, Könönen M, Savolainen A. Perceived stress, pain and work performance among non-patient working personnel with clinical signs of temporomandibular or neck pain. J Oral Rehabil. 2004;31(8):733–7.
49. Dolbier CL, Smith SE, Steinhardt MA. Relationships of protective factors to stress and symptoms of illness. Am J Health Behav. 2007;31(4):423–33.
50. Levy BR, Slade MD, Kunkel SR, Kasl SV. Longevity increased by positive self-perceptions of aging. J Pers Soc Psychol. 2002;83(2):261–70.
51. West CP, Dyrbye LN, Sinsky C, et al. Resilience and burnout among physicians and the general US working population. JAMA Netw Open. 2020;3(7):e209385. Published 2020 Jul 1
52. Karnatovskaia LV, Johnson MM, Varga K, et al. Stress and fear: clinical implications for providers and patients (in the time of COVID-19 and beyond). Mayo Clin Proc. 2020;95(11):2487–98.

6 Depression

Mandana Modirrousta

Prevalence and Comorbidity

Depression frequently co-occurs with functional illness. As many as two-thirds of patients with functional illness have some comorbid psychiatric disease, with a history of depression being the most common [1]. Lifetime comorbidity of Major Depressive Disorder (MDD) in adults with functional illness has been estimated to be anywhere from 35% to 86%, with a current prevalence of 22–40% [2–5]. This strong comorbidity is seen across all domains of functional illness: from functional pain to movement disorders to voice dysfunction.

Numerous studies have documented the high rates of depression in patients with movement and paretic expressions of Functional Neurological Disorders, with the lifetime prevalence of MDD estimated at 35–42% in this population [4]. A review of 31 articles reporting psychiatric comorbidities in individuals with psychogenic non-epileptic seizures (PNES) found that—although the reported prevalence varies from study to study—some groups showed depression in almost 4 out of every 5 individuals [2]. These exceptionally high rates of depression are also seen in people with functional pain, as 90% of patients with fibromyalgia show depressive symptoms at some point in their lifetime, with 50–86% of individuals experiencing a major depressive episode [3, 6]. Indeed, the odds of patients with fibromyalgia having depression are roughly three times higher than the healthy population, even when controlling for important socio-demographic characteristics [5]. Functional voice dysfunction is similarly impacted; a study of 61 individuals with functional dysphonia found that 57% of the group met clinical criteria for a mood disorder, and patients had significantly higher depression scores than healthy, matched controls [7].

M. Modirrousta (✉)
Department of Psychiatry, University of Manitoba, Winnipeg, MB, Canada
e-mail: mandana.modirrousta@umanitoba.ca

© The Author(s), under exclusive license to Springer Nature Switzerland AG 2023

B. W. Blakley, J. E. Blakley (eds.), *Functional Illness of the Head and Neck*,
https://doi.org/10.1007/978-3-031-12998-8_6

Depression as a Risk Factor for Functional Illness

Clearly, functional illness and depression are strongly tied to one another. Indeed, not only is there a strong comorbidity, but the presence of depression can affect the severity of a functional illness. For instance, depression scores have been found to positively correlate with the severity of functional motor symptoms [8]. The question becomes, then, to what extent do depression and functional illness influence one another? Does depression precede or precipitate functional illness, or vice versa? Or are these two sets of symptoms linked to a common underlying mechanism which causes and/or modifies the severity of both in tandem? While there are no definitive answers to these questions—the causality of the relationship between depression and functional illness has yet to be fully discovered—there are observations and models that are beginning to explore the potential mechanisms of this comorbidity.

There is evidence for a genetic connection between depression and functional disorders, in that genetic factors may predispose certain individuals to develop both depression and functional symptoms in response to precipitating events such as injury or psychosocial stressors [3]. For instance, a polymorphism in the serotonin transporter (5-HHT) gene has been implicated in both MDD and fibromyalgia [9, 10], and MDD is predicted nearly equally by the presence of familial MDD or fibromyalgia, reinforcing the biological link between the two [11]. Functional pain and depression have also both been associated with the consequences of an abnormally persistent stress response, leading to disturbed cortisol levels and their effects on neurotransmitter systems, especially the hypothalamic–pituitary–adrenal axis [3, 12]. Gracely and colleagues [3] suggest that depression and functional pain likely share a mutual predisposition through a combination of genetic and environmental factors. However, they argue that the differing response of depression and fibromyalgia to certain pharmacological treatments indicates that they are "mediated by largely independent mechanisms with mutual modulation of specific symptoms" [3].

Functional illness is often explained using a biopsychosocial model in which characteristics such as depression may act as predisposing or triggering factors and may contribute to the chronicity of functional symptoms [13–15]. A link between depression and functional illness has also been suggested with regard to underlying deficits in emotional processing. It is well known that MDD is characterized by the presence of disturbed emotional processing [16], and it has been proposed that this deficit may also result in some individuals experiencing emotions more somatically; for instance, producing physical tension that impacts the voice leading to functional dysphonia [17, 18]. Under this model, high stress situations may produce both depression and functional symptoms in individuals with deficits in emotional processing.

Impact of Depression on Prognosis

The influence of comorbid depression on treatment outcomes is difficult to ascertain, and studies have produced conflicting results. For instance, some studies have observed that the presence of depression correlates with favorable prognosis in patients with functional motor symptoms [19, 20], with one recent study finding that higher depression scores actually predicted better clinical outcomes [21]. However, not all reports concur with this observation, and other studies have found comorbid depression to be associated with poor clinical outcomes [22, 23].

Treatment

Functional illnesses often require an integrated multidisciplinary approach to treatment which targets the presenting symptoms with an understanding that neurological and psychological symptoms influence one another and may even share an underlying etiology [1, 15]. As we have seen, depression and low mood can influence prognosis, so it is important to consider these symptoms in treatment selection. Where a straightforward presentation of depression is identified, treatment according to established guidelines for depression may be appropriate [24]. However, the selection of therapeutic intervention must also take into account comorbidities, so clinical judgement should be used to maximize efficacy in treating depression while avoiding the potential exacerbation of functional symptoms [1]. Furthermore, a physician's approach to treatment is important; patients may benefit simply from validation and normalization of their concerns, and effective communication with the patient as well as between treating physicians may aid in treatment adherence and with the efficacy of interventions such as psychotherapy [25].

Medication

Antidepressant medications for the treatment of functional illness or depression and anxiety will be discussed in more detail in other sections. Here we discuss certain general considerations when selecting pharmaceutical treatments for functional symptoms in the face of comorbid depression. Evidence is scarce with regards to pharmaceutical intervention specifically for depression in functional illness, as there are few randomized controlled trials assessing the efficacy of any given antidepressant [1, 26, 27]. As such, pharmacological therapy is often primarily guided by the predominant symptoms that accompany functional complaints [1, 24, 28].

With regard to functional pain, tricyclic antidepressants (TCA), such as amitriptyline, have frequently been employed for their ability to improve both pain and depression. Serotonin–norepinephrine reuptake inhibitors (SNRIs), such as duloxetine, are also useful for this dual purpose. It is interesting to note that the dosage of TCAs used to treat pain is often much lower than that employed in the treatment of depression, and pain relief is usually achieved in a much shorter time compared with changes in depression symptoms [3, 29, 30]. These observations, paired with reports of independent symptom improvement with SNRIs, suggest the presence of independent mechanisms underlying these two disorders [3, 31]. Care should be taken in the use of opioids or cannabinoids for the treatment of functional pain, as they may exacerbate depression [13].

Psychotherapy

Psychological therapies are one of the most prevalent and effective forms of intervention in the care of depression [32, 33], and psychotherapies have also proven useful for reducing symptoms of functional illness. For instance, a variety of psychotherapies, including psychodynamic psychotherapy, mindfulness-based interventions, and group psychoeducation, have all been shown useful in the management of functional movement disorders [34–36]. O'Neal and Baslet [1] recommend having patients keep a diary of the things which precipitate their symptoms, helping create new behaviors to break unconscious patterns which may be leading to the expression of functional symptoms, and teaching strategies to reduce the tendency to express distress through physical symptoms.

Cognitive behavioral therapy (CBT) is a form of psychotherapy that involves efforts to pinpoint irrational or distorted thinking, identify emotions associated with this thinking, and restructure these thought patterns to affect positive changes in mood and behavior [37]. CBT is widely used in the treatment of depression, and its use in conjunction with pharmacotherapy is significantly more effective than medication alone [37, 38]. CBT is also beneficial in the treatment and management of functional illnesses and may even be superior to standard medical care in reducing symptom burden in certain populations [1]. In relation to functional disorders, CBT may focus on identifying thought patterns that are reinforcing symptoms while introducing stress management techniques and beneficial behavioral responses [1].

Given the widespread use of CBT for the treatment of depression and its demonstrated efficacy for both depression and certain functional symptoms, CBT represents a very promising modality for the unified treatment of comorbid psychiatric and functional symptoms. One study found that CBT alone and CBT + sertraline in combination were effective in reducing functional seizure frequency, but patients who received CBT alone reported a greater improvement of secondary outcomes including depression [24, 39]. Indeed, for patients with episodic symptoms, such as functional seizures, CBT has been suggested as the preferred treatment modality [1].

Brain Stimulation

Non-invasive brain stimulation, including repetitive transcranial magnetic stimulation (rTMS), has shown some early promise in the treatment of symptoms associated with functional illness. For instance, stimulation of motor cortex can reduce pain, whereas temporal–parietal junction stimulation may improve psychogenic seizure frequency [40, 41]. rTMS for the treatment of MDD typically targets the dorsolateral prefrontal cortex, and there is preliminary evidence to indicate that this target site is also effective at alleviating depression in individuals with comorbid functional pain [40]. Thus, although it is too early to establish optimal stimulation parameters in functional illness, rTMS and other non-invasive stimulation techniques—such as transcranial direct current stimulation (tDCS)—may represent an effective treatment alternative [24].

References

1. O'Neal MA, Baslet G. Treatment for patients with a functional neurological disorder (conversion disorder): an integrated approach. Am J Psychiatry. 2018;175(4):307–14.
2. Baslet G, Bajestan SN, Aybek S, Modirrousta M, Price JD, Cavanna A, et al. Evidence-based practice for the clinical assessment of psychogenic nonepileptic seizures: a report from the American neuropsychiatric association committee on research. J Neuropsychiatry Clin Neurosci. 2021;33(1):27–42.
3. Gracely RH, Ceko M, Bushnell MC. Fibromyalgia and depression. Pain Res Treat. 2012;2012:486590.
4. Perez DL, Aybek S, Popkirox S, Kozlowska K, Stephen CD, Anderson J, et al. A review and expert opinion on the neuropsychiatric assessment of motor functional neurological disorders. J Neuropsychiatry Clin Neurosci. 2021. Winter;33(1):14–26.
5. Fuller-Thomson E, Nimigon-Young J, Brennenstuhl S. Individuals with fibromyalgia and depression: findings from a nationally representative Canadian survey. Rheumatol Int. 2012;32(4):853–62.
6. Alciati A, Atzeni F, Caldirola D, Perna G, Sarzi-Puttini P. The co-morbidity between bipolar and panic disorder in fibromyalgia syndrome. J Clin Med. 2020;9(11):3619.
7. Willinger U, Völkl-Kernstock S, Aschauer HN. Marked depression and anxiety in patients with functional dysphonia. Psychiatry Res. 2005;134(1):85–91.
8. Ricciardi L, Demartini B, Morgante F, Parees I, Nielsen G, Edwards MJ. Symptom severity in patients with functional motor symptoms: patient's perception and doctor's clinical assessment. Parkinsonism Relat Disord. 2015;21(5):529–32.
9. Lotrich FE, Pollock BG. Meta-analysis of serotonin transporter polymorphisms and affective disorders. Psychiatr Genet. 2004;14(3):121–9.
10. Cohen H, Buskila D, Neumann L, Ebstein RP. Confirmation of an association between fibromyalgia and serotonin transporter promoter region (5- HTTLPR) polymorphism, and relationship to anxiety-related personality traits. Arthritis Rheum. 2002;46(3):845–7.
11. Raphael KG, Janal MN, Nayak S, Schwartz JE, Gallagher RM. Familial aggregation of depression in fibromyalgia: a community-based test of alternate hypotheses. Pain. 2004;110(1-2):449–60.
12. Gold PW, Gabry KE, Yasuda MR, Chrousos GP. Divergent endocrine abnormalities in melancholic and atypical depression: clinical and pathophysiologic implications. Endocrinol Metab Clin N Am. 2002;31(1):37–62. vi
13. Fitzcharles MA, Ste-Marie PA, Goldenberg DL, Pereira JX, Abbey S, Choinière M, et al. 2012 Canadian Guidelines for the diagnosis and management of fibromyalgia syndrome: executive summary. Pain Res Manag. 2013;18(3):119–26.
14. Pick S, Goldstein LH, Perez DL, Nicholson TR. Emotional processing in functional neurological disorder: a review, biopsychosocial model and research agenda. J Neurol Neurosurg Psychiatry. 2019;90(6):704–11.
15. Pun P, Frater J, Broughton M, Dob R, Lehn A. Psychological profiles and clinical clusters of patients diagnosed with functional neurological disorder. Front Neurol. 2020;11:580267.
16. Ritchey M, Dolcos F, Eddington KM, Strauman TJ, Cabeza R. Neural correlates of emotional processing in depression: changes with cognitive behavioral therapy and predictors of treatment response. J Psychiatr Res. 2011;45(5):577–87.
17. Baker J. Women's voices: lost or mislaid, stolen or strayed? Int J Speech Lang Pathol. 2010;12(2):94–106.
18. Deary V, Miller T. Reconsidering the role of psychosocial factors in functional dysphonia. Curr Opin Otolaryngol Head Neck Surg. 2011;19(3):150–4.
19. Thomas M, Vuong KD, Jankovic J. Long-term prognosis of patients with psychogenic movement disorders. Parkinsonism Relat Disord. 2006;12(6):382–7.
20. Crimlisk HL, Bhatia K, Cope H, David A, Marsden CD, Ron MA. Slater revisited: 6 year follow up study of patients with medically unexplained motor symptoms. BMJ. 1998;316(7131):582–6.

21. Jalilianhasanpour R, Ospina JP, Williams B, Mello J, MacLean J, Ranford J, et al. Secure attachment and depression predict 6-month outcome in motor functional neurological disorders: a prospective pilot study. Psychosomatics. 2019;60(4):365–75.
22. Ibrahim NM, Martino D, van de Warrenburg BP, Quinn NP, Bhatia KP, Brown RJ, et al. The prognosis of fixed dystonia: a follow-up study. Parkinsonism Relat Disord. 2009;15(8):592–7.
23. Feinstein A, Stergiopoulos V, Fine J, Lan AE. Psychiatric outcome in patients with a psychogenic movement disorder: a prospective study. Neuropsychiatry Neuropsychol. Behav Neurol. 2001;14(3):169–76.
24. Gilmour GS, Nielsen G, Teodoro T, Yogarajah M, Coebergh JA, Dilley MD, et al. Management of functional neurological disorder. J Neurol. 2020;267(7):2164–72.
25. Adams C, Anderson J, Madva EN, LaFrance WC Jr, Perez DL. You've made the diagnosis of functional neurological disorder: now what? Pract Neurol. 2018;18(4):323–30.
26. Voon V, Lang AE. Antidepressant treatment outcomes of psychogenic movement disorder. J Clin Psychiatry. 2005;66(12):1529–34.
27. Kleinstäuber M, Witthöft M, Steffanowski A, van Marwijk H, Hiller W, Lambert MJ. Pharmacological interventions for somatoform disorders in adults. Cochrane Database Syst Rev. 2014;11:CD010628.
28. Clauw DJ. Fibromyalgia: a clinical review. JAMA. 2014;311(15):1547–55.
29. Mudyanadzo TA, Hauzaree C, Yerokhina O, Architha NN, Ashqar HM. Irritable bowel syndrome and depression: a shared pathogenesis. Cureus. 2018;10(8):e3178.
30. Wilmes L, Collins JM, O'Riordan KJ, O'Mahony SM, Cryan JF, Clarke G. Of bowels, brain and behavior: a role for the gut microbiota in psychiatric comorbidities in irritable bowel syndrome. Neurogastroenterol Motil. 2021;33(3):e14095.
31. Marangell LB, Clauw DJ, Choy E, Wang F, Shoemaker S, Bradley L, et al. Comparative pain and mood effects in patients with comorbid fibromyalgia and major depressive disorder: secondary analyses of four pooled randomized controlled trials of duloxetine. Pain. 2011;152(1):31–7.
32. Cuijpers P, Quero S, Dowrick C, Arroll B. Psychological treatment of depression in primary care: recent developments. Curr Psychiatry Rep. 2019;21(12):129.
33. Cuijpers P, Karyotaki E, Eckshtain D, Ng MY, Corteselli KA, Noma H, et al. Psychotherapy for depression across different age groups: a systematic review and meta-analysis. JAMA Psychiat. 2020;77(7):694–702.
34. Kompoliti K, Wilson B, Stebbins G, Bernard B, Hinson V. Immediate vs. delayed treatment of psychogenic movement disorders with short term psychodynamic psychotherapy: randomized clinical trial. Parkinsonism Relat Disord. 2014;20(1):60–3.
35. Baslet G, Dworetzky B, Perez DL, Oser M. Treatment of psychogenic nonepileptic seizures: updated review and findings from a mindfulness-based intervention case series. Clin EEG Neurosci. 2015;46(1):54–64.
36. Zaroff CM, Myers L, Barr WB, Luciano D, Devinsky O. Group psychoeducation as treatment for psychological nonepileptic seizures. Epilepsy Behav. 2004;5(4):587–92.
37. Vasile C. CBT and medication in depression (review). Exp Ther Med. 2020;20(4):3513–6.
38. Gautam M, Tripathi A, Deshmukh D, Gaur M. Cognitive behavioral therapy for depression. Indian J Psychiatry. 2020;62(Suppl 2):S223–9.
39. LaFrance WC Jr, Baird GL, Barry JJ, Blum AS, Frank Webb A, Keitner GI, et al. Multicenter pilot treatment trial for psychogenic nonepileptic seizures. JAMA Psychiat. 2014;71:997–1005.
40. Hou WH, Wang TY, Kang JH. The effects of add-on non-invasive brain stimulation in fibromyalgia: a meta-analysis and meta-regression of randomized controlled trials. Rheumatology (Oxford). 2016;55(8):1507–17.
41. Peterson KT, Kosior R, Meek BP, Ng M, Perez DL, Modirrousta M. Right temporoparietal junction transcranial magnetic stimulation in the treatment of psychogenic nonepileptic seizures: a case series. Psychosomatics. 2018;59(6):601–6.

Chronic Pain Syndromes: Neck Pain

7

George Deng

Introduction

Neck pain is a common source of pain with an overall prevalence of up to 86.6% and a mean of 23.1% [1]. Neck pain was identified as the main cause in 20.4% of chronic pain patients [2]. There are several risk factors for neck pain including female gender, high-income countries, urban location, age, occupation, and previous musculoskeletal pain [1, 3].

The cervical spine is composed of seven vertebrae and eight cervical nerve roots. Each vertebra is connected to the adjacent level via the facet joints, uncinate process, and the intervertebral disc except for the atlantooccipital (C0–C1) articulations and the atlantoaxial (C1–C2) articulation.

Pain referral can pose another challenge in the assessment of neck pain. This phenomenon is attributed to the convergence theory of pain [4]. Neck pain not only refers pain distally but can also refer pain cranially causing cervicogenic headaches [5] via the cervicotrigeminal convergence [6].

Etiology

The differential diagnosis for neck pain can be either categorized from an anatomical perspective or from a disease perspective (Table 7.1). Anatomically, innervated structures include the bones, intervertebral discs, facet joint, ligaments, muscles, and nerves can be a source of pain.

G. Deng (✉)
Section of Physical Medicine and Rehabilitation, Department of Clinical Neuroscience, University of Calgary, Calgary, AB, Canada

© The Author(s), under exclusive license to Springer Nature Switzerland AG 2023

B. W. Blakley, J. E. Blakley (eds.), *Functional Illness of the Head and Neck*,
https://doi.org/10.1007/978-3-031-12998-8_7

Table 7.1 Differential diagnosis for neck pain

Mechanical	• Osteoarthritis • Cervical strain and sprain • Adjacent level arthritis post-spinal fusion • Radiculopathy and radiculitis • Superficial cervical plexopathy
Inflammatory	• Seronegative spondyloarthropathy • Connective tissue disease • Rheumatoid arthritis (atlantoaxial) • Diffuse idiopathic skeletal hyperostosis • Longus colli tendinitis
Infectious	• Vertebral osteomyelitis • Diskitis • Cervical Pott's disease from tuberculosis • Granulomatous process • Epidural, intradural, and subdural abscesses • Retropharyngeal abscess
Tumors	• Benign osseus tumors • Malignant tumors • Metastasis • Intradural and extradural tumors
Congenital	• Down's syndrome • Ehrler's Danlos syndrome • Chiari malformation
Syndromes	• Myofascial pain syndrome • Fibromyalgia and widespread pain syndrome • Hypermobility syndrome

Clinical Evaluation

History

The evaluation for neck pain includes a thorough history and physical examination. The history should include details about the pain. Aggravating or alleviating features that are not activity related or positional should prompt the physician to consider nonmechanical sources of pain. Associated features such as headaches or dizziness are commonly reported and would necessities further characterization of these symptoms. Red flags should be elicited to rule out potentially devastating etiologies of pain which includes neurologic compromise, vertebrobasilar insufficiency, craniovertebral ligament instability, infections, and malignancy.

There is a bidirectional effect of pain with mood [7] and sleep [8]. Identification and treatment of these concurrent issues are important in helping a patient with pain. Additionally, many of the pain-modulating medications can also affect mood and sleep.

Certain medical conditions may be pertinent in the patient with neck pain. For example, cervical instability may be present in patients with Down's syndrome [9], Rheumatoid Arthritis [10], and among others [11–16] and patients with hypermobility syndrome [17] or fibromyalgia may present with generalized pain include pain in the cervical region. There are several inherited conditions that may predispose a patient to neck pain. These include rheumatological [10, 12, 14], hypermobility [16–18], and cervical dystonia [15] to name a few. Lastly, a history of bleeding diathesis and anticoagulation use may limit neuroaxial interventional options [19].

One must be mindful of drug–drug interactions (see Pharmacology chapter). Although commonly used for pain management, cannabis is only recommended for use in specific pain conditions [20, 21]. Antidepressants and gabapentinoids used for pain modulation can also increase the risks of suicidality.

Previous neck surgeries may provide a clue to current neck pain. A history of cervical spinal surgery may lead to acceleration of adjacent level spondylosis and pain [22]. Additionally, previous anterior neck dissections may predispose a patient to superficial cervical plexus neuropathic pain [23].

Approaching chronic pain from the psychosocial perspective is important. Components of the social history include occupation, living situation, and ongoing litigation and worker's compensation. It is also important to elicit a history of alcohol, smoking, and illicit drug use. A functional history includes how the pain is affecting their activities of daily living, instrumental activities of daily living, vocational demands, and avocational pursuits. Treatment of pain can also lead to improvement of function which can be a more objective measure of improvement than a pain numeric rating scale.

Outcome Measures

Outcome measures can use to help the physician better characterize and communicate the patient's symptoms and severity in a more objective and validated manner. Common outcome measures include the brief pain inventory, Patient Reported Outcome Measurement Information System, Numeric Pain Rating Scale, Neck Disability Index, and the Neck Pain and Disability scale.

Physical Examination

The goal of the physical examination is to determine the main structural source of the pain, rule out neurologic deficits, and to help guide treatment. The components of a physical examination would include both musculoskeletal and neurologic maneuvers.

Musculoskeletal examination includes observation, range of motion, palpation, and special tests. The examination should include not only the cervical spine but also the joint above and below, which includes the temporomandibular joint and the shoulder joint.

Special testing of the neck includes cervical flexion rotation test (while patient is supine, the head is supported by the examiner and the cervical spine is rotated to end range with the cervical spine passively fully flexed) and Spurling's test (axial load with neck in extension, rotation, and lateral flexion). Cervical flexion rotation test is considered positive for C1–C2 involvement with reduction of rotation range and pain provocation. Spurling's test is considered positive for cervical nerve root involvement with reproduction of radicular arm pain.

Neurologic examination includes the cranial nerve evaluation, Horner's syndrome, as well as assessing for tone, bulk, power, deep tendon reflexes, Hoffman's, plantar response, and sensation in the limbs.

Laboratory Studies

Laboratory studies ordered should be guided by the patient's history and physical examination. The goal of laboratory studies is to rule out systemic causes of pain. For example, a patient presenting with systemic features of malignancy or infection would benefit from a complete blood count with differential and C-reactive protein/erythrocyte sedimentation rate. Prolonged morning stiffness, polyarthralgias, and rashes may warrant a rheumatologic workup.

Imaging Studies

Although imaging studies are commonly ordered for the evaluation of neck pain, one must be mindful of its poor sensitivity and specificity. There is good evidence that the location and degree of degenerative changes seen on imaging does not always correlate with the patient's symptoms [24].

When traumatic fractures, osteoporotic fracture, infection, or malignancy is suspected, a plain radiograph can be a helpful initial modality. Additional flexion and extension view helpful in identifying ligamentous injuries or segmental instability.

CTs or MRIs can be helpful in further evaluation of the cervical spine to assess for alternative reasons for neck pain other than spondylosis. Additionally, bone scan can be helpful in identifying pathological fractures, and inflammatory sources of pain.

Common Disorders

Chronic Primary Cervical Pain

The International Association For the Study of Pain published the new ICD 11 classification in 2019 [25]. Previously, chronic primary cervical pain was known as nonspecific neck pain or mechanical neck pain. This new language in labeling attempts to be inclusive of the pain regardless of its complex biopsychosocial origins.

From a biomechanical approach, there are many structures in the neck that are innervated by nociceptive neurons and can be implicated in pain. Cervical facet mediated pain is the most implicated anatomical structure in neck pain with an estimated prevalence of 60% [26]. The most common levels implicated is the C2–3 level, followed by C5–C7 [27]. There are no pathognomonic features on history that can help the clinician differentiate facet joint pain from other sources of pain [28]. Clinically, there may be restrictions in range and pain provocation. Palpable tenderness over the suspected facet joint levels can be as diagnostically accurate as local anesthetic blocks [29]. Imaging studies can rule out other serious sources of pain.

Another structure that is implicated in primary cervical pain is the cervical disks. This structure typically refer pain to the posterior neck in the midline with pain radiation into a wider area [30]. Physical exam signs are similar to those of cervical facet-mediated pain. As most interventional pain procedures are targeted at the facet joint due to safety, local anesthetic blockade of the facet joint without any pain relief likely points to involvement of the disc. Similar to facet-mediated pain, imaging modalities are used to rule out more serious pathology rather than to rule in the disc as a pain generator as imaging changes can occur in asymptomatic population [24].

Management of primary neck pain must be approached systematically and involve the patient's own preferences to maximize success. Management options can be divided into conservative, pharmacologic, and interventional options.

Conservative options for chronic primary cervical pain are associated with limited side effects and risks. Allied health providers including physiotherapy, occupational therapy, and pain psychology can be enlisted to help. There is heterogeneity in the literature which limits the level of evidence for rehabilitation [31]. Activity modification, pacing, and ergonomic adjustments are basic first steps. Modalities and passive treatments include, thermotherapy or cryotherapy [32–36], various manual therapies [37–41], transcutaneous electrical nerve stimulation [42–45], therapeutic ultrasound [43, 46–48], and needle intramuscular stimulation [49–51] can be helpful for short-term pain management. However, current management paradigms prefer a focus on active based rehabilitation and self-management options [52–54]. This can include, but is not limited to, pain neuroscience education [55–58], various exercise therapies [31, 59–62], and mind-body exercises (e.g., yoga, tai-chi, and qi gong) [25, 31, 63–66]. There is also evidence for the use of psychological therapies in the management of chronic neck pain [67–74].

Pharmacologic options include simple analgesics such as acetaminophen or nonsteroidal anti-inflammatory drugs (NSAIDs). One must be careful about underlying health conditions that may preclude the use of these medications. Escalation to opioids is rarely needed and often contraindicated due to the potential for dependency and the social implications of such. Pain modulating medications, although not well studied, can also provide longer duration of relief. These pain modulating medications include serotonin norepinephrine reuptake inhibitor (SNRI's), tricyclic antidepressants (TCAs), or gabapentinoids. Additionally, cannabis products may provide relief in certain patients. This includes nabilone, Sativex, or other plant-based products. Lastly, topical compounded options may serve a middle ground for patients who want to decrease their pill burden. There is limited evidence of such, but some patients do report relief. Many medications can be compounded into a topical formulation, including diclofenac, ketoprofen, cyclobenzaprine, gabapentin, lidocaine, and amitriptyline to name a few.

There has been a dramatic increase in interventional options in the management of pain [75]. Although, steroid injections are commonly used, the evidence supporting its use is limited [76, 77] and has risks [78, 79]. Radiofrequency ablation has the strongest interventional evidence in patients with neck predominant pain [80, 81]. This involves cauterization of the medial branch of the dorsal rami that innervates the facet joints. The main potential risk of this procedure is pain aggravation as well as, very rarely post radiofrequency neuritis [81, 82]. Lastly, there is interest in the use of platelet rich plasma therapy in the management of facet mediated pain in the lumbar spine [83–85] but evidence in the neck does not exist. This procedure involves centrifuging the patient's own platelets to concentrate the various growth factors and signaling proteins and injecting it into the putative painful facet joint. Lastly, one must be careful with maintaining a patient's expectation after interventional procedures as these procedures can potentially cause complications such as pain aggravation, failure for pain relief, hematoma formation, nerve injury, and theoretically stroke and death.

Neuromodulation is a growing field that involves either chemical or electrical modulation of the central or peripheral nervous system. One option is spinal cord stimulators which has evidence in neuropathic pain [86] and persistent post-operative spinal surgery axial or radicular pain [87, 88]. It does have a high initial cost to the healthcare system but economic studies do indicate that they are beneficial when accounting for the overall reduced healthcare utilization [89].

Lastly, there is some evidence that surgery can be used for recalcitrant axial cervical pain thought to be discogenic in origin [90–92]. If pursued, typically provocative discography is used to demonstrate that the targeted level is the main pain generator [91].

Cervical Radiculopathy

Cervical radiculopathy is a pathology of the cervical nerve roots. Symptoms are typically radicular in a dermatomal pattern and can be associated with a somatic referral pattern in the neck and in the periscapular regions. Patients may report neuropathic quality of pain associated with a myotomal distribution of weakness. Physical examination may identify the pattern of weakness following a myotome, but rarely sensory abnormalities are found due to the overlap of dermatomes. Deep tendon reflexes can be helpful if the nerve root pathology involves the C5, C6, or C7 nerve roots which are tested with biceps, brachioradialis, and triceps deep tendon reflexes. One must also rule out any upper motor neuron findings in both the upper and lower limbs which can be suggestive of spinal cord involvement. This includes spasticity, hyperreflexia, clonus, Hoffmann's, and plantar response. Spurling's maneuver and Bakody's hyperabduction signs are other physical examination maneuvers useful in identifying cervical radiculopathy. Bakody's hyperabduction sign is positive for cervical radiculitis if the radicular pain is improved with the ipsilateral hand placed over the patient's own head.

Cervical spine X-rays can identify potential areas of neural foraminal stenosis due to bony spondylosis. However, MRIs are better suited at defining the structures surrounding the nerve root and to rule out underlying cervical myelopathy. Electrodiagnostic evaluation with nerve conduction studies and electromyography can also localize nerve injuries to the root and help with clarifying prognosis.

The typical natural history of cervical radiculopathy is gradual resolution of symptoms with conservative care [93]. Education and reassurance are important part of the management. Activity modification and ergonomic adjustments can be helpful in avoiding re-aggravation of the nerve root. Modalities used in primary neck pain can also be used but evidence of such is lacking. Thermotherapy is often used to help with pain [94] but one study indicates that its use in cervical radiculopathy is associated with poorer outcomes [95]. A number of studies have shown that traction is helpful temporarily [95–103].

Additionally, neuropathic medications can be helpful in controlling some of the neuropathic radicular pain [20]. As mentioned in the previous section, the choice of medication should take into account a patient's expectations, medical history, and concomitant medications. Occasionally, the pain from radiculopathy can be so severe that opioids may be needed.

Surgery is indicated for patients with severe symptoms, neurologic deficits, progressive symptoms, or after failing conservative care. Decompression surgery has satisfactory results in up to 96% of patients [92, 104–106]. There is an estimated complication rate of around 10% with a less than 1% risk of clinical worsening [107–110].

Conclusion

Axial cervical pain is a very common complaint that all physicians may encounter in their clinical practice. The biomechanical source of axial cervical pain is broad with cervical facets and disks being most studied in the literature. One must also consider the patient as a whole and consider the biopsychosocial factors to best help the patient in achieving their goals and meeting their expectations.

References

1. Hoy DG, Protani M, De R, Buchbinder R. The epidemiology of neck pain. Best Pract Res Clin Rheumatol. Bailliere Tindall Ltd. 2010;24:783–92.
2. Schopflocher D, Taenzer P, Jovey R. The prevalence of chronic pain in Canada. Pain Res Manag. 2011;16(6):445–50.
3. Côté P, van der Velde G, Cassidy JD, Carroll LJ, Hogg-Johnson S, Holm LW, et al. The burden and determinants of neck pain in workers. Results of the bone and joint decade 2000-2010 task force on neck pain and its associated disorders. J Manip Physiol Ther. 2009;32(2 SUPPL)
4. Bogduk N. The anatomy and pathophysiology of neck pain. Vol. 14, physical medicine and rehabilitation clinics of North America. W.B. Saunders; 2003. p. 455–72.
5. Olesen J, Bes A, Kunkel R, Lance JW, Nappi G, Pfaffenrath V, et al. The international classification of headache disorders, 3rd edition (beta version). Cephalalgia. 2013;33(9):629–808.
6. Piovesan EJ, Kowacs PA, Oshinsky ML. Convergence of cervical and trigeminal sensory afferents. Curr Pain Headache Rep. Current Medicine Group LLC 1. 2003;7:377–83.

7. Lumley MA, Cohen JL, Borszcz GS, Cano A, Radcliffe AM, Porter LS, et al. Pain and emotion: a biopsychosocial review of recent research. J Clin Psychol. 2011;67:942–68. NIH Public Access
8. Finan PH, Goodin BR, Smith MT. The association of sleep and pain: an update and a path forward. J Pain. NIH Public Access. 2013;14:1539–52.
9. Tredwell SJ, Newman DE, Lockitch G. Instability of the upper cervical spine in down syndrome. J Pediatr Orthop. 1990;10(5):602–6.
10. Da Côrte FC, Neves N. Cervical spine instability in rheumatoid arthritis. Eur J Orthop Surg Traumatol. Springer-Verlag France. 2014;24
11. Isu T, Miyasaka K, Abe H, Ito T, Iwasaki Y, Tsuru M, et al. Atlantoaxial dislocation associated with neurofibromatosis: report of three cases. J Neurosurg. 1983;58(3):451–3.
12. Liu J, Zhu L, Jiang E, Zou S, Xu G. Ankylosing spondylitis manifested by extensive cervical erosions with spontaneous anterior atlantoaxial subluxation. World Neurosurg. 2019;122:583–9.
13. Shunmugam M, Poonnoose S. Spontaneous atlantoaxial subluxation associated with tonsillitis. Asian J Neurosurg. 2015;10(2):139.
14. Elgafy H, Liu X, Herron J. Spinal gout: a review with case illustration. World J Orthop. 2016;7:766–75. Baishideng Publishing Group Co
15. Charles PD, Adler CH, Stacy M, Comella C, Jankovic J, Manack Adams A, et al. Cervical dystonia and pain: characteristics and treatment patterns from CD PROBE (cervical dystonia patient registry for observation of OnabotulinumtoxinA efficacy). J Neurol. 2014;261(7):1309–19.
16. Levander B, Mellström A, Grepe A. Atlantoaxial instability in marfans syndrome. Diagnosis and treatment—a case report. Neuroradiology. 1981;21(1):43–6.
17. Tobias JH, Deere K, Palmer S, Clark EM, Clinch J. Joint hypermobility is a risk factor for musculoskeletal pain during adolescence: findings of a prospective cohort study. Arthritis Rheum. 2013;65(4):1107–15.
18. Castori M, Morlino S, Ghibellini G, Celletti C, Camerota F, Grammatico P. Connective tissue, Ehlers-Danlos syndrome(s), and head and cervical pain. Am J Med Genet Part C Semin Med Genet. 2015;169(1):84–96.
19. Narouze S, Benzon HT, Provenzano D, Buvanendran A, De Andres J, Deer T, et al. Interventional spine and pain procedures in patients on antiplatelet and anticoagulant medications (Second Edition): Guidelines from the American Society of Regional Anesthesia and Pain Medicine, the European Society of Regional Anaesthesia and Pain Therapy, the American Academy of Pain Medicine, the International Neuromodulation Society, the North American Neuromodulation Society, and the World Institute of Pain. Reg Anesthesia Pain Med. Lippincott Williams and Wilkins. 2018;43:225–62.
20. De Moulin D, Boulanger A, Clark AJ, Clarke H, Dao T, Finley GA, et al. Pharmacological management of chronic neuropathic pain: revised consensus statement from the Canadian Pain Society. Pain Res Manag. 2014;19(6):328–35.
21. Allan GM, Ramji J, Perry D, Ton J, Beahm NP, Crisp N, et al. Simplified guideline for prescribing medical cannabinoids in primary care. Can Fam Physician. 2018;64(2):111.
22. Alhashash M, Shousha M, Boehm H. Adjacent segment disease after cervical spine fusion. Spine (Phila Pa 1976). 2018;43(9):605–9.
23. Sist T, Miner M, Lema M. Characteristics of postradical neck pain syndrome: a report of 25 cases. J Pain Symptom Manag. 1999;18(2):95–102.
24. Kato F, Yukawa Y, Suda K, Yamagata M, Ueta T. Normal morphology, age-related changes and abnormal findings of the cervical spine. Part II: magnetic resonance imaging of over 1,200 asymptomatic subjects. Eur Spine J. 2012;21(8):1499–507.
25. Nicholas M, Vlaeyen JWS, Rief W, Barke A, Aziz Q, Benoliel R, et al. The IASP classification of chronic pain for ICD-11: chronic primary pain. Pain. 2019;160:28–37. Lippincott Williams and Wilkins
26. Manchikanti L, Singh V, Rivera J, Pampati V. ## M. prevalence of cervical facet joint pain in chronic neck pain. Pain Physician. 5(3):243–9.

27. Cooper G, Bailey B, Bogduk N. Cervical zygapophysial joint pain maps. Pain Med. 2007;8(4):344–53.
28. Bogduk N, Marsland A. The cervical zygapophysiai joints as a source of neck pain. Spine (Phila Pa 1976). 1988;13(6):610–7.
29. Jull G, Bogduk N, Marsland A. The accuracy of manual diagnosis for cervical zygapophysial joint pain syndromes. Med J Aust. 1988;148(5):233–6.
30. Slipman CW, Plastaras C, Patel R, Isaac Z, Chow D, Garvan C, et al. Provocative cervical discography symptom mapping. Spine J. 2005;5(4):381–8.
31. Gross A, Kay TM, Paquin JP, Blanchette S, Lalonde P, Christie T, et al. Exercises for mechanical neck disorders. Cochrane Database Syst Rev. 2015;2017. John Wiley and Sons Ltd
32. Garra G, Singer AJ, Leno R, Taira BR, Gupta N, Mathaikutty B, et al. Heat or cold packs for neck and back strain: a randomized controlled trial of efficacy. Acad Emerg Med. 2010;17(5):484–9.
33. Lizis P, Kobza W, Manko G, Jaszczur-Nowicki J, Perlinski J, Para B. Cryotherapy with mobilization versus cryotherapy with mobilization reinforced with home stretching exercises in treatment of chronic neck pain: a randomized trial. J Manip Physiol Ther. 2020;43(3):197–205.
34. Cramer H, Baumgarten C, Choi KE, Lauche R, Saha FJ, Musial F, et al. Thermotherapy self-treatment for neck pain relief-a randomized controlled trial. Eur J Integr Med. 2012;4(4):e371–8.
35. Petrofsky JS, Laymon M, Alshammari F, Khowailed IA, Lee H. Use of low level of continuous heat and ibuprofen as an adjunct to physical therapy improves pain relief, range of motion and the compliance for home exercise in patients with nonspecific neck pain: a randomized controlled trial. J Back Musculoskelet Rehabil. 2017;30(4):889–96.
36. Shin HJ, Kim SH, Hahm SC, Cho HY. Thermotherapy plus neck stabilization exercise for chronic nonspecific neck pain in elderly: a single-blinded randomized controlled trial. Int J Environ Res Public Health. 2020;17(15):1–12.
37. Kim JH, Lee HS, Park SW. Effects of the active release technique on pain and range of motion of patients with chronic neck pain. J Phys Ther Sci. 2015;27(8):2461–4.
38. Hidalgo B, Hall T, Bossert J, Dugeny A, Cagnie B, Pitance L. The efficacy of manual therapy and exercise for treating non-specific neck pain: a systematic review. J Back Musculoskelet Rehabil. 2017;30:1149–69. IOS Press
39. Costello M, Puentedura E, Louie J, Cleland J, Ciccone CD. The immediate effects of soft tissue mobilization versus therapeutic ultrasound for patients with neck and arm pain with evidence of neural mechanosensitivity: a randomized clinical trial. J Man Manip Ther. 2016;24(3):128–40.
40. Sasso RC, Smucker JD, Hacker RJ, Heller JG. Artificial disc versus fusion: a prospective, randomized study with 2-year follow-up on 99 patients. Spine (Phila Pa 1976). 2007;32(26):2933–40.
41. D'Sylva J, Miller J, Gross A, Burnie SJ, Goldsmith CH, Graham N, et al. Manual therapy with or without physical medicine modalities for neck pain: a systematic review. Man Ther. 2010;15:415–33.
42. Martimbianco ALC, Porfírio GJM, Pacheco RL, Torloni MR, Riera R. Transcutaneous electrical nerve stimulation (TENS) for chronic neck pain. Cochrane Database Syst Rev. 2019;2019. John Wiley and Sons Ltd
43. Sayilir S. The short-term effects of TENS plus therapeutic ultrasound combinations in chronic neck pain. Complement Ther Clin Pract. 2018;31:278–81.
44. Chiu TTW, Hui-Chan CWY, Cheing G. A randomized clinical trial of TENS and exercise for patients with chronic neck pain. Clin Rehabil. 2005;19(8):850–60.
45. Maayah M. Evaluation of transcutaneous electrical nerve stimulation as a treatment of neck pain due to musculoskeletal disorders. J Clin Med Res. 2010;2(3):127.
46. Noori SA, Rasheed A, Aiyer R, Jung B, Bansal N, Chang KV, et al. Therapeutic ultrasound for pain management in chronic low back pain and chronic neck pain: a systematic review. Pain Medicine (United States). 2020;21:1482–93. Oxford University Press

47. Matijević-Mikelić V, Crnković M, Matijević M, Leović D, Demarin V. The effectiveness of the therapeutic ultrasound on the psycho-physiological functioning in patients who presented with neck pain. Coll Antropol. 2012;36(3):921–8.
48. Qing W, Shi X, Zhang Q, Peng L, He C, Wei Q. Effect of therapeutic ultrasound for neck pain: a systematic review and meta-analysis. Arch Phys Med Rehabil. 2021;
49. Lee SH, Chen CC, Lee CS, Lin TC, Chan RC. Effects of needle electrical intramuscular stimulation on shoulder and cervical myofascial pain syndrome and microcirculation. J Chin Med Assoc. 2008;71(4):200–6.
50. Karakurum B, Karaalin O, Coskun Ö, Dora B, Üçler S, Inan L. The 'dry-needle technique': intramuscular stimulation in tension-type headache. Cephalalgia. 2001;21(8):813–7.
51. Navarro-Santana MJ, Sanchez-Infante J, Fernández-de-las-Peñas C, Cleland JA, Martín-Casas P, Plaza-Manzano G. Effectiveness of dry needling for myofascial trigger points associated with neck pain symptoms: an updated systematic review and meta-analysis. J Clin Med. 2020;9(10):3300.
52. Gustavsson C, von Koch L. A 9-year follow-up of a self-management group intervention for persistent neck pain in primary health care: a randomized controlled trial. J Pain Res. 2016;10:53–64.
53. Gustavsson C, Denison E, Von Koch L. Self-management of persistent neck pain: two-year follow-up of a randomized controlled trial of a multicomponent group intervention in primary health care. Spine (Phila Pa 1976). 2011;36(25):2105–15.
54. Escolar-Reina P, Medina-Mirapeix F, Gascón-Cánovas JJ, Montilla-Herrador J, Valera-Garrido JF, Collins SM. Self-Management of Chronic Neck and low Back Pain and relevance of information provided during clinical encounters: an observational study. Arch Phys Med Rehabil. 2009;90(10):1734–9.
55. Andias R, Neto M, Silva AG. The effects of pain neuroscience education and exercise on pain, muscle endurance, catastrophizing and anxiety in adolescents with chronic idiopathic neck pain: a school-based pilot, randomized and controlled study. Physiother Theory Pract. 2018;34(9):682–91.
56. Willaert W, Malfliet A, Coppieters I, Lenoir D, De Pauw R, Danneels L, et al. Does pain neuroscience education and cognition-targeted motor control training improve cervical motor output? Secondary analysis of a randomized clinical trial. Pain Pract. 2020;20(6):600–14.
57. Malfliet A, Kregel J, Coppieters I, De Pauw R, Meeus M, Roussel N, et al. Effect of pain neuroscience education combined with cognition-targeted motor control training on chronic spinal pain a randomized clinical trial. JAMA Neurol. 2018;75(7):808–17.
58. Brage K, Ris I, Falla D, Søgaard K, Juul-Kristensen B. Pain education combined with neck- and aerobic training is more effective at relieving chronic neck pain than pain education alone—a preliminary randomized controlled trial. Man Ther. 2015;20(5):686–93.
59. Fredin K, Lorås H. Manual therapy, exercise therapy or combined treatment in the management of adult neck pain—a systematic review and meta-analysis. Musculoskelet Sci Pract. Elsevier Ltd. 2017;31:62–71.
60. Louw S, Makwela S, Manas L, Meyer L, Terblanche D, Brink Y. Effectiveness of exercise in office workers with neck pain: a systematic review and meta-analysis. South African J Physiother. 2017;73:1.
61. Martin-Gomez C, Sestelo-Diaz R, Carrillo-Sanjuan V, Navarro-Santana MJ, Bardon-Romero J, Plaza-Manzano G. Motor control using cranio-cervical flexion exercises versus other treatments for non-specific chronic neck pain: a systematic review and meta-analysis. Musculoskelet Sci Pract. 2019;42:52–9.
62. Chen X, Coombes BK, Sjøgaard G, Jun D, O'Leary S, Johnston V. Workplace-based interventions for neck pain in office workers: systematic review and meta-analysis. Phys Ther. Oxford University Press. 2018;98:40–62.
63. Lauche R, Stumpe C, Fehr J, Cramer H, Cheng YW, Wayne PM, et al. The effects of tai chi and Neck exercises in the treatment of chronic nonspecific Neck pain: a randomized controlled trial. J Pain. 2016;17(9):1013–27.

64. Zhang F. Tai chi as a potentially effective treatment for neck pain. J Formos Med Assoc. Elsevier Ltd. 2014;113:199–200.
65. Li Y, Li S, Jiang J, Yuan S. Effects of yoga on patients with chronic nonspecific neck pain; a PRISMA systematic review and meta-analysis. Medicine (United States). Lippincott Williams and Wilkins. 2019;98
66. Kim SD. Effects of yoga on chronic neck pain: a systematic review of randomized controlled trials. J Phys Ther Sci. Society of Physical Therapy Science (Rigaku Ryoho Kagakugakkai). 2016;28:2171–4.
67. Guerrero AVS, Maujean A, Campbell L, Sterling M. A systematic review and meta-analysis of the effectiveness of psychological interventions delivered by physiotherapists on pain, disability and psychological outcomes in musculoskeletal pain conditions. Clin J Pain. Lippincott Williams and Wilkins. 2018;34:838–57.
68. Sterling M, Smeets R, Keijzers G, Warren J, Kenardy J. Physiotherapist-delivered stress inoculation training integrated with exercise versus physiotherapy exercise alone for acute whiplash-associated disorder (StressModex): a randomised controlled trial of a combined psychological/physical intervention. Br J Sports Med. 2019;53:19.
69. Monticone M, Cedraschi C, Ambrosini E, Rocca B, Fiorentini R, Restelli M, et al. Cognitive-behavioural treatment for subacute and chronic neck pain, Cochrane Database Syst Rev. John Wiley and Sons Ltd; 2015 2015.
70. Jeitler M, Brunnhuber S, Meier L, Lüdtke R, Büssing A, Kessler C, et al. Effectiveness of Jyoti meditation for patients with chronic neck pain and psychological distress—a randomized controlled clinical trial. J Pain. 2015;16(1):77–86.
71. Rosenzweig S, Greeson JM, Reibel DK, Green JS, Jasser SA, Beasley D. Mindfulness-based stress reduction for chronic pain conditions: variation in treatment outcomes and role of home meditation practice. J Psychosom Res. 2010;68(1):29–36.
72. Vowles KE, Fink BC, Cohen LL. Acceptance and commitment therapy for chronic pain: a diary study of treatment process in relation to reliable change in disability. J Context Behav Sci. 2014;3(2):74–80.
73. McCracken LM, Sato A, Taylor GJ. A trial of a brief group-based form of acceptance and commitment therapy (ACT) for chronic pain in general practice: pilot outcome and process results. J Pain. 2013;14(11):1398–406.
74. Probst T, Baumeister H, McCracken L, Lin J. Baseline psychological inflexibility moderates the outcome pain interference in a randomized controlled trial on internet-based acceptance and commitment therapy for chronic pain. J Clin Med. 2018;8(1):24.
75. Manchikanti L, Pampati V, Hirsch JA. Utilization of interventional techniques in managing chronic pain in Medicare population from 2000 to 2014: an analysis of patterns of utilization. Pain Physician. 2016;19(4):E531–46.
76. Barnsley L, Lord SM, Wallis BJ, Bogduk N. Lack of effect of intraarticular corticosteroids for chronic pain in the cervical zygapophyseal joints. N Engl J Med. 1994;330(15):1047–50.
77. Falco FJE, Manchikanti L, Datta S, Wargo BW, Geffert S, Bryce DA, et al. Systematic review of the therapeutic effectiveness of cervical facet joint interventions: an update. Pain Physician. 2012;15
78. Habib GS. Systemic effects of intra-articular corticosteroids. Clin Rheumatol. 2009;28:749–56.
79. Stout A, Friedly J, Standaert CJ. Systemic absorption and side effects of locally injected glucocorticoids, vol. 11. PM and R. John Wiley and Sons Inc.; 2019. p. 409–19.
80. Burnham T, Conger A, Salazar F, Petersen R, Kendall R, Cunningham S, et al. The effectiveness of cervical medial branch radiofrequency ablation for chronic facet joint syndrome in patients selected by a practical medial branch block paradigm. Pain Med (United States). 2020;21(10):2071–6.
81. Engel AJ, Rappard G, King W, Kennedy DJ. The effectiveness and risks of fluoroscopically-guided cervical medial branch thermal radiofrequency neurotomy: a systematic review with comprehensive analysis of the published data. Pain Med (United States). Oxford University Press. 2016;17:658–69.

82. Gazelka HM, Knievel S, Mauck WD, Moeschler SM, Pingree MJ, Rho RH, et al. Incidence of neuropathic pain after radiofrequency denervation of the third occipital nerve. J Pain Res. 2014;7:195.
83. Navani A, Manchikanti L, Albers SL, Latchaw RE, Sanapati J, Kaye AD, et al. Responsible, safe, and effective use of biologics in the Management of low Back Pain: American Society of Interventional Pain Physicians (ASIPP) guidelines. Pain Physician. 2019;22(1S):S1–74.
84. Wu J, Du Z, Lv Y, Zhang J, Xiong W, Wang R, et al. A new technique for the treatment of lumbar facet joint syndrome using intra-articular injection with autologous platelet rich plasma. Pain Physician. 2016;19(8):617–25.
85. Wu J, Zhou J, Liu C, Zhang J, Xiong W, Lv Y, et al. A prospective study comparing platelet-rich plasma and local Anesthetic (LA)/corticosteroid in intra-articular injection for the treatment of lumbar facet joint syndrome. Pain Pract. 2017;17(7):914–24.
86. Wolter T, Kieselbach K. Cervical spinal cord stimulation: an analysis of 23 patients with long-term follow-up. Pain Physician. 15(3):203–12.
87. Vallejo R, Kramer J, Benyamin R. Neuromodulation of the cervical spinal cord in the treatment of chronic intractable neck and upper extremity pain: a case series and review of the literature. Pain Physician. 2007;10(2):305–11.
88. Hunter CW, Carlson J, Yang A, Deer T. Spinal cord stimulation for the treatment of failed neck surgery syndrome: outcome of a prospective case series. Neuromodulation. 2018;21(5):495–503.
89. Deer TR, Skaribas IM, Haider N, Salmon J, Kim C, Nelson C, et al. Effectiveness of cervical spinal cord stimulation for the management of chronic pain. Neuromodulation. 2014;17(3):265–71.
90. Palit M, Schofferman J, Goldthwaite N, Reynolds J, Kerner M, Keaney D, et al. Anterior discectomy and fusion for the management of neck pain. Spine (Phila Pa 1976). 1999;24(21):2224–8.
91. Whitecloud TS, Seago RA. Cervical discogenic syndrome. Results of operative intervention in patients with positive discography. Spine (Phila Pa 1976). 1987;12(4):313–6.
92. Gore DR, Sepic SB. Anterior cervical fusion for degenerated or protruded discs-a review of one hundred forty-six patients. Spine (Phila Pa 1976). 1984;9(7):667–71.
93. Heckmann JG, Lang CJ, Zöbelein I, Laumer R, Druschky A, Neundörfer B. Herniated cervical intervertebral discs with radiculopathy: an outcome study of conservatively or surgically treated patients. J Spinal Disord. 1999;12(5):396–401.
94. Malanga GA, Yan N, Stark J. Mechanisms and efficacy of heat and cold therapies for musculoskeletal injury. Postgrad Med. Taylor and Francis Inc. 2015;127:57–65.
95. Jette DU, Jette AM. Physical therapy and health outcomes in patients with spinal impairments. Phys Ther. 1996;76(9):930–45.
96. Swezey RL, Swezey AM, Warner K. Efficacy of home cervical traction therapy. Am J Phys Med Rehabil. 1999;78(1):30–2.
97. Valtonen EJ, Kiuru E. Cervical traction as a therapeutic tool. A clinical analysis based on 212 patients. Scand J Rehabil Med. 1970;2(1):29–36.
98. Van der Heijden GJMG, Beurskens AJHM, Koes BW, Assendelft WJJ, De Vet HCW, Bouter LM. The efficacy of traction for back and neck pain: a systematic, blinded review of randomized clinical trial methods. Phys Ther. 1995;75(2):93–104.
99. Wong AMK, Lee MY, Chang WH, Tang FT. Clinical trial of a cervical traction modality with electromyographic biofeedback. Am J Phys Med Rehabil. 1997;76(1):19–25.
100. Romeo A, Vanti C, Boldrini V, Ruggeri M, Guccione AA, Pillastrini P, et al. Cervical radiculopathy: effectiveness of adding traction to physical therapy-a systematic review and meta-analysis of randomized controlled trials. Phys Ther. Oxford University Press. 2018;98:231–42.
101. Constantoyannis C, Konstantinou D, Kourtopoulos H, Papadakis N. Intermittent cervical traction for cervical radiculopathy caused by large-volume herniated disks. J Manip Physiol Ther. 2002;25(3):188–92.
102. Jellad A, Ben Salah Z, Boudokhane S, Migaou H, Bahri I, Rejeb N. The value of intermittent cervical traction in recent cervical radiculopathy. Ann Phys Rehabil Med. 2009;52(9):638–52.

103. Garg P. Home care neck traction for a patient with neck pain and cervical radiculopathy symptoms: a case report. J Chiropr Med. 2019;18(2):127–30.
104. Aldrich F. Posterolateral microdiscectomy for cervical monoradiculopathy caused by posterolateral soft cervical disc sequestration. J Neurosurg. 1990;72(3):370–7.
105. Herkowitz HN, Kurz LT, Overholt DP. Surgical management of cervical soft disc herniation: a comparison between the anterior and posterior approach. Spine (Phila Pa 1976). 1990;15(10):1026–30.
106. Klein GR, Vaccaro AR, Albert TJ. Health outcome assessment before and after anterior cervical discectomy and fusion for radiculopathy: a prospective analysis. Spine (Phila Pa 1976). 2000;25(7):801–3.
107. Tasiou A, Giannis T, Brotis AG, Siasios I, Georgiadis I, Gatos H, et al. Anterior cervical spine surgery-associated complications in a retrospective case-control study. J Spine Surg. 2017;3(3):444–59.
108. Cheung JPY, Luk KDK. Complications of anterior and posterior cervical spine surgery. Asian Spine J. 2016;10:385–400. Korean Society of Spine Surgery
109. Bernstein DN, Thirukumaran C, Saleh A, Molinari RW, Mesfin A. Complications and readmission after cervical spine surgery in elderly patients: an analysis of 1786 patients. World Neurosurg. 2017;103:859–68.e8
110. Yee TJ, Swong K, Park P. Complications of anterior cervical spine surgery: a systematic review of the literature. J Spine Surg. AME Publishing Company. 2020;6:302–22.

8 Chronic Pain Syndromes: Shoulder Pain

George Deng

Introduction

Shoulder pain affects almost 50% of the population [1]. The shoulder is involved in many activities of daily living as well as vocational and a vocational pursuit as part of the larger change. Therefore, persistent shoulder pain can substantially limit the patient's quality of life and health.

The shoulder joint complex consists of the interplay between the glenohumeral (GH), acromioclavicular (AC), scapulothoracic, and the sternoclavicular joints. Additionally, there is a balance of stability and mobility that must be achieved to allow for function without dysfunction.

The glenohumeral joint is considered the main joint of the shoulder. It is a ball and socket joint held in place by dynamic and static stabilizers. The innervation of the glenohumeral joint is mainly supplied by the suprascapular nerve and to a lesser degree the axillary nerve and the lateral pectoral nerve.

The acromioclavicular joint is a saddle joint that is located at the cephalad and lateral portion of the shoulder. Along with the sternoclavicular joints, it helps with allowing the mobility of the clavicle with shoulder movements. Additionally, the scapulothoracic joint is a contact point between the scapula and the thorax. The scapulothoracic joint plays a role in allowing gliding of the scapula along the posterior thoracic wall.

G. Deng (✉)
Section of Physical Medicine and Rehabilitation, Department of Clinical Neuroscience, University of Calgary, Calgary, AB, Canada

© The Author(s), under exclusive license to Springer Nature Switzerland AG 2023

B. W. Blakley, J. E. Blakley (eds.), *Functional Illness of the Head and Neck*,
https://doi.org/10.1007/978-3-031-12998-8_8

Table 8.1 Differential diagnosis of shoulder pain

Categorical differential of shoulder pain	Common mechanical causes of shoulder pain	Less common mechanical causes of shoulder pain
1. Mechanical 2. Malignant 3. Visceral referral pain (diaphragm, gall bladder, ulcer, duodenum, heart, spleen, apex of lungs) 4. Neurologic (brachial neuritis, neuropraxia, post-hepatic neuropathy) 5. Cervical referral pain 6. Chronic pain syndromes (chronic regional pain syndrome, fibromyalgia, myofascial pain, thoracic outlet syndrome)	1. Subacromial pain syndrome (rotator cuff tendinosis, rotator cuff tear, subacromial impingement, rotator cuff strain, bicipital tendinosis) 2. Glenohumeral instability 3. Acromioclavicular joint sprain	1. Adhesive capsulitis 2. Fractures 3. Glenohumeral joint arthritis

Etiology

The differential for shoulder pain is broad but, most shoulder pain is mechanical and musculoskeletal in origin (Table 8.1).

Clinical Evaluation

The history of a patient with shoulder pain involve characterization of the pain including the onset, pattern of change, characterization of pain, location, radiation, intensity, aggravating, and alleviating features. Additionally, one must inquire if the pain changes with head and neck movements. Red flags for shoulder pain include symptoms suggesting of an underlying malignancy, visceral, and neurologic etiologies.

As part of the comprehensive assessment, the patient's past medical history, medications, and allergies needs to be elicited. Patient's handedness, occupation, and avocational pursuits are also important to document.

The physical examination of the shoulder includes inspection, range of motion, palpation, and special tests. It begins with inspection and includes how the patient carries their arm and neck as well as any skin changes, soft tissue changes and any malalignment of the bony structures. Typically, people with or without shoulder pain may have a protracted shoulder. There are limited association of poor posture and pain [2–6]. Capsular pattern of restriction first occurs in shoulder external rotation and abduction and could point to adhesive capsulitis. Surface anatomy would be important in identifying the tender structure with palpation. See Table 8.2 for

Table 8.2 Common orthopedic special tests

Condition tested	Orthopedic specialty test
Shoulder impingement	• Nears • Hawkins Kennedy
Rotator cuff tendinopathy or tear	• Supraspinatus: Empty can (Jobe's), full can • Infraspinatus: resisted shoulder external rotation with elbow against the body • Teres minor: Resisted shoulder external rotation in the Hornblower's position • Subscapularis: Liftoff test, belly press test
Bicipital tendinopathy	• Uppercut test • Speed's test • Yergason's test
Acromioclavicular joint	• Scarf's test • AC joint shear test
Shoulder instability	• Sulcus sign • Load-and-shift test • Anterior and posterior apprehension test

commonly used orthopedic specialty testing. Although these tests have limited sensitivity and specificity [7–9] they are nevertheless helpful in narrowing down the differential diagnosis.

Diagnostic Testing

Imaging

Basic imaging includes shoulder radiograph and ultrasound. The X-ray can help identify underlying bony fractures, infiltrative lesions, or malignancy. Additionally, a high riding humeral head with decreased subacromial height can be suggestive of rotator cuff tears [10, 11]. Shoulder ultrasound is better at identifying pathology of the soft tissue [12, 13]. One caveat is musculoskeletal ultrasound is highly user dependent [14–16]. Shoulder MRIs can also better help identifying underlying soft tissue pathology and bony or joint pathology. MR arthrograms has the added benefit of being more sensitive for labral tears. A negative bone scan can be helpful in ruling out chronic regional pain syndrome [17].

Electrodiagnostic Testing

Electrodiagnostic testing with nerve conduction studies and electromyography can be helpful in identifying underlying neurologic causes and characterizing the pattern of involvement if the patient presents with neurological symptoms or signs. Conditions that electrodiagnostic testing can help define in patients with shoulder pain includes axillary neuropathy, neuralgic amyotrophy, and radiculopathy.

Outcome Measures and Psychosocial Testing

Shoulder Pain and Disability Index is a common outcome measure that can be used to better characterize patients with shoulder pain to monitor response to treatment and the less subjective manner. Other pain outcome measures including the brief pain inventory are also helpful.

Common Shoulder Conditions

Subacromial Pain Syndrome

Subacromial pain syndrome is defined as non-traumatic shoulder pain related to the structures of the subacromial space. This new term, subacromial pain syndrome, has been proposed to include conditions such as rotator cuff tendinosis which can occur concurrently, and impingement which is a mechanistic description [18].

Typically, patients will report pain in the anterolateral shoulder with a referral pattern down the lateral arm to the level of the elbow. This pain is aggravated mostly with overhead activities, repetitive activities, or sleeping at night. The pain is described typically as an achy or dull pain with sharp characteristics when aggravated. Palpation of the rotator interval and over the distal portion of the acromion may be tender. Range of motion may be limited with a painful arc between 60 and 120° in abduction. Shoulder impingement testing may be positive and resisted rotator cuff tendon testing may reproduce pain and giveaway weakness. A drop arm sign occurs when the patient suddenly drops their arm when asked to gradually lower the arm from a fully shoulder abducted position. A positive test suggests a rotator cuff tear.

This condition responds very favorably to active based rehabilitation program with loading of the rotator cuff tendons and building strength of the periscapular muscles [19, 20]. Additionally, education regarding pacing, and activity modification can be helpful. Medications with simple analgesics can help control incidental pain. Pain modulating analgesics, although having limited evidence, are often used with persistent pain.

There are several interventional options. Steroid injections in the subacromial space have shown mixed results [21–23]. There are limited evidence with subacromial ketorolac injections [24, 25]. Barbotage can be helpful if there is calcific tendinosis [26]. Interest in orthobiologic options has been growing with mixed evidence for the use of platelet rich plasma therapy [27–31]. Platelet-rich plasma therapy involves the injection of autologous platelets into the painful structure to deliver a supraphysiologic concentration of the growth factors and signaling proteins found within the granules of the platelets.

Glenohumeral Joint Instability

There are dynamic and static stabilizers of the shoulder that maintains GH joint stability. It is important to differentiate between the terms of laxity, which is increased joint flexibility that is normal and asymptomatic, and instability which unlike laxity is pathological. Instability can be post-traumatic, atraumatic, or mixed in etiology. Additionally, it can be unidirectional or multidirectional.

Clinically, it can present with symptoms of vague pain, history of recurrent subluxation or dislocations, popping, catching, and stiffness. A history of antecedent trauma with shoulder subluxation or dislocation is often recalled. Atraumatic instability is usually in patients who participate in overhead sports or have underlying connective tissue disorder.

Physical examination with observation, palpation, range of motion, and special tests is still important to rule out concomitant pathology. Special tests for shoulder instability include sulcus sign (presence of a divot below the acromion upon downward traction of the arm), anterior apprehension test (patient apprehension with slow shoulder external rotation with the shoulder at 90° abduction and elbow at 90° flexion while supine), and relocation test (resolution of apprehension with posteriorly directed pressure on the anterior shoulder after patient displays apprehension with anterior apprehension test). Additionally, posterior apprehension test (patient apprehension with posterior force on the elbow and shoulder adduction with the shoulder at 90° anterior flexion, neutral shoulder rotation, and elbow at 90° flexion while supine with the scapula supported) can be indicative of posterior shoulder instability. Examination of the joint above and below as well as neurological examination is part of the comprehensive shoulder examination.

Plain radiographs may demonstrate a dislocated shoulder. Additionally, Bankart fractures or Hill-Sach lesions are indicative of previous shoulder dislocations. MR arthrograms have the added benefit of identifying underlying labral, cartilage, and joint capsule injuries.

Conservative management under the guidance of physiotherapy includes strengthening the dynamic stabilizers, addressing kinetic chain deficits, improving scapulothoracic mechanics, and optimizing neuromuscular control. Immobilization can be helpful for comfort but does not change the rate of recurrence [32, 33]. Surgical stabilization is considered if conservative management fails. Some clinicians do pursue surgical stabilization after initial shoulder dislocation [34] due to the high rates of recurrence [35].

Conclusion

There are many causes for shoulder pain with local musculoskeletal sources being most common. Accurate diagnosis and appropriate therapy while considering the patient's goals and expectations are important in the management of shoulder pain.

References

1. Pope DP, Croft PR, Pritchard CM, Silman AJ. Prevalence of shoulder pain in the community: the influence of case definition. Ann Rheum Dis. 1997;56(5):308–12.
2. Mahmoud NF, Hassan KA, Abdelmajeed SF, Moustafa IM, Silva AG. The relationship between forward head posture and neck pain: a systematic review and meta-analysis. Curr Rev Musculoskelet Med. Springer. 2019;12:562–77.
3. Martinez-Merinero P, Nuñez-Nagy S, Achalandabaso-Ochoa A, Fernandez-Matias R, Pecos-Martin D, Gallego-Izquierdo T. Relationship between forward head posture and tissue mechanosensitivity: a cross-sectional study. J Clin Med. 2020;9(3):634.
4. Griegel-Morris P, Larson K, Mueller-Klaus K, Oatis CA. Incidence of common postural abnormalities in the cervical, shoulder, and thoracic regions and their association with pain in two age groups of healthy subjects. Phys Ther. 1992:425–31.
5. Bullock MP, Foster NE, Wright CC. Shoulder impingement: the effect of sitting posture on shoulder pain and range of motion. Man Ther. 2005;10(1):28–37.
6. Kim EK, Kim JS. Correlation between rounded shoulder posture, neck disability indices, and degree of forward head posture. J Phys Ther Sci. 2016;28(10):2929–32.
7. Boettcher CE, Ginn KA, Cathers I. The "empty can" and "full can" tests do not selectively activate supraspinatus. J Sci Med Sport. 2009;12(4):435–9.
8. Hegedus EJ, Wright AA, Cook C. Orthopaedic special tests and diagnostic accuracy studies: house wine served in very cheap containers. Br J Sports Med. BMJ Publishing Group. 2017;51:1578–9.
9. Cook C. The lost art of the clinical examination: an overemphasis on clinical special tests. J Man Manip Ther . Taylor & Francis. 2010;18:3–4.
10. Moosikasuwan JB, Miller TT, Burke BJ. Rotator cuff tears: clinical, radiographic, and US findings. Radiographics. 2005:1591–607.
11. Hussain A, Muzzammil M, Butt F, Valsamis EM, Dwyer AJ. Effectiveness of plain shoulder radiograph in detecting degenerate rotator cuff tears. J Ayub Med Coll Abbottabad. 30(1):8–11.
12. Singh J. Shoulder ultrasound: what you need to know. Indian J Radiol Imaging. 2012;22(4):284–92.
13. Amoo-Achampong K, Nwachukwu BU, McCormick F. An orthopedist's guide to shoulder ultrasound: a systematic review of examination protocols. Phys Sports Med. 2016;44:407–16. Taylor and Francis Ltd.
14. Le Corroller T, Cohen M, Aswad R, Pauly V, Champsaur P. Sonography of the painful shoulder: role of the operator's experience. Skelet Radiol. 2008;37(11):979–86.
15. O'Connor PJ, Rankine J, Gibbon WW, Richardson A, Winter F, Miller JH. Interobserver variation in sonography of the painful shoulder. J Clin Ultrasound. 2005;33(2):53–6.
16. Day M, Phil M, McCormack RA, Nayyar S, Jazrawi L. Physician training ultrasound and accuracy of diagnosis in rotator cuff tears. Bull Hosp Jt Dis. 2016;74(3):207–11.
17. Wertli MM, Brunner F, Steurer J, Held U. Usefulness of bone scintigraphy for the diagnosis of complex regional pain syndrome 1: a systematic review and Bayesian meta-analysis. PLoS One. 2017;12:3.
18. Diercks R, Bron C, Dorrestijn O, Meskers C, Naber R, De Ruiter T, et al. Guideline for diagnosis and treatment of subacromial pain syndrome. Acta Orthop. Informa Healthcare. 2014;85:314–22.
19. Michener LA, Walsworth MK, Burnet EN. Effectiveness of rehabilitation for patients with subacromial impingement syndrome: a systematic review. J Hand Ther. 2004;17(2):152–64.
20. Hanratty CE, McVeigh JG, Kerr DP, Basford JR, Finch MB, Pendleton A, et al. The effectiveness of physiotherapy exercises in subacromial impingement syndrome: a systematic review and meta-analysis. Semin Arthritis Rheum. 2012;42(3):297–316.
21. Naredo E, Cabero F, Beneyto P, Cruz A, Mondéjar B, Uson J, et al. A randomized comparative study of short term response to blind injection versus sonographic-guided injection of local corticosteroids in patients with painful shoulder. J Rheumatol. 2004;31(2):308–14.

22. McInerney JJ, Dias J, Durham S, Evans A. Randomised controlled trial of single, subacromial injection of methylprednisolone in patients with persistent, post-traumatic impingement of the shoulder. Emerg Med J. 2003;20(3):218–21.
23. Hay EM, Thomas E, Paterson SM, Dziedzic K, Croft PR. A pragmatic randomised controlled trial of local corticosteroid injection and physiotherapy for the treatment of new episodes of unilateral shoulder pain in primary care. Ann Rheum Dis. 2003;62(5):394–9.
24. Taheri P, Dehghan F, Mousavi S, Solouki R. Comparison of subacromial ketorolac injection versus corticosteroid injection in the treatment of shoulder impingement syndrome. J Res Pharm Pract. 2017;6(4):223.
25. Min KS, St. Pierre P, Ryan PM, Marchant BG, Wilson CJ, Arrington ED. A double-blind randomized controlled trial comparing the effects of subacromial injection with corticosteroid versus NSAID in patients with shoulder impingement syndrome. J Shoulder Elb Surg. 2013;22(5):595–601.
26. Gatt DL, Charalambous CP. Ultrasound-guided barbotage for calcific tendonitis of the shoulder: a systematic review including 908 patients. Arthroscopy. Journal of Arthroscopic and Related Surgery. W.B. Saunders. 2014;30:1166–72.
27. Pasın T, Ataoğlu S, Pasın Ö, Ankarali H. Comparison of the effectiveness of platelet-rich plasma, corticosteroid, and physical therapy in subacromial impingement syndrome. Arch Rheumatol. 2019;34(3):308–16.
28. Kesikburun S, Tan AK, Yilmaz B, Yaşar E, Yazicioğlu K. Platelet-rich plasma injections in the treatment of chronic rotator cuff tendinopathy: a randomized controlled trial with 1-year follow-up. Am J Sports Med. 2013;41(11):2609–15.
29. Rha DW, Park GY, Kim YK, Kim MT, Lee SC. Comparison of the therapeutic effects of ultrasound-guided platelet-rich plasma injection and dry needling in rotator cuff disease: a randomized controlled trial. Clin Rehabil. 2013;27(2):113–22.
30. Shams A, El-Sayed M, Gamal O, Ewes W. Subacromial injection of autologous platelet-rich plasma versus corticosteroid for the treatment of symptomatic partial rotator cuff tears. Eur J Orthop Surg Traumatol. 2016;26(8):837–42.
31. Barnsley L, Lord SM, Wallis BJ, Bogduk N. Lack of effect of intraarticular corticosteroids for chronic pain in the cervical zygapophyseal joints. N Engl J Med. 1994;330(15):1047–50.
32. Whelan DB, Kletke SN, Schemitsch G, Chahal J. Immobilization in external rotation versus internal rotation after primary anterior shoulder dislocation: a meta-analysis of randomized controlled trials. Am J Sports Med. 2016;44(2):521–32.
33. Liavaag S, Brox JI, Pripp AH, Enger M, Soldal LA, Svenningsen S. Immobilization in external rotation after primary shoulder dislocation did not reduce the risk of recurrence: a randomized controlled trial. J Bone Jt Surg Ser A. 2011;93(10):897–904.
34. Rugg CM, Hettrich CM, Ortiz S, Wolf BR, Baumgarten KM, Bishop JY, et al. Surgical stabilization for first-time shoulder dislocators: a multicenter analysis. J Shoulder Elb Surg. 2018;27(4):674–85.
35. Hovelius L, Olofsson A, Sandström B, Augustini BG, Krantz L, Fredin H, et al. Nonoperative treatment of primary anterior shoulder dislocation in patients forty years of age and younger: a prospective twenty-five-year follow up. J Bone Jt Surg Ser A. 2008;90(5):945–52.

Fibromyalgia

9

George Deng

Introduction

Fibromyalgia is commonly seen by physicians in all fields. Due to the various diagnostic criteria used, fibromyalgia has been estimated between 2% and as high as 15% in certain populations [1–3]. This condition is often associated with several other painful and chronic conditions such as headaches, temporal mandibular joint disorder, irritable bowel syndrome, and endometriosis [4, 5].

Pain can be classified as nociceptive, neuropathic, or nociplastic as per the International Association for the Study of Pain [6, 7]. Fibromyalgia falls within the nociplastic classification. Nociplastic pain is defined as "arises from altered nociception despite no clear evidence of actual or threatened tissue damage causing the activation of peripheral nociceptors or evidence for disease or lesion of the somatosensory system causing the pain" [6, 7].

The exact etiology and pathophysiology are unknown as patients often do not have a structural source of pain but describe debilitating pain [8]. The prevailing theory is that fibromyalgia is the result of abnormal pain processing resulting from central sensitization with multiple contributing factors [8, 9]. Studies in the peripheral nervous system have also found that a proportion of patients who was initially labeled as having fibromyalgia have abnormal sodium channels in their nociceptors or have small fiber neuropathy [10–12]. Additionally, there is a strong family history for fibromyalgia. Twin studies suggest a 50% contribution from genes [13, 14]. On the other hand, early life adversity and adverse childhood events have been shown to be associated with several negative heath consequences including pain [15, 16]. Additionally, stress and exposure to war and persecution has also been associated with fibromyalgia [17, 18].

G. Deng (✉)
Section of Physical Medicine and Rehabilitation, Department of Clinical Neuroscience, University of Calgary, Calgary, AB, Canada

© The Author(s), under exclusive license to Springer Nature Switzerland AG 2023

B. W. Blakley, J. E. Blakley (eds.), *Functional Illness of the Head and Neck*,
https://doi.org/10.1007/978-3-031-12998-8_9

Clinical Evaluation

The diagnosis of fibromyalgia has evolved through the years. Previous versions have relied on physical examination identifying 11 tender points [19]. However, the most recent diagnostic criteria moved away from relying on physical examination and uses a physician administered checklist with the 2010 update [20]. The current, 2016 modification [21], diagnostic criteria require the presence of widespread pain, reaching threshold for a widespread pain index and symptom severity scale, and a duration lasting for at least 3 months [21].

As a part of the comprehensive pain evaluation, sleep [22–24] and mood [24, 25] dysfunction should be identified and managed due to their bidirectional influence with pain. Eliciting psychosocial factors can be helpful in better understanding the patient's pain and to address the patient's pain from a biopsychosocial perspective [26, 27]. Patients may also have other functional somatic symptoms that should be screened [4, 5, 28].

Past treatments and their response are important to elicit to help guide further management.

The physical examination includes a comprehensive neurological and musculoskeletal examination. The tender point examination is no longer part of the fibromyalgia diagnostic criteria and is associated with its own challenges in standardization and training [19, 21].

Diagnostic Testing

Additional investigations should be undertaken with care and while balancing the pre-test probability and limiting the risk of excessive investigations. The Canadian fibromyalgia guidelines recommend the following blood work to rule out common treatable painful conditions: complete blood count (CBC), C-reactive protein/erythrocyte sedimentation rate (CRP/ESR), creatine kinase (CK), and thyroid stimulating hormone (TSH) [29]. Further investigations of bloodwork or imaging should be guided by the patient's symptoms [29]. Other investigations, for example, are electrodiagnostic testing, sleep study, and imaging. Electrodiagnostic testing can be helpful in ruling out large fiber polyneuropathy, mononeuropathy, or radiculopathies which can present with pain and neuropathic symptoms. Non-restorative sleep correlates with psychological variables, somatic symptoms, and pain severity [30–32].

Management

Although there is no cure for fibromyalgia, there are several management options to help with symptoms and to optimize function. Management should be patient centered and goal directed focusing on self-management from a multi-modal approach [33–36].

Non-pharmacological Options

Pain neuroscience education has been shown to have a positive effect in numerous chronic pain conditions [37–40]. Education needs to be patient tailored to maximize understanding. Components of pain neuroscience education include topics such as neuroanatomy, function of pain, definition of pain, pain processing, central sensitization, descending inhibition of pain, as well as the different dimensions of pain to name a few. Additionally, consistent messages and approach from health care providers including reassurance regarding patient's symptoms, the difference between harm and hurt, and the avoidance of over-medicalization is important. Fibromyalgia support groups or chronic pain clinics often can help organize a structured education program. The benefit of education includes improving attitudes, coping skills, and self-efficacy, all of which can influence response to treatment [29]. Specifically, multicomponent therapy which is the combination of education or physiological therapy with exercise has been found to be helpful for fibromyalgia management [41, 42].

There is a bidirectional correlation between pain and mood with increased psychological and substance use comorbidities in patients with fibromyalgia [24, 25, 43–45]. Even if the patient does not meet criteria for a psychological pathology, various traditional psychological interventions can be helpful. Psychological treatments that have evidence in the management of chronic pain include operant behavior therapy [46–48], cognitive behavior therapy [42, 48–50], acceptance and commitment therapy (ACT) [51–55], as well as mindfulness-based stress relaxation (MBSR) [55–57]. ACT and MBSR are considered third wave treatments that have been gaining evidence in the treatment of chronic pain [58].

Exercise has also been shown to be helpful in fibromyalgia and various other chronic pain conditions [41, 42, 59–71]. The mechanism is likely multifactorial including upregulation of the endogenous opioid system, endogenous cannabinoid system, immune system, and the descending noxious inhibitory system [72–75]. When counseling patients on exercise, one must be mindful of the risk of pain aggravation associated with increasing physical activity which may discourage a patient in pain from continuing with exercise. Generally, starting slow and building upon positive goals would be helpful in maintaining a positive lifestyle change.

Complementary and alternative medicines are commonly used by fibromyalgia patients [76]. This includes Chinese medicine [77], homeopathy [78], nutraceuticals [79], acupuncture [77, 80, 81], and chiropractic treatments [82]. These treatments may have some immediate effects in pain relief, but evidence is lacking for a sustained effect.

Pharmacological Therapies

Medications can help augment the above mentioned non-pharmacological treatments. The current paradigm in pharmacological therapy includes starting with simple analgesics such as acetaminophen or nonsteroidal anti-inflammatory drugs as needed. Additional pain modulating medications can be considered. Many of these medications have side effects or dual indications that may be beneficial in a fibromyalgia patient and therefore treatment from a symptom based approach can help more than one of the patient's symptoms [33, 83]. Only duloxetine and pregabalin have Health Canada approval for the treatment of fibromyalgia, and the FDA has also approved milnacipran, whereas the other medications are used off label. Classes of medications includes serotonin norepinephrine reuptake inhibitor, tricyclic antidepressant, gabapentinoids, cyclobenzaprine, and cannabinoids [29, 84].

Drug	Potential beneficial effects	Potential negative effects
Serotonin norepinephrine reuptake inhibitor	Antidepressant Anxiolytic	Suicidal ideation Worsens sleep Gastrointestinal side effects
Tricyclic antidepressant	Sedating	Increases fatigue
Gabapentinoids	Sedating anxiolytic	Increases fatigue Increases weight
Cyclobenzaprine	Sedating	Increases fatigue
Cannabis	Sedating Improves anxiety	Increases fatigue

Although opioids have a strong analgesic effect, careful consideration for its indication is recommended prior to an opioid trial. There are multiple comorbidities with high-risk factors for opioid abuse in patients with fibromyalgia. These include history of physical, sexual, and substance abuse as well as history of mental health disorders. This can be better elucidated with validated tools such as the opioid risk tool. Of the opioids, only tramadol has been studied in fibromyalgia and provides a positive effect on the pain and improve quality of life [85, 86]. Guidelines recommend starting with weak opioids if an opioid trial is to be initiated [29, 84].

Although there is biological possibility for the effect of cannabis on pain, its clinical utility for pain remains controversial [87, 88]. Reviews found that cannabis can be helpful in neuropathic pain and fibromyalgia [88, 89]. There is a recent interest in using low-dose naltrexone for management of fibromyalgia [90–92].

Other Treatments

There are several other therapies with limited evidence used for the management of fibromyalgia. Lidocaine and ketamine infusions are used clinically to treat chronic pain but the evidence for its use is sparse [93–95]. There is emerging evidence that transcranial direct current stimulation and repetitive transcranial magnetic stimulation is helpful in fibromyalgia patients [96, 97].

Conclusion

Generalized pain is a chronic condition and a definitive cure is challenging to achieve. A biopsychosocial approach can be the most pragmatic path to pain management. Involvement of allied health members in an interdisciplinary model of care can help address the pain from a variety of directions.

References

1. Marques AP, Santo A d S d E, Berssaneti AA, Matsutani LA, SLK Y. Prevalence of fibromyalgia: literature review update. Rev Bras Reumatol (English Ed). 2017;57(4):356–63.
2. Gran JT. The epidemiology of chronic generalized musculoskeletal pain. Best Pract Res Clin Rheumatol. Bailliere Tindall Ltd. 2003;17:547–61.
3. Wolfe F, Ross K, Anderson J, Russell IJ, Hebert L. The prevalence and characteristics of fibromyalgia in the general population. Arthritis Rheum. 1995;38(1):19–28.
4. Aaron LA, Buchwald D. A review of the evidence for overlap among unexplained clinical conditions. Ann Intern Med. 2001;134(9 II SUPPL):868–81.
5. Hudson JI, Pope HG. The concept of affective spectrum disorder: relationship to fibromyalgia and other syndromes of chronic fatigue and chronic muscle pain. Baillieres Clin Rheumatol. 1994;8(4):839–56.
6. Kosek E, Cohen M, Baron R, Gebhart GF, Mico JA, Rice ASC, et al. Do we need a third mechanistic descriptor for chronic pain states? Pain. Lippincott Williams and Wilkins. 2016;157:1382–6.
7. Raja SN, Carr DB, Cohen M, Finnerup NB, Flor H, Gibson S, et al. The revised International Association for the Study of Pain definition of pain: concepts, challenges, and compromises. Pain. 2020;161(9):1976–82.
8. Clauw DJ. Fibromyalgia: A clinical review. JAMA. American Medical Association. 2014;311:1547–55.
9. Pomares FB, Funck T, Feier NA, Roy S, Daigle-Martel A, Ceko M, et al. Histological underpinnings of grey matter changes in fibromyalgia investigated using multimodal brain imaging. J Neurosci. 2017;37(5):1090–101.
10. Grayston R, Czanner G, Elhadd K, Goebel A, Frank B, Üçeyler N, et al. A systematic review and meta-analysis of the prevalence of small fiber pathology in fibromyalgia: implications for a new paradigm in fibromyalgia etiopathogenesis. Semin Arthritis Rheum. 2019;48(5):933–40.
11. Giannoccaro MP, Donadio V, Incensi A, Avoni P, Liguori R. Small nerve fiber involvement in patients referred for fibromyalgia. Muscle Nerve. 2014;49(5):757–9.
12. Lawson VH, Grewal J, Hackshaw KV, Mongiovi PC, Stino AM. Fibromyalgia syndrome and small fiber, early or mild sensory polyneuropathy. Muscle Nerve. 2018;58(5):625.
13. Kato K, Sullivan PF, Evengård B, Pedersen NL. A population-based twin study of functional somatic syndromes. Psychol Med. 2009;39(3):497–505.
14. Markkula RA, Kalso EA, Kaprio JA. Predictors of fibromyalgia: a population-based twin cohort study. BMC Musculoskelet Disord. 2016;17(1):29.
15. Beveridge JK, Dobson KS, Madigan S, Yeates KO, Stone AL, Wilson AC, et al. Adverse childhood experiences in parents of youth with chronic pain: prevalence and comparison with a community-based sample. PAIN Rep. 2020;5(6):e866.
16. Low LA, Schweinhardt P. Early life adversity as a risk factor for fibromyalgia in later life. Pain Res Treat. Hindawi Limited. 2012;2012:15.

17. Kivimäki M, Leino-Arjas P, Virtanen M, Elovainio M, Keltikangas-Jarvinen L, Puttonen S, et al. Work stress and incidence of newly diagnosed fibromyalgia: prospective cohort study. J Psychosom Res. 2004;57(5):417–22.
18. Ablin JN, Cohen H, Eisinger M, Buskila D. Holocaust survivors: the pain behind the agony. Increased prevalence of fibromyalgia among Holocaust survivors. Clin Exp Rheumatol. 28(6 Suppl 63):S51-6.
19. Wolfe F, Smythe HA, Yunus MB, Bennett RM, Bombardier C, Goldenberg DL, et al. The American College of Rheumatology 1990 criteria for the classification of fibromyalgia. Arthritis Rheum. 1990;33(2):160–72.
20. Wolfe F, Clauw DJ, Fitzcharles M-A, Goldenberg DL, Katz RS, Mease P, et al. The American College of Rheumatology Preliminary Diagnostic Criteria for Fibromyalgia and Measurement of Symptom Severity. 2010.
21. Wolfe F, Clauw DJ, Fitzcharles MA, Goldenberg DL, Häuser W, Katz RL, et al. 2016 revisions to the 2010/2011 fibromyalgia diagnostic criteria. Semin Arthritis Rheum. 2016;46(3):319–29.
22. Keskindag B, Karaaziz M. The association between pain and sleep in fibromyalgia. Saudi Med J. Saudi Arabian Armed Forces Hospital. 2017;38:465–75.
23. Finan PH, Goodin BR, Smith MT. The association of sleep and pain: an update and a path forward. J Pain. NIH Public Access. 2013;14:1539–52.
24. Consoli G, Marazziti D, Ciapparelli A, Bazzichi L, Massimetti G, Giacomelli C, et al. The impact of mood, anxiety, and sleep disorders on fibromyalgia. Compr Psychiatry. 2012;53(7):962–7.
25. Arnold LM, Hudson JI, Keck PE, Auchenbach MB, Javaras KN, Hess EV. Comorbidity of fibromyalgia and psychiatric disorders. J Clin Psychiatry. 2006;67(8):1219–25.
26. Wolfe F, Hawley DJ. Psychosocial factors and the fibromyalgia syndrome. In: Zeitschrift fur Rheumatologie. D. Steinkopff-Verlag; 1998. 88–91.
27. Eich W, Hartmann M, Müller A, Fischer H. The role of psychosocial factors in fibromyalgia syndrome. Scand J Rheumatol Suppl. 2000:30–1.
28. Donnachie E, Schneider A, Enck P. Comorbidities of patients with functional somatic syndromes before, during and after first diagnosis: a population-based study using Bavarian routine data. Sci Rep. 2020;1:1–10.
29. Fitzcharles MA, Ste-Marie PA, Goldenberg DL, Pereira JX, Abbey S, Choinière M, et al. 2012 Canadian guidelines for the diagnosis and management of fibromyalgia syndrome: executive summary. Pain Res Manage. Hindawi Limited. 2013;18:119–26.
30. Terauchi M, Hiramitsu S, Akiyoshi M, Owa Y, Kato K, Obayashi S, et al. Associations between anxiety, depression and insomnia in peri- and post-menopausal women. Maturitas. 2012;72(1):61–5.
31. Liedberg GM, Björk M, Börsbo B. Self-reported nonrestorative sleep in fibromyalgia—relationship to impairments of body functions, personal function factors, and quality of life. J Pain Res. 2015;8:499–505.
32. Bigatti SM, Hernandez AM, Cronan TA, Rand KL. Sleep disturbances in fibromyalgia syndrome: relationship to pain and depression. Arthritis Care Res. 2008;59(7):961–7.
33. Boomershine CS, Crofford LJ. A symptom-based approach to pharmacologic management of fibromyalgia. Nat Rev Rheumatol. 2009;5(4):191–9.
34. Rossy LA, Buckelew SP, Dorr N, Hagglund KJ, Thayer JF, McIntosh MJ, et al. A meta-analysis of fibromyalgia treatment interventions. Ann Behav Med. 1999;21(2):180–91.
35. Dobkin PL, Liu A, Abrahamowicz M, Ionescu-Ittu R, Bernatsky S, Goldberger A, et al. Predictors of disability and pain six months after the end of treatment for fibromyalgia. Clin J Pain. 2010;26(1):23–9.
36. Becker H, Stuifbergen A, Taxis C, Beal CC, Pierini DM. The use of goal attainment scaling to facilitate and assess individualized change in a wellness intervention for women with fibromyalgia syndrome. J Holist Nurs. 2009;27(4):232–40.
37. Amer-Cuenca JJ, Pecos-Martín D, Martínez-Merinero P, Girbés EL, Nijs J, Meeus M, et al. How much is needed? Comparison of the effectiveness of different pain education dosages in patients with fibromyalgia. Pain Med (United States). 2020;21(4):782–93.

38. Louw A, Zimney K, Puentedura EJ, Diener I. The efficacy of pain neuroscience education on musculoskeletal pain: a systematic review of the literature. Physiother Theory Pract. Taylor and Francis Ltd. 2016;32:332–55.
39. Watson JA, Ryan CG, Cooper L, Ellington D, Whittle R, Lavender M, et al. Pain neuroscience education for adults with chronic musculoskeletal pain: a mixed-methods systematic review and meta-analysis. J Pain. Churchill Livingstone Inc. 2019;20:1140.e1–1140.e22.
40. Nicassio PM, Radojevic V, Weisman MH, Schuman C, Kim J, Schoenfeld-Smith K, et al. A comparison of behavioral and educational interventions for fibromyalgia. J Rheumatol. 1997;24(10):2000–7.
41. Häuser W, Bernardy K, Arnold B, Offenbächer M, Schiltenwolf M. Efficacy of multicomponent treatment in fibromyalgia syndrome: a meta-analysis of randomized controlled clinical trials. Arthritis Care Res. 2009;61(2):216–24.
42. Suman AL, Biagi B, Biasi G, Carli G, Gradi M, Prati E, et al. One-year efficacy of a 3-week intensive multidisciplinary non-pharmacological treatment program for fibromyalgia patients. Clin Exp Rheumatol. 27(1):7–14.
43. Bondesson E, Larrosa Pardo F, Stigmar K, Ringqvist PIF, Jöud A, et al. Comorbidity between pain and mental illness—evidence of a bidirectional relationship. Eur J Pain (United Kingdom). 2018;22(7):1304–11.
44. Tsang A, Von Korff M, Lee S, Alonso J, Karam E, Angermeyer MC, et al. Common chronic pain conditions in developed and developing countries: gender and age differences and comorbidity with depression-anxiety disorders. J Pain. 2008;9(10):883–91.
45. Roughan WH, Campos AI, García-Marín LM, Cuéllar-Partida G, Lupton MK, Hickie IB, et al. Comorbid chronic pain and depression: shared risk factors and differential antidepressant effectiveness. Front Psych. 2021;12:12.
46. Thieme K, Turk DC. Cognitive-behavioral and operant-behavioral therapy for people with fibromyalgia. Reumatismo. Page Press Publications. 2012;64:275–85.
47. Thieme K, Gromnica-Ihle E, Flor H. Operant behavioral treatment of fibromyalgia: a controlled study. Arthritis Care Res. 2003;49(3):314–20.
48. Bernardy K, Füber N, Köllner V, Häuser W. Efficacy of cognitive-behavioral therapies in fibromyalgia syndrome—a systematic review and metaanalysis of randomized controlled trials. J Rheumatol. 2010;37:1991–2005.
49. Falcao DM, Sales L, Leite JR, Feldman D, Valim V, Natour J. Cognitive behavioral therapy for the treatment of fibromyalgia syndrome: a randomized controlled trial. J Musculoskelet Pain. 2008;16(3):133–40.
50. Bennett R, Nelson D. Cognitive behavioral therapy for fibromyalgia. Nat Clin Pract Rheumatol. 2006;2:416–24.
51. Wicksell RK, Kemani M, Jensen K, Kosek E, Kadetoff D, Sorjonen K, et al. Acceptance and commitment therapy for fibromyalgia: a randomized controlled trial. Eur J Pain (United Kingdom). 2013;17(4):599–611.
52. Simister HD, Tkachuk GA, Shay BL, Vincent N, Pear JJ, Skrabek RQ. Randomized controlled trial of online acceptance and commitment therapy for fibromyalgia. J Pain. 2018;19(7):741–53.
53. Luciano JV, Guallar JA, Aguado J, López-Del-Hoyo Y, Olivan B, Magallón R, et al. Effectiveness of group acceptance and commitment therapy for fibromyalgia: a 6-month randomized controlled trial (EFFIGACT study). Pain. 2014;155(4):693–702.
54. Aytur SA, Ray KL, Meier SK, Campbell J, Gendron B, Waller N, et al. Neural mechanisms of acceptance and commitment therapy for chronic pain: a network-based fMRI approach. Front Hum Neurosci. 2021;5:15.
55. Haugmark T, Hagen KB, Smedslund G, Zangi HA. Mindfulness- and acceptance-based interventions for patients with fibromyalgia—a systematic review and meta-analyses. PLoS One. 2019;14:9.
56. Sanabria-Mazo JP, Montero-Marin J, Feliu-Soler A, Gasión V, Navarro-Gil M, Morillo-Sarto H, et al. Mindfulness-based program plus amygdala and insula retraining (MAIR) for the treatment of women with fibromyalgia: a pilot randomized controlled trial. J Clin Med. 2020;9(10):3246.

57. Lauche R, Cramer H, Dobos G, Langhorst J, Schmidt S. A systematic review and meta-analysis of mindfulness-based stress reduction for the fibromyalgia syndrome. J Psychosom Res. Elsevier Inc. 2013;75:500–10.
58. Morley S, Williams A. New developments in the psychological management of chronic pain. Can J Psychiatry. Canadian Psychiatric Association. 2015;60:168–75.
59. Mannerkorpi K, Nordeman L, Cider Å, Jonsson G. Does moderate-to-high intensity Nordic walking improve functional capacity and pain in fibromyalgia? A prospective randomized controlled trial. Arthritis Res Ther. 2010;12:5.
60. Thomas EN, Blotman F. Aerobic exercise in fibromyalgia: a practical review. Rheumatol Int. 2010;30:1143–50.
61. Busch AJ, Webber SC, Richards RS, Bidonde J, Schachter CL, Schafer LA, et al. Resistance exercise training for fibromyalgia. Cochrane Database Syst Rev. John Wiley and Sons Ltd. 2013;2013
62. Busch AJ, Barber KAR, Overend TJ, Peloso PMJ, Schachter CL. Exercise for treating fibromyalgia syndrome. Cochrane Database Syst Rev. John Wiley and Sons Ltd. 2007;
63. Berardi G, Senefeld JW, Hunter SK, Bement MKH. Impact of isometric and concentric resistance exercise on pain and fatigue in fibromyalgia. Eur J Appl Physiol. 2021;121(5):1389–404.
64. Da Silva GD, Lorenzi-Filho G, Lage LV. Effects of yoga and the addition of Tui Na in patients with fibromyalgia. J Altern Complement Med. 2007;13(10):1107–13.
65. Chen KW, Hassett AL, Hou F, Staller J, Lichtbroun AS. A pilot study of external qigong therapy for patients with fibromyalgia. J Altern Complement Med. 2006;12(9):851–6.
66. Taggart HM, Arslanian CL, Bae S, Singh K. Effects of t'ai chi exercise on fibromyalgia symptoms and health-related quality of life. Orthop Nurs. 2003;22(5):353–60.
67. Altan L, Korkmaz N, Bingol Ü, Gunay B. Effect of Pilates training on people with fibromyalgia syndrome: a pilot study. Arch Phys Med Rehabil. 2009;90(12):1983–8.
68. Sauch Valmaña G, Vidal-Alaball J, Poch PR, Peña JM, Panadés Zafra R, Cantero Gómez FX, et al. Effects of a physical exercise program on patients affected with fibromyalgia. J Prim Care Community Heal. 2020;11
69. Kim SY, Busch AJ, Overend TJ, Schachter CL, van der Spuy I, Boden C, et al. Flexibility exercise training for adults with fibromyalgia. Cochrane Database Syst Rev. John Wiley and Sons Ltd. 2019;2019
70. Mannerkorpi K, Nordeman L, Ericsson A, Arndorw M. Pool exercise for patients with fibromyalgia or chronic widespread pain: a randomized controlled trial and subgroup analyses. J Rehabil Med. 2009;41(9):751–60.
71. Larsson A, Palstam A, Löfgren M, Ernberg M, Bjersing J, Bileviciute-Ljungar I, et al. Resistance exercise improves muscle strength, health status and pain intensity in fibromyalgia-a randomized controlled trial. Arthritis Res Ther. 2015;17:1.
72. Lesnak JB, Sluka KA. Mechanism of exercise-induced analgesia: what we can learn from physically active animals. PAIN Rep. 2020;5(5):e850.
73. Sluka KA, Frey-Law L, Hoeger BM. Exercise-induced pain and analgesia? Underlying mechanisms and clinical translation. Pain NLM (Medline). 2018;159:S91–7.
74. Rice D, Nijs J, Kosek E, Wideman T, Hasenbring MI, Koltyn K, et al. Exercise-induced hypoalgesia in pain-free and chronic pain populations: state of the art and future directions. J Pain. 2019;20(11):1249–66.
75. Koltyn KF, Brellenthin AG, Cook DB, Sehgal N, Hillard C. Mechanisms of exercise-induced hypoalgesia. J Pain. 2014;15(12):1294–304.
76. Pioro-Boisset M, Esdaile JM, Fitzcharles MA. Alternative medicine use in fibromyalgia syndrome. Arthritis Rheum. 1996;9(1):13–7.
77. Cao H, Liu JP, Lewith GT. Traditional Chinese medicine for treatment of fibromyalgia: a systematic review of randomized controlled trials. J Altern Complement Med. 2010;16(4):397–409.
78. Perry R, Terry R, Ernst E. A systematic review of homoeopathy for the treatment of fibromyalgia. Clin Rheumatol. 2010;29:457–64.

79. Lowry E, Marley J, McVeigh JG, McSorley E, Allsopp P, Kerr D. Dietary interventions in the management of fibromyalgia: a systematic review and best-evidence synthesis. Nutrients. MDPI AG. 2020;12:1–18.
80. Mayhew E, Ernst E. Acupuncture for fibromyalgia—a systematic review of randomized clinical trials. Rheumatology (Oxford). 2007;46:801–4.
81. Martin-Sanchez E, Torralba E, Diaz-Dominguez E, Barriga A, R.Martin JL. Efficacy of acupuncture for the treatment of fibromyalgia: systematic review and meta-analysis of randomized trials. Open Rheumatol J. 2009;3(1):25–9.
82. Ernst E. Chiropractic treatment for fibromyalgia: a systematic review. Clin Rheumatol. 2009;28:1175–8.
83. Perrot S, Dickenson AH, Bennett RM. Fibromyalgia: harmonizing science with clinical practice considerations. Pain Pract. 2008;8:177–89.
84. Macfarlane GJ, Kronisch C, Dean LE, Atzeni F, Häuser W, Flub E, et al. EULAR revised recommendations for the management of fibromyalgia. Ann Rheum Dis. 2017;76(2):318–28.
85. Biasi G, Manca S, Manganelli S, Marcolongo R. Tramadol in the fibromyalgia syndrome: a controlled clinical trial versus placebo. Int J Clin Pharmacol Res. 1998;18(1):13–9.
86. Bennett RM, Kamin M, Karim R, Rosenthal N. Tramadol and acetaminophen combination tablets in the treatment of fibromyalgia pain: a double-blind, randomized, placebo-controlled study. Am J Med. 2003;114(7):537–45.
87. Campbell FA, Tramèr MR, Carroll D, Reynolds DJM, Moore RA, Mcquay HJ. Are cannabinoids an effective and safe treatment option in the management of pain? A qualitative systematic review. BMJ. 2001;323(7303):13.
88. Lynch ME, Campbell F. Cannabinoids for treatment of chronic non-cancer pain; a systematic review of randomized trials. Br J Clin Pharmacol. 2011;72(5):735–44.
89. Allan GM, Ramji J, Perry D, Ton J, Beahm NP, Crisp N, et al. Simplified guideline for prescribing medical cannabinoids in primary care. Can Fam Physician. 2018;64(2):111.
90. Younger J, Noor N, McCue R, MacKey S. Low-dose naltrexone for the treatment of fibromyalgia: findings of a small, randomized, double-blind, placebo-controlled, counterbalanced, crossover trial assessing daily pain levels. Arthritis Rheum. 2013;65(2):529–38.
91. Metyas SK, Chen CL, Yeter K, Solyman J, Arkfeld D. Low dose naltrexone in the treatment of fibromyalgia. Curr Rheumatol Rev. 2018;14(2):177–80.
92. Younger J, Mackey S. Fibromyalgia symptoms are reduced by low-dose naltrexone: a pilot study. Pain Med. 2009;10(4):663–72.
93. Wilderman I, Pugacheva O, Perelman V, Wansbrough MCT, Voznyak Y, Zolnierczyk L. Repeated intravenous lidocaine infusions for patients with fibromyalgia: higher doses of lidocaine have a stronger and longer-lasting effect on pain reduction. Pain Med (United States). 2020;21(6):1230–9.
94. Cohen SP, Bhatia A, Buvanendran A, Schwenk ES, Wasan AD, Hurley RW, et al. Consensus Guidelines on the Use of Intravenous Ketamine Infusions for Chronic Pain From the American Society of Regional Anesthesia and Pain Medicine, the American Academy of Pain Medicine, and the American Society of Anesthesiologists. Reg Anesth Pain Med. Lippincott Williams and Wilkins. 2018;43:521–46.
95. Sörensen J, Bengtsso A, Bäckman E, Henriksson KG, Bengtsson M. Pain analysis in patients with fibromyalgia: effects of intravenous morphine, lidocaine, and ketamine. Scand J Rheumatol. 1995;24(6):360–5.
96. Short EB, Borckardt JJ, Anderson BS, Frohman H, Beam W, Reeves ST, et al. Ten sessions of adjunctive left prefrontal rTMS significantly reduces fibromyalgia pain: a randomized, controlled pilot study. Pain. 2011;152(11):2477–84.
97. Lloyd DM, Wittkopf PG, Arendsen LJ, Jones AKP. Is transcranial direct current stimulation (tDCS) effective for the treatment of pain in fibromyalgia? A systematic review and meta-analysis. J Pain. Churchill Livingstone Inc. 2020;21:1085–100.

Myofascial Pain

10

George Deng

Introduction

Pain localized over particular muscles is commonly seen in clinical practice. However, the existence of myofascial pain is debated due to the paucity of convincing biological plausibility. It may be better conceptualized as central and peripheral sensitization. The definition of myofascial pain is "a hyperirritable spot in skeletal muscle that is associated with a hypersensitive palpable nodule in a taut band. The spot is painful on manual compression and can give rise to characteristic referred pain, referred tenderness, motor dysfunction, and autonomic phenomena" [1]. Key features in the presentation of myofascial pain include taut bands, trigger points, referred pain, and local twitch response [1].

Myofascial pain and fibromyalgia are similar in that both are pain syndromes arising from altered nociception without evidence of actual or threatened tissue damage. In contrast to the widespread pain seen in fibromyalgia, myofascial pain is a localized chronic pain syndrome [2]. Other contrasting features of myofascial pain from fibromyalgia include referral pain with palpation and the lower prevalence of somatic symptoms [2].

The pathogenesis of myofascial pain is controversial and incompletely understood. Simmons' "integrated hypothesis" later expanded by Gerwin is perhaps the most widely accepted theory for the pathogenesis of myofascial pain [3]. The theory postulates that myofascial pain begins with abnormal acetylcholine release leading to increased tension in the muscle fiber with blood flow constriction and muscle hypoxia, disrupted mitochondrial function and the subsequent release of sensitizing substances [3]. This creates a cycle of additional abnormal acetylcholine release and

G. Deng (✉)
Section of Physical Medicine and Rehabilitation, Department of Clinical Neuroscience, University of Calgary, Calgary, AB, Canada

© The Author(s), under exclusive license to Springer Nature Switzerland AG 2023

B. W. Blakley, J. E. Blakley (eds.), *Functional Illness of the Head and Neck*,
https://doi.org/10.1007/978-3-031-12998-8_10

further sensitization of the local muscle tissues [3]. Additionally, neurogenic inflammation, sensitization, and limbic system dysfunction can play a role [4].

Clinical Evaluation

As with clinical evaluation of patients with pain, it starts with a thorough history. Characterization of the pain is important. Additionally, it is important to rule out an underlying neuromuscular condition with signs and symptoms of muscle cramping, pigmenturia, weakness, atrophy, and fasciculations.

It is also important to elicit any sleep and mood symptoms, given the bidirectional nature of sleep, mood, and pain [5–8].

A functional history is also important. It is not only important to elicit what can and cannot be done but also the tolerance of activities that is limiting a patient's function. This can include things like sitting and walking tolerance, or tolerance while working on the computer. This can also serve as a measure of response to treatment.

A neurological examination with particular attention to ruling out an upper motor neuron syndrome is important which includes assessing for tone, deep tendon reflexes, plantar response, and Hoffman's response. Assessment of power may be difficult to interpret as there may be antalgic weakness due to the pain.

The examination for myofascial pain follows the musculoskeletal examination approach of look, move, feel, and special tests. On inspection, it is important to look for malalignment that may be indicative of contributing factors, but one must be mindful that alterations in posture does not necessarily mean pain [9]. Additionally, information can be gleaned from how the patient moves during the whole of the clinical encounter. With myofascial pain, a patient's range of motion may be restricted due to the underlying myofascial pain. Identifications of the myofascial restrictions of range can help a clinician prescribe targeted therapy of those muscles. Palpation is needed for the diagnosis of myofascial pain. Palpation can localize taut bands and trigger points that may be amenable to treatment. It is also important to ask about referral pain patterns during palpation of the tender points. Orthopedic special testing can be included to further evaluate any other common underlying musculoskeletal pathology such as rotator cuff dysfunction, lateral epicondylosis, and radiculopathy for example.

Diagnostic Testing

Although there is no bloodwork that can give the diagnosis of myofascial pain, it is still important to rule out other diagnosis on the differential. Blood work according to the Canadian Fibromyalgia guidelines is a good place to start including, complete blood count, creatine kinase, thyroid stimulating hormone, c-reactive progein, and erythrocyte sedimentation rate as these abnormalities can suggest an underlying painful treatable condition [10].

Electrodiagnostic studies can be helpful to rule out underlying myopathic or neurogenic causes of pain, but again cannot diagnoses myofascial pain syndrome. Similarly, imaging studies cannot diagnose myofascial pain. Its use is to rule out other diagnosis on the differential and must be undertaken at the clinician's discretion. Novel imaging techniques still under investigation that has not yet gained clinical adoption include sonographic assessment [11], and magnetic resonance elastography [12].

Treatment

Research on the treatment for myofascial pain is sparse and the evidence for various treatments are mixed and is based on lower evidence recommendations. Treatment options can be broadly classified under conservative, pharmacological, and interventional options.

Several conservative options exist. Although pain neuroscience education has shown to be beneficial in chronic pain with central sensitization [13–16], this has not been well studied in myofascial pain syndrome [17, 18].

Several allied health professionals can help with the management of myofascial pain. Their tools include thermotherapy [19], spray and stretch techniques [19, 20], electrotherapy [20, 21], laser therapy [21, 22], muscle energy technique [23], spinal manipulation [21], massage [20], and post-isometric relaxation [24] to name a few. Although these modalities can bring short-term pain relief, as they are passive treatments, they do not serve to build patient self-efficacy in the management of chronic pain conditions such as myofascial pain.

Exercise-based treatments for chronic pain are shown to be helpful in various conditions including myofascial pain. Exercise has been known to increase pain thresholds, induce endogenous opioid production, and stimulate endogenous anti-inflammatory response [25]. Randomized control trials have shown an effect with exercise [26]. Additionally, resistance exercise has some evidence in its management as well [27, 28]. There is also evidence with stretching-based exercises [27, 29].

Other more invasive conservative treatment options commonly employed includes dry needling sometimes also called intramuscular stimulation [30–32], and acupuncture [21]. Likewise, these treatment options are passive and has a concern of not bolstering patient self-efficacy.

The evidence for pharmacological management of myofascial pain is very sparse. Simple analgesics can be an initial option using a stepwise approach. Additionally, topical compounded medications can be helpful in delivering therapeutic to localized areas of tenderness. The evidence of topical compounded medications is limited, and the exact compounds is often guided by expert's opinion and local practice patterns. Compounded medications can include lidocaine [33, 34], nonsteroidal anti-inflammatories such as diclofenac [35] or ketoprofen, muscle relaxers such as cyclobenzaprine, pain-modulating neuropathic medications such as gabapentin, amitriptyline, and NMDA antagonists such as ketamine. Additionally, topical menthol [36] and capsaicin [37] can also be used to induce certain sensory receptors.

Other pharmacological options include pain modulating antidepressants and antiepileptic medications. These include tricyclic antidepressants [38, 39], serotonin norepinephrine reuptake inhibitors, and gabapentinoids [39]. Given that myofascial pain is typically a chronic condition, opioid trials should be taken only after very careful consideration and with specific functional goals [40, 41]. The evidence for cannabis in the management of pain is mixed and controversial [42].

Interventional options for the management of myofascial pain include trigger point injections [32, 43, 44]. These injections deliver local anesthetic into the trigger points to interrupt the pain cycle. Although the expected duration of the local anesthetic effect is a few hours, patients often report benefits lasting for days to weeks. Additionally, some practitioners may include corticosteroids or botulinum toxin [44–46] into the trigger point injections to prolong the duration of response from these injections with mixed evidence. Nevertheless, long-term benefit is difficult to achieve with trigger point injections and the patient's self-efficacy is often neglected with this treatment modality. Additionally, there is some evidence that suggests that it does not matter what substance is used for the injection [43].

Conclusion

Myofascial pain is a poorly understood clinical entity that is commonly encountered by clinicians. The diagnosis of this condition is still controversial and the evidence for treatments are mixed. One must be mindful of any underlying pain generators that may be perpetuating myofascial pain. Principles of using interdisciplinary and comprehensive pain treatments are helpful for the management of this chronic pain condition.

References

1. Fernández-de-las-Peñas C, Dommerholt J. International consensus on diagnostic criteria and clinical considerations of myofascial trigger points: a Delphi study. Pain Med (United States). 2018;19(1):142–50.
2. Han SC, Harrison P. Myofascial pain syndrome and trigger-point management. Reg Anesth. 1997;22(1):89–101.
3. Gerwin RD, Dommerholt J, Shah JP. An expansion of Simons' integrated hypothesis of trigger point formation. Curr Pain Headache Rep. 2004;8:468–75.
4. Shah JP, Thaker N, Heimur J, Aredo JV, Sikdar S, Gerber L. Myofascial trigger points then and now: a historical and scientific perspective. PM and R. Elsevier Inc. 2015;7:746–61.
5. Keskindag B, Karaaziz M. The association between pain and sleep in fibromyalgia. Saudi Med J. Saudi Arabian Armed Forces Hospital. 2017;38:465–75.
6. Finan PH, Goodin BR, Smith MT. The association of sleep and pain: An update and a path forward. J Pain. NIH Public Access. 2013;14:1539–52.
7. Consoli G, Marazziti D, Ciapparelli A, Bazzichi L, Massimetti G, Giacomelli C, et al. The impact of mood, anxiety, and sleep disorders on fibromyalgia. Compr Psychiatry. 2012;53(7):962–7.

8. Arnold LM, Hudson JI, Keck PE, Auchenbach MB, Javaras KN, Hess EV. Comorbidity of fibromyalgia and psychiatric disorders. J Clin Psychiatry. 2006;67(8):1219–25.
9. Swain CTV, Pan F, Owen PJ, Schmidt H, Belavy DL. No consensus on causality of spine postures or physical exposure and low back pain: a systematic review of systematic reviews. J Biomech. Elsevier Ltd. 2020;102
10. Fitzcharles MA, Ste-Marie PA, Goldenberg DL, Pereira JX, Abbey S, Choinière M, et al. 2012 Canadian guidelines for the diagnosis and management of fibromyalgia syndrome: executive summary. Pain Res Manage. Hindawi Limited. 2013;18:119–26.
11. Gerwin RD, Duranleau D. Ultrasound identification of the myofascial trigger point. Muscle Nerve. 1997;20(6):767–8.
12. Chen Q, Bensamoun S, Basford JR, Thompson JM, An KN. Identification and quantification of myofascial taut bands with magnetic resonance elastography. Arch Phys Med Rehabil. 2007;88(12):1658–61.
13. Amer-Cuenca JJ, Pecos-Martín D, Martínez-Merinero P, Girbés EL, Nijs J, Meeus M, et al. How much is needed? Comparison of the effectiveness of different pain education dosages in patients with fibromyalgia. Pain Med (United States). 2020;21(4):782–93.
14. Louw A, Zimney K, Puentedura EJ, Diener I. The efficacy of pain neuroscience education on musculoskeletal pain: a systematic review of the literature. Physiother Theory Pract. Taylor and Francis Ltd. 2016;32:332–55.
15. Watson JA, Ryan CG, Cooper L, Ellington D, Whittle R, Lavender M, et al. Pain neuroscience education for adults with chronic musculoskeletal pain: a mixed-methods systematic review and meta-analysis. J Pain. Churchill Livingstone Inc. 2019;20:1140.e1–1140.e22.
16. Nicassio PM, Radojevic V, Weisman MH, Schuman C, Kim J, Schoenfeld-Smith K, et al. A comparison of behavioral and educational interventions for fibromyalgia. J Rheumatol. 1997;24(10):2000–7.
17. Michelotti A, Steenks MH, Farella M, Parisini F, Cimino R, Martina R. The additional value of a home physical therapy regimen versus patient education only for the treatment of myofascial pain of the jaw muscles: short-term results of a randomized clinical trial. J Orofac Pain. 2004;18(2):114–25.
18. Lin SY, Neoh CA, Huang YT, Wang KY, Ng HF, Shi HY. Educational program for myofascial pain syndrome. J Altern Complement Med. 2010;16(6):633–40.
19. Hong CZ, Chen YC, Pon CH, Yu J. Immediate effects of various physical medicine modalities on pain threshold of an active myofascial trigger point. J Musculoskelet Pain. 1993;1(2):37–53.
20. Hou CR, Tsai LC, Cheng KF, Chung KC, Hong CZ. Immediate effects of various physical therapeutic modalities on cervical myofascial pain and trigger-point sensitivity. Arch Phys Med Rehabil. 2002;83(10):1406–14.
21. Vernon H, Schneider M. Chiropractic Management of Myofascial Trigger Points and Myofascial Pain Syndrome: a systematic review of the literature. J Manip Physiol Ther. 2009;32:14–24.
22. Ceylan Y, Hizmetli S, Siliğ Y. The effects of infrared laser and medical treatments on pain and serotonin degradation products in patients with myofascial pain syndrome. A controlled trial. Rheumatol Int. 2004;24(5):260–3.
23. Thomas E, Cavallaro AR, Mani D, Bianco A, Palma A. The efficacy of muscle energy techniques in symptomatic and asymptomatic subjects: a systematic review. Chiropr Man Ther. BioMed Central Ltd. 2019;27
24. Lewit K, Simons DG. Myofascial pain: relief by post-isometric relaxation. Arch Phys Med Rehabil. 1984;65(8):452–6.
25. Ahmed S, Khattab S, Haddad C, Babineau J, Furlan A, Kumbhare D. Effect of aerobic exercise in the treatment of myofascial pain: a systematic review. J Exerc Rehabil. Korean Society of Exercise Rehabilitation. 2018;14:902–10.
26. Cantarero-Villanueva I, Fernández-Lao C, Fernández-de-las-Peñas C, López-Barajas IB, Del-Moral-Ávila R, de la-Llave-Rincón AI, et al. Effectiveness of water physical therapy on pain, pressure pain sensitivity, and myofascial trigger points in breast cancer survivors: a randomized, controlled clinical trial. Pain Med (United States). 2012;13(11):1509–19.

27. Mata Diz JB, de Souza JRLM, Leopoldino AAO, Oliveira VC. Exercise, especially combined stretching and strengthening exercise, reduces myofascial pain: a systematic review. J Physiother. 2017;63(1):17–22.
28. Kim W, Hur MH. Effect of resistance exercise program for middle-aged women with myofascial pain syndrome on shoulder pain, angle of shoulder range of motion, and body composition randomized controlled trial. RCT J Korean Acad Nurs. 2020;50(2):286–97.
29. Mansoori SS, Moustafa IM, Ahbouch A, Harrison DE. Optimal duration of stretching exercise in patients with chronic myofascial pain syndrome: a randomized controlled trial. J Rehabil Med. 2021;53:1.
30. Navarro-Santana MJ, Sanchez-Infante J, Fernández-de-las-Peñas C, Cleland JA, Martín-Casas P, Plaza-Manzano G. Effectiveness of dry needling for myofascial trigger points associated with neck pain symptoms: an updated systematic review and meta-analysis. J Clin Med. 2020;9(10):3300.
31. Edwards J, Knowles N. Superficial dry needling and active stretching in the treatment of myofascial pain—a randomised controlled trial. Acupunct Med. 2003;21(3):80–6.
32. Hong CZ. Lidocaine injection versus dry needling to myofascial trigger point: the importance of the local twitch response. Am J Phys Med Rehabil. 1994;73(4):256–63.
33. Dalpiaz AS, Dodds TA. Myofascial pain response to topical lidocaine patch therapy: case report. J Pain Palliat Care Pharmacother. 2002;16(1):99–104.
34. Dalpiaz AS, Lordon SP, Lipman AG. Topical lidocaine patch therapy for myofascial pain. J Pain Palliat Care Pharmacother. 2004;18(3):15–34.
35. Hsieh LF, Hong CZ, Chern SH, Chen CC. Efficacy and side effects of diclofenac patch in treatment of patients with myofascial pain syndrome of the upper trapezius. J Pain Symptom Manag. 2010;39(1):116–25.
36. Avrahami D, Hammond A, Higgins C, Vernon H. A randomized, placebo-controlled double-blinded comparative clinical study of five over-the-counter non-pharmacological topical analgesics for myofascial pain: single session findings. Chiropr Man Ther. 2012;20(01):7.
37. Romero V, Lara JR, Otero-Espinar F, Salgado MH, Modolo NSP, de Barros GAM. Capsaicin topical cream (8%) for the treatment of myofascial pain syndrome. Braz J Anesthesiol. 2019;69(5):432–8.
38. Bendtsen L, Jensen R. Amitriptyline reduces myofascial tenderness in patients with chronic tension-type headache. Cephalalgia. 2000;20(6):603–10.
39. Haviv Y, Rettman A, Aframian D, Sharav Y, Benoliel R. Myofascial pain: An open study on the pharmacotherapeutic response to stepped treatment with tricyclic antidepressants and gabapentin. J Oral Facial Pain Headache. 2015;29(2):144–51.
40. Dowell D, Haegerich TM, Chou R. CDC guideline for prescribing opioids for chronic pain-United States, 2016. JAMA J Am Med Assoc. 2016;315(15):1624–45.
41. Busse JW, Craigie S, Juurlink DN, Buckley DN, Li W, Couban RJ, et al. Guideline for opioid therapy and chronic noncancer pain. CMAJ. 2017;189(18):E659–66.
42. Lynch ME, Campbell F. Cannabinoids for treatment of chronic non-cancer pain; a systematic review of randomized trials. Br J Clin Pharmacol. 2011;72(5):735–44.
43. Cummings TM, White AR. Needling therapies in the management of myofascial trigger point pain: a systematic review. Arch Phys Med Rehabil. 2001;82(7):986–92.
44. Kamanli A, Kaya A, Ardicoglu O, Ozgocmen S, Zengin FO, Bayık Y. Comparison of lidocaine injection, botulinum toxin injection, and dry needling to trigger points in myofascial pain syndrome. Rheumatol Int. 2005;25(8):604–11.
45. Nicol AL, Wu II, Ferrante FM. Botulinum toxin type a injections for cervical and shoulder girdle myofascial pain using an enriched protocol design. Anesth Analg. 2014;118(6):1326–35.
46. Graboski CL, Shaun Gray D, Burnham RS. Botulinum toxin a versus bupivacaine trigger point injections for the treatment of myofascial pain syndrome: a randomised double blind crossover study. Pain. 2005;118(1–2):170–5.

Chronic Sore Throat

11

Kevin Fung and Andrew James MacDonald

Chronic Pain Syndromes—Chronic Sore Throat

Sore throat is a common presentation in otolaryngology that almost everyone will experience multiple times over their lifespan. It is a seemingly benign complaint; however, there are a wide range of etiologies. These are most often infectious causes with viral infection being the most common. The diagnosis is relatively simple, and the acute sore throat is usually self-resolving with a relatively low risk for complications outside of true Group A streptococcal pharyngitis [1]. The management and recommended investigations for acute sore throat differ between countries, although most involve some combination of conservative management and antibiotics [2]. Chronic sore throat is more complicated to diagnose and before concluding with a functional diagnosis, there are a number of differentials that need to be considered.

Consider the Differential

Viral is the most common infectious etiology. Common pathogens include influenza, rhinovirus, and coronavirus. Due to the difficulty of testing and the self-resolving nature of these infections, specific viral testing is not employed [3]. Bacterial pharyngitis is less common, but tends to be more severe. Common causes

K. Fung (✉)
Department of Otolaryngology-Head and Neck Surgery, Western University, London, ON, Canada
e-mail: kevin.fung@lhsc.on.ca

A. J. MacDonald
PGY1, Department of Family Medicine, Schulich School of Medicine and Dentistry, London, ON, Canada

© The Author(s), under exclusive license to Springer Nature Switzerland AG 2023

B. W. Blakley, J. E. Blakley (eds.), *Functional Illness of the Head and Neck*,
https://doi.org/10.1007/978-3-031-12998-8_11

include Group A beta-hemolytic streptococci, Group C streptococci, and *Neisseria Gonorrhoeae*. Fungal infections should be considered in certain immunocompromised individuals [3].

Non-infectious contributors to sore throat can be physiological, chemical, and environmental. Physiological and chemical factors include cigarette smoke inhalation (including second-hand smoke), snoring, tracheal intubation, phonotrauma, and drug effects, including angiotensin-converting enzyme inhibitors [4], chemotherapy agents, and inhaled corticosteroids [5, 6].

Certain diseases are linked with pharyngitis as well. Gastroesophageal reflux disease [7], Kawasaki disease [8], and thyroid disease [9] can all cause symptoms of sore throat throughout their pathological course. Rare presentations can include epipharyngitis from IgA nephropathy [10], and throat pain caused by cervical spondylosis [11, 12]. In pediatric populations, adenitis periodic fever, aphthous ulcers, pharyngitis, and adenitis (PFAPA) should be considered when the cardinal symptoms described in its name are present [13].

Environmental factors should also be considered when determining a differential of chronic sore throat. Ambient air pollution, urban living/traffic fumes, occupational irritants (including pulp mills, woodworking, biowaste, and factory exhaust emissions), gas pollution, machine coolants, nitrogen trichloride from indoor swimming pools, sulfur dioxide from volcano eruptions, indoor air pollution, low humidity, and cold temperature can all contribute as environmental causes of sore throat [14].

When inflammation and pathology remain undetectable after examination of the patient with chronic sore throat, there is still a differential to consider. It is most important to rule out a concealed malignancy, for example in the base of the tongue, tonsils, or hypopharynx. Additionally, one should inspect anatomically adjacent areas for sources of pain such as submandibular gland pathology and temporomandibular joint arthritis. Once proper investigations are made to rule these out, various functional diseases can be considered in the diagnosis.

Functional Causes of Chronic Sore Throat (Table 11.1)

Table 11.1 Functional diseases causing sore throat, key investigations for their diagnosis, and potential management

Functional disease	Clinical picture and pearls	Key investigations	Potential management
Burning mouth syndrome	Burning oropharyngeal pain; taste alterations; oral dryness; exacerbated by hot foods, relieved by cold foods	History and oral examination for reactive oral appliances	Medical management (e.g., gabapentin, alpha lipoic acid); CBT
Chronic fatigue syndrome	Adolescents with profound fatigue in addition to sore throat	History	CBT; exercise therapy

Table 11.1 (continued)

Functional disease	Clinical picture and pearls	Key investigations	Potential management
Glossopharyngeal neuralgia	Intermittent, unilateral, sharp shooting pain in oropharynx	Imaging to rule out secondary glossopharyngeal nerve compression	Medical management +/− local analgesic injection; surgery if unresponsive to treatment
Eagle syndrome	Unilateral pain in oropharynx; possible radiation to neck and referred otalgia	CT	Medical management +/− local analgesic injection; surgery if unresponsive to treatment
Hyoid syndrome	Sore throat with anterior neck pain	–	Medical analgesia; surgery if unresponsive to treatment
Functional globus sensation	Non-painful "lump in the throat" feeling	History	PPI; antidepressants; psychotherapy
Muscle tension dysphonia	Chronic sore throat with hoarseness	History	Vocal therapy; manual therapy; TENS
Psychogenic sore throat	Psychologic comorbidity	History	CBT

Burning Mouth Syndrome

Burning mouth syndrome is a chronic pain disorder that can present as pharyngeal pain, although it classically involves almost all areas of the oral mucosa, most often affecting the anterior two thirds of the tongue. Many patients report taste alterations, oral dryness, and that pain is exacerbated by hot or spicy foods and relieved by cold foods. The disease can be secondary to a medical condition, like a nutritional deficiency, or a reaction to an oral appliance [15]. Pain without any predisposing cause is considered primary burning mouth syndrome [16]. The condition is most commonly found in older adults [17] and is found more frequently in women than men. Due to its association with postmenopausal women, it has been theorized that hormonal factors could contribute to the condition [15]..

Management should involve ruling out and addressing the root cause of burning mouth syndrome in the case of secondary disease. This includes managing systemic disease such as diabetes, treating a nutritional deficiency (e.g., vitamin B12) [18], or addressing an ill-fitting or reactive oral appliance. Next, management for primary disease can be considered. Strong evidence from clinical trials is lacking for primary burning mouth syndrome treatment, but certain modalities hold some success and show promise. Clonazepam has been demonstrated to relieve pain topically [19, 20] and systemically in low doses, however, the latter has mixed results [20–22]. Combination therapy of gabapentin and alpha lipoic acid has also shown to reduce symptoms [23]. Other interventions with lower evidence of effectiveness include anticonvulsants, electromagnetic radiation, and physical barriers [22]. Burning mouth syndrome can be associated with psychiatric conditions including depression and anxiety [17, 24], and psychotherapy interventions such as cognitive behavioral therapy (CBT) have had success in reducing pain symptoms [25]..

Chronic Fatigue Syndrome

Chronic fatigue syndrome is a functional disease found in children, adolescence, and adults that is primarily characterized by new, severe, and disabling fatigue, co-presenting with sore throat among other symptoms; specifically, impaired memory/concentration, tender cervical/axillary lymph nodes, muscle pain, multi-joint pain, headaches, non-restorative sleep, and/or post-exertion malaise have been associated with chronic fatigue syndrome [26]. Although not every patient with chronic fatigue syndrome will present with sore throat, it is consistently part of multiple diagnostic criteria for the disease [27]..

There are several biological and psychosocial predisposing factors to chronic fatigue syndrome, most which center around trauma and are precipitated by stress [26]. The idea of a chronic viral infectious etiology has been proposed and studied, but the data remain controversial and inconclusive [28]. The strongest evidence for treatment of this disease is for CBT [29–31]. Exercise therapy has also demonstrated potential for treatment [32]. Prognosis is generally favorable and is more effective the earlier the treatment is initiated [33]. However, diagnosis must be certain as intervention on persistently fatigued children and adolescents without full chronic fatigue syndrome criteria can reduce motivation and increase persistence of fatigue [34]. If a patient presents with chronic sore throat secondary to profound fatigue, physicians should keep chronic fatigue syndrome within their differential diagnosis.

Glossopharyngeal Neuralgia

Glossopharyngeal neuralgia (GPN) is characterized as sharp, shooting pain in the oropharynx, often unilateral and aggravated by mandibular functions and swallowing [35]. The pain tends to be fleeting, lasting seconds to minutes, and can also involve the tonsillar fossa, ear canal, and the base of the tongue [35]. Rarely, patients can experience vagal symptoms with the pain including cough, hoarseness, syncope and/or bradycardia [36]. Following an acute attack, it is possible for patients to have GPN-related discomfort episodes for weeks to months [36]. The disease is fairly uncommon, estimated 0.8 per 100,000 populations a year [37]..

Secondary causes of GPN include trauma, radiation, neoplasm, infection, surgery, vascular malformations, and demyelinating diseases [35]. Idiopathic causes can be due to compression via vessels or compression of the glossopharyngeal at anatomic constrictions, such as entering or exiting the brainstem [38].. Diagnosis is clinical and determined by the presence of neuralgic pain characteristics and pain distribution [38]..

Treatment for GPN begins with pharmacotherapy and can be treated surgically if initial management fails. Carbamazepine, gabapentin, and pregabalin are considered first line treatment [35], and glossopharyngeal nerve block can work as a safe adjunct to medication [39]. Microvascular decompression of nerve roots has established itself as an effective surgical option for GPN [40]. Although there is no evidence for treating GPN with psychiatric therapies, it is possible patients with significant quality of life effects can benefit from psychopharmacology or psychotherapy [16].

Stylalgia/Eagle Syndrome

Eagle's syndrome, or stylalgia, is classically described by recurrent unilateral throat pain, neck pain, pharyngeal foreign body sensation, dysphagia, and referred otalgia [41]. Similar to glossopharyngeal neuralgia, pain symptoms can be exacerbated by swallowing and mandibular functions. It is typically associated with the elongation of the styloid process to a length of greater than 3 cm, however relatively few individuals with elongated styloid processes will be symptomatic [42]. This anatomic variance is associated with increased risk of carotid artery dissection [43, 44]. There are two identified forms of Eagle syndrome: the classic type associated with irritation of the trigeminal, facial, glossopharyngeal, and vagus nerves, and the carotid artery type which is linked to irritation of the carotid nerve plexus [45].

Gold standard for diagnosis is CT scan, but angiography and 3D reconstructive imaging both have roles for diagnosis as well. The relief of symptoms upon injection of lidocaine into the tonsillar fossa can also be diagnostic for Eagle syndrome [46].

Medical management is advocated to be the first-line treatment, although no single optimal treatment has yet been identified. This is typically an analgesic such as an NSAID, and an alternative conjunct such as anti-convulsants, anti-depressants, local injections, and manual manipulation [47]. When medical management fails, surgical interventions can be considered. Both extra- and intra-oral surgical options exist, each with their own benefits and drawbacks [48]. Other therapies, such as manual therapy and exercise, have been studied as alternatives, but with mixed results [49].

Hyoid Syndrome/Anterior Neck Pain Syndrome

Although hyoid syndrome classically presents as anterior neck pain, it is possible for pharyngeal pain to be part of the presentation [50]. The pain can also spread to the supraclavicular region, the sternocleidomastoid, the ear and the temporal region [50]. Similar to other chronic throat pains, swallowing and head movement can exacerbate symptoms [51]. Treatment includes medical analgesia, such as NSAIDs, or local anesthetic to the greater cornu of the hyoid bone. Alternatively, surgical excision of the greater cornu of hyoid bone has demonstrated to be effective management [50].

Functional Globus Sensation

If a patient describes their chronic sore throat as non-painful, globus pharyngeus should be considered on the differential. It is described as a "lump in the throat" feeling and most commonly affects women under the age of 50 [52]. The etiology is currently unknown. It is generally considered to have psychological components, however, there are theories that physiological factors such as GERD and other esophageal pathologies also play a role [52, 53]. Small studies have suggested that anti-depressants may have some benefit [54]. Proton pump inhibitors have been advocated as treatment, but studies have demonstrated mixed results for its efficacy [55–57]. Given the psychological components of globus sensation, CBT may play a role in treatment [55]. A small study has also suggested hypnotically assisted relaxation therapy may also have some benefit to patients [58].

Muscle Tension Dysphonia

Suspect muscle tension dysphonia (MTD) if the chronic sore throat is accompanied with a history of dysphonia. MTD is a relatively common functional voice disorder that specifically involves excess tension in laryngeal and paralaryngeal muscles, with throat pain or discomfort as a common symptom. Etiology of this disease has a number of contributors, including psychological factors, voice misuse, and compensation for underlying disease [59]. As with other functional voice disorders, voice therapy is highly recommended in management [60, 61]. Studies have suggested that manual manipulations of the larynx such as laryngeal manual therapy or manual circumlaryngeal therapy have short-term [62] and long-term [63] pain reducing effects. Transcutaneous electrical stimulation (TENS) was also found to be effective in treating pain from MTD [64, 65].

Psychogenic Sore Throat

A psychogenic sore throat should only be diagnosed after all other potential diagnoses have been excluded. It is possible that true psychogenic chronic sore throat may be rare, as a recent two year study found only 48 out of 1580 patients presenting to a clinic with chronic sore throat were diagnosed with psychogenic sore throat [66]. As with other somatizing disease, CBT can be effective for reducing pain symptoms [25].

Conclusion

There is a wide differential for functional causes of chronic sore throat, however they do not have time-sensitive mortality nor morbidities. Thus, it is important to take the time to rule out organic causes first, especially concealed malignancies.

Once the diagnosis is confidently narrowed down to functional disease, a multidisciplinary approach is important for management. There are important roles for exercise therapy, voice therapy, and CBT or psychotherapy in certain diagnoses. Additionally, although there are invasive interventions for some diseases, such as surgery, it is important to begin with conservative management first.

References

1. Stephenson KN. Acute and chronic pharyngitis across the lifespan. Lippincotts Prim Care Pract. 2000;4(5):471–89.
2. Chiappini E, Regoli M, Bonsignori F, Sollai S, Parretti A, Galli L, et al. Analysis of different recommendations from international guidelines for the management of acute pharyngitis in adults and children. Clin Ther. 2011;33(1):48–58.
3. Weber R. Pharyngitis. Prim Care. 2014;41(1):91–8.
4. Fletcher AE, Palmer AJ, Bulpitt CJ. Cough with angiotensin converting enzyme inhibitors: how much of a problem? J Hypertens Suppl. 1994;12(2):S43–7.
5. Pinto CR, Almeida NR, Marques TS, Yamamura LLL, Costa LA, Souza-Machado A. Local adverse effects associated with the use of inhaled corticosteroids in patients with moderate or severe asthma. J Bras Pneumol. 2013;39(4):409–17.
6. Bhalla RK, Taylor W, Jones AS, Roland NJ. The inflammation produced by corticosteroid inhalers in the pharynx in asthmatics. Clin Otolaryngol. 2008;33(6):581–6.
7. Murray RC, Chennupati SK. Chronic streptococcal and non-streptococcal pharyngitis. Infect Disord Drug Targets. 2012;12(4):281–5.
8. Wolff AE, Hansen KE, Zakowski L. Acute Kawasaki disease: not just for kids. J Gen Intern Med. 2007;22(5):681–4.
9. Rotman-Pikielny P, Borodin O, Zissin R, Ness-Abramof R, Levy Y. Newly diagnosed thyrotoxicosis in hospitalized patients: clinical characteristics. QJM. 2008;101(11):871–4.
10. Hotta O, Tanaka A, Oda T. Chronic epipharyngitis: a missing background of IgA nephropathy. Autoimmun Rev. 2019;18(8):835–6.
11. Alaani A, Hogg R, Johnson AP. Chronic throat symptoms cured by osteophyte excision. J R Soc Med. 2004;97(4):181–2.
12. Fan ZT, Wang XX, Liang H, Liu CB. Cervical pharyngeal syndrome: a case report. Lin Chuang Er Bi Yan Hou Tou Jing Wai Ke Za Zhi J Clin Otorhinolaryngol Head Neck Surg. 2018;32(16):1275–6.
13. Manthiram K, Nesbitt E, Morgan T, Edwards KM. Family history in periodic fever, aphthous stomatitis, pharyngitis, adenitis (PFAPA) syndrome. Pediatrics [Internet]. 2016;138:3. [cited 2021 Jan 3] https://www.ncbi.nlm.nih.gov/pmc/articles/PMC5005017/
14. Renner B, Mueller CA, Shephard A. Environmental and non-infectious factors in the aetiology of pharyngitis (sore throat). Inflamm Res. 2012;61(10):1041–52.
15. Jääskeläinen SK. Pathophysiology of primary burning mouth syndrome. Clin Neurophysiol. 2012;123(1):71–7.
16. Tait RC, Ferguson M, Herndon CM. Chronic orofacial pain: burning mouth syndrome and other neuropathic disorders. J Pain Manag Med [Internet]. 2017;3:1. [cited 2021 Jan 2] https://www.ncbi.nlm.nih.gov/pmc/articles/PMC5475277/
17. Gurvits GE, Tan A. Burning mouth syndrome. World J Gastroenterol. 2013;19(5):665–72.
18. Ducasse D, Courtet P, Olie E. Burning mouth syndrome: current clinical, physiopathologic, and therapeutic data. Reg Anesth Pain Med. 2013;38(5):380–90.
19. Gremeau-Richard C, Woda A, Navez ML, Attal N, Bouhassira D, Gagnieu MC, et al. Topical clonazepam in stomatodynia: a randomised placebo-controlled study. Pain. 2004;108(1–2):51–7.

20. Amos K, Yeoh S-C, Farah CS. Combined topical and systemic clonazepam therapy for the management of burning mouth syndrome: a retrospective pilot study. J Orofac Pain. 2011;25(2):125–30.
21. Heckmann SM, Kirchner E, Grushka M, Wichmann MG, Hummel T. A double-blind study on clonazepam in patients with burning mouth syndrome. Laryngoscope. 2012;122(4):813–6.
22. McMillan R, Forssell H, Buchanan JA, Glenny A, Weldon JC, Zakrzewska JM. Interventions for treating burning mouth syndrome. Cochrane Database Syst Rev [Internet]. 2016;2016:11. [cited 2021 Jan 1] https://www.ncbi.nlm.nih.gov/pmc/articles/PMC6464255/
23. López-D'alessandro E, Escovich L. Combination of alpha lipoic acid and gabapentin, its efficacy in the treatment of burning mouth syndrome: a randomized, double-blind, placebo controlled trial. Med Oral Patol Oral Cirugia Bucal. 2011;16(5):e635-640.
24. Bogetto F, Maina G, Ferro G, Carbone M, Gandolfo S. Psychiatric comorbidity in patients with burning mouth syndrome. Psychosom Med. 1998;60(3):378–85.
25. Noma N, Watanabe Y, Shimada A, Usuda S, Iida T, Shimada A, et al. Effects of cognitive behavioral therapy on orofacial pain conditions. J Oral Sci. 2020;63(1):4–7.
26. Werker CL, Nijhof SL, van de Putte EM. Clinical practice: chronic fatigue syndrome. Eur J Pediatr. 2013;172(10):1293–8.
27. Twisk FN. Accurate diagnosis of myalgic encephalomyelitis and chronic fatigue syndrome based upon objective test methods for characteristic symptoms. World J Methodol. 2015;5(2):68–87.
28. Rasa S, Nora-Krukle Z, Henning N, Eliassen E, Shikova E, Harrer T, et al. Chronic viral infections in myalgic encephalomyelitis/chronic fatigue syndrome (ME/CFS). J Transl Med [Internet]. 2018:16. [cited 2021 Jan 1] https://www.ncbi.nlm.nih.gov/pmc/articles/PMC6167797/
29. Knoop H, Stulemeijer M, de Jong LWAM, Fiselier TJW, Bleijenberg G. Efficacy of cognitive behavioral therapy for adolescents with chronic fatigue syndrome: long-term follow-up of a randomized, controlled trial. Pediatrics. 2008;121(3):e619–25.
30. Knight SJ, Scheinberg A, Harvey AR. Interventions in pediatric chronic fatigue syndrome/myalgic encephalomyelitis: a systematic review. J Adolesc Health. 2013;53(2):154–65.
31. Nijhof SL, Priesterbach LP, Uiterwaal CSPM, Bleijenberg G, Kimpen JLL, van de Putte EM. Internet-based therapy for adolescents with chronic fatigue syndrome: long-term follow-up. Pediatrics. 2013;131(6):e1788-1795.
32. Larun L, Brurberg KG, Odgaard-Jensen J, Price JR. Exercise therapy for chronic fatigue syndrome. Cochrane Database Syst Rev. 2017;4:CD003200.
33. Burns D. Chronic fatigue syndrome or myalgic encephalomyelitis. Nurs Stand R Coll Nurs G B. 2012;26(25):48–56. 1987 quiz 58
34. Bakker RJ, van de Putte EM, Kuis W, Sinnema G. Effects of an educational video film in fatigued children and adolescents: a randomised controlled trial. Arch Dis Child. 2011;96(5):457–60.
35. Khan M, Nishi SE, Hassan SN, Islam MA, Gan SH. Trigeminal neuralgia, glossopharyngeal neuralgia, and myofascial pain dysfunction syndrome: an update. Pain Res Manag [Internet]. 2017:2017. [cited 2021 Jan 2] https://www.ncbi.nlm.nih.gov/pmc/articles/PMC5554565/
36. Headache Classification Committee of the International Headache Society (IHS) The International Classification of Headache Disorders, 3rd. Cephalalgia 2018;38(1):1–211.
37. Koopman JSHA, Dieleman JP, Huygen FJ, de Mos M, Martin CGM, Sturkenboom MCJM. Incidence of facial pain in the general population. Pain. 2009;147(1–3):122–7.
38. Singh PM, Kaur M, Trikha A. An uncommonly common: glossopharyngeal neuralgia. Ann Indian Acad Neurol. 2013;16(1):1–8.
39. Liu Q, Zhong Q, Tang G, He G. Ultrasound-guided glossopharyngeal nerve block via the styloid process for glossopharyngeal neuralgia: a retrospective study. J Pain Res. 2019;12:2503–10.
40. Kandan SR, Khan S, Jeyaretna DS, Lhatoo S, Patel NK, Coakham HB. Neuralgia of the glossopharyngeal and vagal nerves: long-term outcome following surgical treatment and literature review. Br J Neurosurg. 2010;24(4):441–6.
41. Mayrink G, Figueiredo EP, Sato FRL, Moreira RWF. Cervicofacial pain associated with Eagle's syndrome misdiagnosed as trigeminal neuralgia. Oral Maxillofac Surg. 2012;16(2):207–10.

42. Murtagh RD, Caracciolo JT, Fernandez G. CT findings associated with eagle syndrome. AJNR Am J Neuroradiol. 2001;22(7):1401–2.
43. Hebant B, Guegan-Massardier E, Macaigne V, Triquenot-Bagan A. Ischemic stroke due to internal carotid artery dissection associated with an elongated styloid process (eagle syndrome). J Neurol Sci. 2017;372:466–7.
44. Ogawa M, Inohara H. Is voice therapy effective for the treatment of dysphonic patients with benign vocal fold lesions? Auris Nasus Larynx. 2018;45(4):661–6.
45. Kim E, Hansen K, Frizzi J. Eagle syndrome: case report and review of the literature. Ear Nose Throat J. 2008;87(11):631–3.
46. Badhey A, Jategaonkar A, Anglin Kovacs AJ, Kadakia S, De Deyn PP, Ducic Y, et al. Eagle syndrome: a comprehensive review. Clin Neurol Neurosurg. 2017;159:34–8.
47. Piagkou M, Anagnostopoulou S, Kouladouros K, Piagkos G. Eagle's syndrome: a review of the literature. Clin Anat N Y N. 2009;22(5):545–58.
48. Costantinides F, Vidoni G, Bodin C, Di Lenarda R. Eagle's syndrome: signs and symptoms. Cranio. 2013;31(1):56–60.
49. Wong ML, Rossi MD, Groff W, Castro S, Powell J. Physical therapy management of a patient with eagle syndrome. Physiother Theory Pract. 2011;27(4):319–27.
50. Lim RY. Carotodynia exposed: hyoid bone syndrome. South Med J. 1987;80(4):444–6.
51. Aydil U, Kizil Y, Köybaşioğlu A. Less known non-infectious and neuromusculoskeletal system-originated anterolateral neck and craniofacial pain disorders. Eur Arch Oto-Rhino-Laryngol. 2012;269(1):9–16.
52. Järvenpää P, Arkkila P, Aaltonen L-M. Globus pharyngeus: a review of etiology, diagnostics, and treatment. Eur Arch Oto-Rhino-Laryngol. 2018;275(8):1945–53.
53. Moser G, Wenzel-Abatzi TA, Stelzeneder M, Wenzel T, Weber U, Wiesnagrotzki S, et al. Globus sensation: pharyngoesophageal function, psychometric and psychiatric findings, and follow-up in 88 patients. Arch Intern Med. 1998;158(12):1365–73.
54. Brown SR, Schwartz JM, Summergrad P, Jenike MA. Globus hystericus syndrome responsive to antidepressants. Am J Psychiatry. 1986;143(7):917–8.
55. Manabe N, Tsutsui H, Kusunoki H, Hata J, Haruma K. Pathophysiology and treatment of patients with globus sensation—from the viewpoint of esophageal motility dysfunction. J Smooth Muscle Res. 2014;50:66–77.
56. Noordzij JP, Khidr A, Evans BA, Desper E, Mittal RK, Reibel JF, et al. Evaluation of omeprazole in the treatment of reflux laryngitis: a prospective, placebo-controlled, randomized, double-blind study. Laryngoscope. 2001;111(12):2147–51.
57. Vaezi MF, Richter JE, Stasney CR, Spiegel JR, Iannuzzi RA, Crawley JA, et al. Treatment of chronic posterior laryngitis with esomeprazole. Laryngoscope. 2006;116(2):254–60.
58. Kiebles JL, Kwiatek MA, Pandolfino JE, Kahrilas PJ, Keefer L. Do patients with globus sensation respond to hypnotically assisted relaxation therapy? A case series report. Dis Esophagus. 2010;23(7):545–53.
59. Van Houtte E, Van Lierde K, Claeys S. Pathophysiology and treatment of muscle tension dysphonia: a review of the current knowledge. J Voice. 2011;25(2):202–7.
60. Stinnett S, Chmielewska M, Akst LM. Update on management of hoarseness. Med Clin North Am. 2018;102(6):1027–40.
61. Mansuri B, Torabinezhad F, Jamshidi A-A, Dabirmoghadam P, Vasaghi-Gharamaleki B, Ghelichi L. Effects of voice therapy on vocal tract discomfort in muscle tension dysphonia. Iran J Otorhinolaryngol. 2019;31(106):297–304.
62. Reimann AP, Siqueira LTD, Rondon AV, Brasolotto AG, Silverio KCA. Immediate effect of laryngeal manual therapy in dysphonic individuals. CoDAS. 2016;28(1):59–65.
63. Dehqan A, Ballard KJ. An evaluation of short-term treatment outcomes of cricothyroid visor maneuver: a proof-of-concept pilot study. J Voice. 2019:24.
64. Siqueira LTD, Silverio KCA, Brasolotto AG, Guirro RR d J, Carneiro CG, Behlau M. Effects of laryngeal manual therapy (LMT) and transcutaneous electrical nerve stimulation (TENS) in vocal folds diadochokinesis of dysphonic women: a randomized clinical trial. Efeitos Ter Man Laringea E Estimul Eletr Nerv Transcutanea TENS Na Diadococinesia Laringea Em Mulh Disfonicas Estudo. Clin Randomizado. 2017;29(3):e20160191.

65. Alves Silverio KC, Brasolotto AG, Thais Donalonso Siqueira L, Carneiro CG, Fukushiro AP, de Jesus R, Guirro R. Effect of application of transcutaneous electrical nerve stimulation and laryngeal manual therapy in dysphonic women: clinical trial. J Voice. 2015;29(2):200–8.
66. Kundu S, Dutta M, Adhikary BK, Ghosh B. Encountering chronic sore throat: how challenging is it for the otolaryngologists? Indian J Otolaryngol Head Neck Surg. 2019;71(Suppl 1):176–81.

Ear Pain and TMJ

12

Brian W. Blakley and Rick Soordhar

Anatomy and Physiology of Ear Pain and Pressure

The neuroanatomy of the ear is complex and varied. Figure 12.1 is a standard depiction of the sensory innervation of the pinna, but many authorities would suggest that the lesser occipital nerve and branches of the glossopharyngeal and facial nerves may innervate portions of the pinna and external auditory canal.

Why is there disagreement? Is there a consistent pattern of sensory innervation of the pinna that some authors do not know about? Clinical observation of patients with well-known nerve lesions often reveals patterns of nerve dysfunction that do not align with a consistent, linear view of innervation. Conflicting descriptions are not "wrong." They illustrate the variability and plasticity that occurs in humans and is one reason why symptoms and findings are not consistent with a single, linear model.

The area surrounding the ear is even more neuroanatomically complex than the pinna (Fig. 12.2) and has the most diverse innervation in the human body. Dysfunction in one nerve causes referred dysfunction in another. Considering that nerves are two-way connections, not just wires, with peripheral and central sensitization, neural plasticity and inherent variability of neuroanatomy, it is not surprising that symptoms and findings often fail to follow a pattern predicted by simple, labelled lines.

Sensory neurons involved in pain include (1) thinly myelinated, high threshold fibers that sense the acute, first wave of pain called Aδ fibers; (2) myelinated, low threshold fibers called Aβ fibers that sense touch, pressure, movement, and vibration; and (3) unmyelinated, high threshold fibers called "C" fibers that act for

B. W. Blakley (✉)
Department of Otolaryngology, University of Manitoba, Winnipeg, MB, Canada

R. Soordhar
Diomate, American Board of Craniofacial Pain (DABCFP), Fellow and Distinguished Fellow, American Board of Craniofacial Pain (FAACP, DFAACP), Private Practice, Milton, ON, Canada

© The Author(s), under exclusive license to Springer Nature Switzerland AG 2023

B. W. Blakley, J. E. Blakley (eds.), *Functional Illness of the Head and Neck*,
https://doi.org/10.1007/978-3-031-12998-8_12

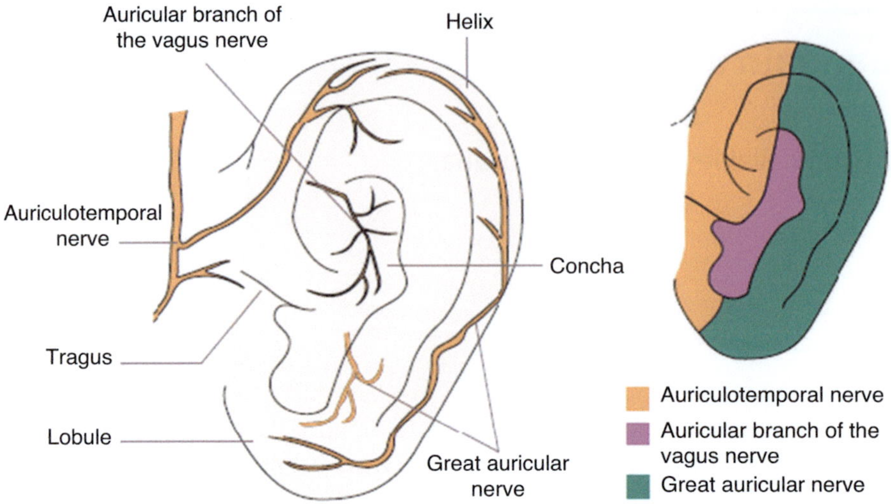

The anterior auricular branches of the auriculotemporal nerve innervates the skin overlying the tragus, as well as the adjacent part of the helix. The auricular branch of the vagus nerve innervates the ear canal, tragus and part of the auricle. The great auricular nerve innervates the skin of the lateral auricle and the skin over both the parotid gland and mastoid process. Source: Roberts 2017. [58] *Reproduced with permission from Elsevier.*

Fig. 12.1 Innervation of the pinna from https://www.aerjournal.com/articles/non-invasive-low-level-tragus-stimulation-cardiovascular-diseases

long duration and cause the sensation of pain to persist (see Chap. 2). Chronic pain that persists in the absence of some stimulus usually results from activation of "C" fibers. When "C" fiber activation occurs chronically in the absence of a stimulus, it can be said that the nervous system is pathological. This is called neuropathic pain, and clinically is the most problematic type of pain. Neuropathic pain responds poorly to NSAIDs. Nociceptors are sensors of unpleasant or nociceptive sensations—pain, pressure, fullness as well as neutral sensations such as the feelings of touch. The thalamus appears to be the site where nociceptive sensations are interpreted as unpleasant. There is growing evidence that aberrant neural processing in the thalamus may result in pain in some cases of neuropathic pain (see Table 12.1). Nociplastic pain is a new pain class consisting of nerve damage caused by ongoing pain [1].

Ear pain can be caused by local, regional, or systemic causes. In all but a few cases the diagnosis can be established by history and physical examination. Some "clinical peals" for evaluation of ear pain include asking:

1. "How is your hearing?" Otitis media is infected fluid in the middle ear so it must have associated hearing loss. A slow or uncertain response will be seen in young children or sometimes in adults with otitis externa which often has altered

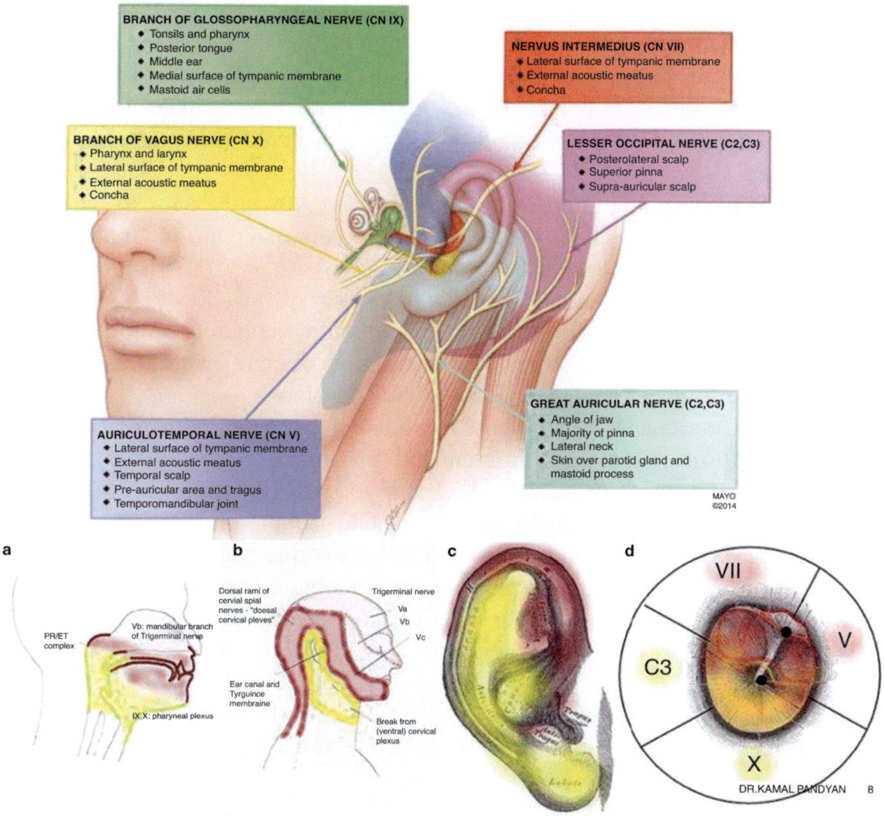

Fig. 12.2 Innervation of the area surrounding the ear. The ear region is a junction point for multiple cranial and peripheral nerves with a variety of sensory functions

Table 12.1 Differentiation of some types of pain

	Nociceptive pain	Neuropathic pain	Myogenic
Cause	Appropriate activation of sensory receptors	Pathology of the nervous system itself; central and peripheral sensitization	Muscle splinting, muscle spasm, myofascial trigger points
Quality descriptors	Sharp, acute	Burning, tingling, electrical shock, stabbing	Dull & achy pain
Time course	Short <3 months	Chronic >3 months	Short or chronic
Treatment	NSAIDs, ASA	Gabapentinoids, SSRIs, SNRIs, TCAs	Muscle relaxant, myofascial trigger point treatment, acupuncture
Examples	Infection, trauma, post-surgical	Herpetic neuralgia, myofascial pain, fibromyalgia	Muscle spasm, myofascial pain dysfunction

hearing or muffling. If the patient quickly answers that his/her hearing is unchanged with pain, otitis media is very unlikely.
2. "Is the ear pain bilateral or unilateral?" The mandible is essentially the only structure that runs from one ear to the other (...well, yes the skull does too, but no muscles do) so bilateral ear pain should be considered TMJ pain until proven otherwise.
3. "Does the pain radiate up the side of the head or down the neck to the shoulders?" Otitis media localizes to the ear. TMJ, myofascial pain, and other muscular pain may center on the ear but radiate.
4. "What makes the pain worse?" Pain that increases with swallowing is suspicious for tonsillar or hypopharyngeal/laryngeal pathology including tumor, and muscle tension dysphonia. Post-tonsillectomy pain is often referred to the ear. Pain induced by biting or chewing suggests dental problems.
5. "Is the pain constant or intermittent?" Pain due to tumors or otitis media is fairly constant. Muscle spasm is intermittent and "spasmodic."
6. "Do you have a lot of headaches?" Migraine and tension headaches are common causes of ear pain. Ask about other migraine symptoms but remember that migraine is common and may exist in addition to other causes.
7. "Do you have muscle or joint pain elsewhere in your body?" Myofascial pain syndrome, fibromyalgia and other rheumatoid disorders often cause ear pain, but patients may not associate the other conditions, so direct questioning is important.

Clinical Evaluation of Ear pain and Pressure

Step 1: Consider Local Causes

History should consider 6 "P's" that cover all ear symptoms:

1. Pain or pressure.
2. Perception of noise (tinnitus).
3. Poor hearing.
4. Pus (drainage or otorrhea).
5. Perturbations of balance (dizziness).
6. Paralysis—or weakness of the facial nerve.

Physical exam should include a general head and neck exam that focuses on whether the tympanic membrane (TM) is normal. For most disorders, the symptom of pressure, rather than pain is present.

Abnormal TM Possibilities.

- Serous otitis media.
- Acute otitis media.
- Retraction.
- Perforation.

- Normal TM.
- Otosclerosis does not cause pain but can cause pressure sensation. Otosclerosis is the presumptive diagnosis for patients with a conductive hearing loss without explanation, with normal tympanic membrane and normal tympanogram. The hearing loss typically starts in young adult years and usually there is a family history consistent with the disorder such as a father who had surgery for hearing loss. The usual therapy is surgical (stapedectomy), but hearing aids also work well for those who do not want surgery.
- Ménière's disease can cause pressure but not pain. Definite Meniere's disease is defined by (1) recurrent attacks of spinning vertigo that last at least half an hour; (2) either fluctuating aural pressure, tinnitus, or fluctuating hearing; and (3) documented hearing loss. Without hearing loss, patients can be told that they may have Meniere's but "probable Meniere's" overlaps with many other ear syndromes and is a non-diagnosis. Treatment for persistent and bothersome Meniere's includes (1) salt restriction and avoiding triggers if these are observed; (2) diuretics; (3) corticosteroids—both systemic and intratympanic; (4) occasional benzodiazepine such as clonazepam or lorazepam if not too frequent; (5) endolymphatic sac surgery or destructive treatments such as (6) intratympanic gentamicin injection; (7) surgical labyrinthectomy; or (9) vestibular nerve section, which is the "gold standard" for eliminating spells of vertigo, but has surgical risks and may result in chronic imbalance.
- Superior semicircular canal dehiscence (SSCD) may cause pressure but not pain. Autophony, aural fullness, hyperacusis without movement of the TM with respiration or sniffing.
- Patulous Eustachian tube (PET) is another possible cause of ear pressure and perhaps mild pain. The typical history includes autophony, aural fullness, often improving when the patient puts his/her head between the knees. PET often follows weight loss or pregnancy. The tympanic membrane moves with respiration or sniffing. Tympanic membrane movement with Valsalva or pinched nostril is normal.
- Stapedius muscle contraction or tensor tympani syndrome may cause pressure, particularly with loud noises. These are difficult to distinguish so a preferred term is the more general "middle ear myoclonus." Symptoms may consist of clicking not synchronous with the pulse or sometimes a muffling or distortion of sound with pressure induced by sound.

Step 2: Consider Regional Causes

Consider TMJ dysfunction first. TMJ dysfunction sometimes called TMD is a common, widely underrecognized cause of ear pain. TMJ dysfunction is associated with a variety of other functional symptoms such as dizziness, tinnitus, neck and facial pain, headaches, and many others so it can be difficult to distinguish from other disorders. The pain of TMJ is variable from constant to intermittent and from mild to severe, although the more severe pain is more likely to radiate.

The physical exam is important for TMJ diagnosis as follows:

- The joints may be tender to palpation. This is strong evidence of TMJ dysfunction.
- Mouth opening is often reduced or there is hesitation to complete opening with TMJ dysfunction. In adults and older children, the distance between upper and lower teeth should be about 50 mm. Clinically the distance between the upper and lower incisors should accommodate the width of three fingers [2].
- Palpate the TMJs while the patient opens and closes the mouth. Fingers can be placed in the external auditory canal during repetitive mouth opening and closing. Often there are clicking, popping, crepitus, or cracking noises which reflect pathology of the intra-articular TMJ disc.

Notice if the TMJs move symmetrically or if the jaw moves from side to side during opening (deviation or deflection). Such movements indicate that one or both TMJ(s) is(are) not moving smoothly. The TMJ is one of the most complex joints of the body, behaving as a ginglymoarthrodial joint, which allows for both rotation and translation to maximize mouth opening. The intra-articular disk of the pathologic TMJ may obstruct translation, sometimes only for a portion of the range of motion, after which it reduces to its normal position (see Fig. 12.3). Observe the incisors during jaw movement to see if there is asymmetric movement as evidence of reduction of the TMJ disk. Displacement with reduction is indicated if the jaw deviates during opening but returns to the midline with complete opening. A unilateral displacement without reduction is found if the jaw deviates to one side and remains displaced with full mouth opening. However, a bilateral disc displacement without reduction is found if the jaw opens straight up and down but the opening is usually less than 45 mm.

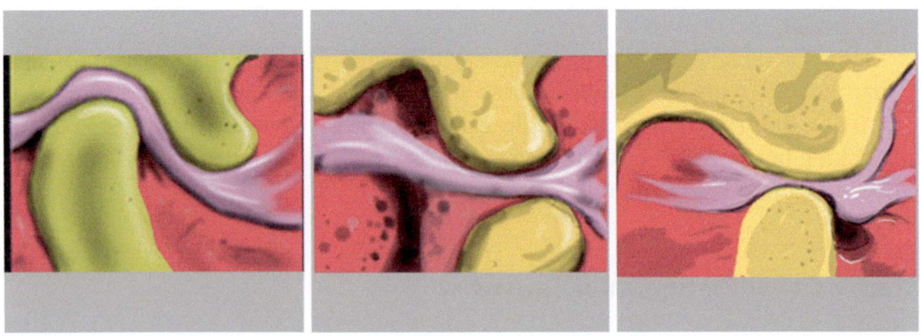

Fig. 12.3 Normal TMJ (left panel) with fibrocartilaginous disc between the condyle and the glenoid fossa. With mouth opening (center panel) the condyle rotates but also slides forward. If the disc is damaged (right panel) movement of the condyle is restricted. It the disc displacement corrects it may do so with a snap or pop. If it does not correct deviation of the jaw with mouth opening may occur

- Palpate the muscles around the TMJ and perform intraoral palpation of the temporalis insertion, lateral pterygoid and medial pterygoid muscles looking for tenderness. Extraorally palpate the temporalis, masseter, sternocleidomastioid, and trapezius for pain, tenderness, or myofascial trigger points.
- The diagnosis of TMJ dysfunction is supported by completing a thorough TMJ examination, TMJ imaging (MRI or cone beam computed tomography (CBCT)) and functional testing. Relief of symptoms can occur if the condyles are decompressed to take the compression of the auriculotemporal nerve by providing a better position of the condyle in the glenoid fossa. Functional testing can be completed by placing a spacer between the incisors and asking if this position relieves some pain and/or a reduction of pain when the clinician is palpating the head and neck muscles. A useful spacer that is usually available is a stack of six tongue blades.

Also, examine the teeth for possible dental problems. Tenderness of molar teeth may indicate dental infection or abscess that can mimic facial and ear pain. Palpate for digastric spasm, tender lymph nodes in the retromandibular area.

If the above examinations are negative, examine the larynx and hypopharynx for pathology causing referred pain.

Step 3: Consider Systemic Causes

These are commonly not considered but are important and can be assessed by most clinical physicians within their specialty [3, 4]. Many patients will think they are irrelevant and not mention these issues unless specifically questioned. The most common systemic causes of ear pain include:

- Migraine.
- Fibromyalgia.
- Myofascial pain.
- Statin-induced myositis.
- Arthritis and connective tissue disorders.

Treatment for ear pain obviously relates to the underlying diagnosis. Infections and tumors have specific treatments. Dental interventions may be helpful for TMJ dysfunction. Occlusal correction and various splints can provide relief [5–7]. Some physiotherapists have a special interest in TMJ disorders [8, 9]. TMJ surgery is occasionally an option for severe cases [10, 11]. If the underlying cause cannot be corrected pharmacological or psychological support may help as discussed in other chapters. Pharmacological support should avoid the chronic use of opioids and benzodiazepines. SNRIs such as venlafaxine may be more helpful than SSRIs but may reflect what has been studied [12]. Good comparisons of SSRIs versus SNRIs are lacking. Of the tricyclics, amitriptyline has the strongest support in the literature

[12]. Sometimes the side-effects of tricyclics such as sleepiness can be helpful but for all these measures the efficacy is only moderate.

References

1. Fitzcharles MA, Cohen SP, Clauw DJ, Littlejohn G, Usui C, Häuser W. Nociplastic pain: towards an understanding of prevalent pain conditions. Lancet. 2021;397(10289):2098–110.
2. Zawawi KH, Al-Badawi EA, Lobo SL, Melis M, Mehta NR. An index for the measurement of normal maximum mouth opening. J Can Dent Assoc. 2003;69(11):737–41.
3. Ranque B, Nardon O. Medically unexplained symptoms' care in internal medicine: a paradigm of doctor-patient relationship in situation of uncertainty. Rev Med Interne. 2017;38(7):458–66.
4. Häuser W, Fitzcharles MA. Facts and myths pertaining to fibromyalgia. Dialogues Clin Neurosci. 2018;20(1):53–62.
5. Luther F, Layton S, McDonald F. Orthodontics for treating temporomandibular joint (TMJ) disorders. Cochrane Database Syst Rev. 2010;7:Cd006541.
6. Türp JC, Greene CS, Strub JR. Dental occlusion: a critical reflection on past, present and future concepts. J Oral Rehabil. 2008;35(6):446–53.
7. Huang MF, Alfi D, Alfi J, Huang AT. The use of patient-specific implants in oral and maxillofacial surgery. Oral Maxillofac Surg Clin North Am. 2019;31(4):593–600.
8. Armijo-Olivo S, Pitance L, Singh V, Neto F, Thie N, Michelotti A. Effectiveness of manual therapy and therapeutic exercise for temporomandibular disorders: systematic review and meta-analysis. Phys Ther. 2016;96(1):9–25.
9. Aggarwal A, Keluskar V. Physiotherapy as an adjuvant therapy for treatment of TMJ disorders. Gen Dent. 2012;60(2):e119–22.
10. Liu F, Steinkeler A. Epidemiology, diagnosis, and treatment of temporomandibular disorders. Dent Clin N Am. 2013;57(3):465–79.
11. Dolwick MF, Widmer CG. Orthognathic surgery as a treatment for temporomandibular disorders. Oral Maxillofac Surg Clin North Am. 2018;30(3):303–23.
12. Clauw DJ, Essex MN, Pitman V, Jones KD. Reframing chronic pain as a disease, not a symptom: rationale and implications for pain management. Postgrad Med. 2019;131(3):185–98.

Functional Dizziness

13

Jason Azzi and Jordan Hochman

Introduction

The vestibular system is formed by a set of paired organs and associated central processing. This sensory system processes head position, motion, and spatial orientation. The processing of these sensory systems allows the stability and fluidity of posture, gaze, and head movements. Dysfunction within this system can result in dizziness; one of the most frequently encountered patient complaints, with a prevalence ranging from 15% to 35% [1]. Vestibular dysfunction frequently causes imbalance or spinning vertigo [2]. However, it is evident that functional disorders can both interact with and imitate vestibular disease.

Dizziness may have a significant impact on an individual's quality of life, productivity, social capacity, may lead to increased use of healthcare resources, and even a reluctance to leave home [3]. These symptoms also contribute to an increased rate of falls and injuries from falls when compared to non-dizzy controls [4]. Given the significant impact on autonomy, production, and healthcare utilization, there is considerable gain from its early diagnosis and management.

The vestibular organs are the semicircular canals and the otolithic organs. Vestibular organs allow the brain to detect accelerations in all directions. The semicircular canals detect angular accelerations while the otolithic organs detect linear accelerations. The semicircular canals are composed of three orthogonally arranged canals—the superior, posterior, and horizontal canal—which communicate with the vestibule. It is this organ system that senses three-dimensional angular acceleration. Semicircular canal dysfunction dominates the vestibular senses after acute inner ear

J. Azzi
Department of Otolaryngology, University of Manitoba, Winnipeg, MB, Canada

J. Hochman (✉)
Department of Otolaryngology, Head and Neck Surgery, Surgical Hearing Implant Program, Rady Faculty of Health Sciences, University of Manitoba, Winnipeg, MB, Canada

© The Author(s), under exclusive license to Springer Nature Switzerland AG 2023

B. W. Blakley, J. E. Blakley (eds.), *Functional Illness of the Head and Neck*,
https://doi.org/10.1007/978-3-031-12998-8_13

damage, resulting in a spinning sensation, but prolonged or chronic inner ear dysfunction may cause imbalance.

The otolithic organs—the utricle and the saccule— sense linear translation and gravity. It is plausible that otolith dysfunction primarily causes imbalance or veering, particularly if the symptom is induced by changes in the head with respect to linear acceleration, head tilt, and gravity.

Hair cells constantly release glutamate in the afferent vestibular neuron synapses, triggering a baseline rate of action potentials. Glutamate is not affected by serotonergic drugs, so selective serotonin reuptake inhibitors (SSRIs) and serotonin and norepinephrine reuptake inhibitors (SNRIs) are not useful in acute dizziness. After a peripheral injury, central compensation occurs over time, so central nervous system and limbic system activation occurs involving serotonin, norepinephrine, and acetylcholine, raising the possibility that SSRIs and SNRIs may be useful for some chronic dizziness, particularly if an emotional component is present.

Reflex disturbances may reflect symptoms. The vestibular system is involved with three main reflexes: the vestibulo-ocular reflex, the vestibulo-spinal reflex, and the vestibulo-collic reflex. The vestibulo-ocular reflex helps stabilize the gaze during movements of the head by coordinating compensatory ocular movements opposite to the head movements. In doing so, the reflex allows for the stabilization of images on the retina of the eye. The vestibulo-spinal reflex modulates the muscle tone and positioning of the body to help maintain posture and gait. Finally, the vestibulo-collic reflex acts on the muscles of the neck to help maintain the stabilization of the position of the head.

Although there are many diagnostic labels for different forms of dizziness, the distinctions between them overlap considerably and are generally "clinical", which means that they are based on a patient's history rather than objective data. Evidence of physiological distinctions is often lacking. For this reason, most dizziness has a functional component. See Fig. 13.1.

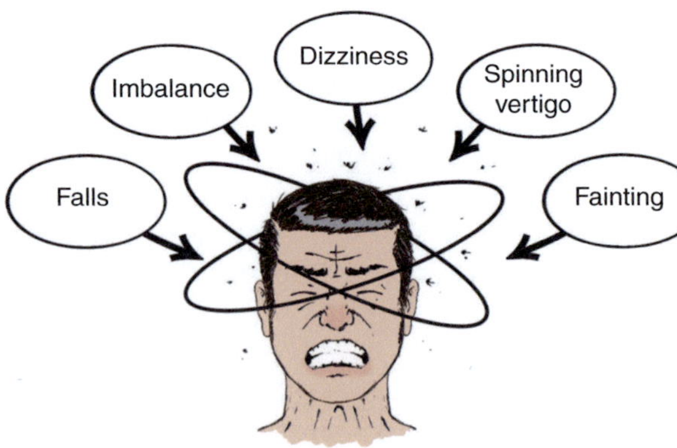

Fig. 13.1 Dizziness has many labels

Pathology

Dysfunction in any of the peripheral or central vestibular structures is common. In a recent survey study, 35.4% of adults in the United States aged 40 years and older reported vestibular dysfunction [5]. In addition to increasing the risk of falls, vestibular dysfunction may have a significant impact on quality of life. In a population survey carried out in Germany, the lifetime prevalence of vertigo was 7.4%, with a one-year prevalence of 4.9% and an incidence of 1.4% [6]. The discrepancy between the rate of vestibular dysfunction and the rate of vertigo suggests that the general population typically compensates for vestibular damage.

Many specific vestibular disorders have been described in the literature, such as benign paroxysmal positional vertigo, Meniere's disease/endolymphatic hydrops, vestibular neuritis, and labyrinthitis. This chapter focuses on functional forms of dizziness.

As opposed to organic diseases, functional diseases are medical conditions that are unexplained by biological processes [7]. Functional dizziness encompasses disorders presenting with symptoms of vertigo, unsteadiness, and imbalance. While quite common, identifying a functional disorder remains challenging. Further, there may be an interplay between a biological process and a maladaptive response. The patient's clinical history, physical examination, and special testing are central to making the diagnosis [7].

Persistent Postural-Perceptual Dizziness

Persistent postural-perceptual dizziness (PPPD) is a recently defined condition characterized by sensations of unsteadiness and non-spinning vertigo. This condition is the result of the amalgamation of diagnostic criteria previously employed for the diagnosis of phobic postural vertigo, visual vertigo, and chronic subjective dizziness.

In 2014, a consensus was reached by the Barany Society in order to officially establish a set of five defining criteria, which must be met to make the diagnosis of PPPD (Table 13.1). In 2017, this condition was officially incorporated into the International Classification of Diseases [9]. PPPD is typically precipitated by an acute vestibular or neurologic event causing dizziness. However, in the case of PPPD, the ensuing adaptation following the acute injury is unsuccessful or maladaptive. The patient then suffers durable symptoms that are challenging to resolve. Recent studies have shown that up to 25% of patients affected by an acute vestibular disorder demonstrate PPPD-like symptoms within the first year of follow-up [8].

While the pathophysiology of this condition remains poorly understood, it is thought that a stiffened postural control, a greater emphasis on visual rather than vestibular input for spatial orientation, and inadequate cortical mechanisms following the initial insult contribute to the onset of this maladaptive behaviour [10]. As a consequence, patients develop an abnormal response to postures, motions, and visual stimuli [11].

Table 13.1 Diagnostic criteria of PPPD from the Bàràny Society [8]

(A)	One or more symptoms of dizziness, unsteadiness, or non-spinning vertigo are present on most days for three months or more. (1) Symptoms last for prolonged (hours long) periods of time but may wax and wane in severity. (2) Symptoms need not be present continuously throughout the entire day.
(B)	Persistent symptoms occur without specific provocation but are exacerbated by three factors: (1) Upright posture, (2) Active or passive motion without regard to direction or position, and (3) Exposure to moving visual stimuli or complex visual patterns.
(C)	The disorder is precipitated by conditions that cause vertigo, unsteadiness, dizziness, or problems with balance, including acute, episodic, or chronic vestibular syndromes, other neurologic or medical illnesses, or psychological distress. (1) When the precipitant is an acute or episodic condition, symptoms settle into the pattern of criterion A as the precipitant resolves, but they may occur intermittently at first and then consolidate into a persistent course. (2). When the precipitant is a chronic syndrome, symptoms may develop slowly at first and worsen gradually.
(D)	Symptoms cause significant distress or functional impairment.
(E)	Symptoms are not better accounted for by another disease or disorder.

The diagnosis of PPPD is made once all the diagnostic criteria are fulfilled based on patient history. This is not a diagnosis of exclusion. These symptoms tend to fluctuate and can often be accompanied by secondary or disparate diagnoses, also causing dizziness [10]. As such, physical examination, vestibular testing, and other investigations may still be indicated to assess for other contributors. Patients may have associated generalized anxiety and should be screened for it, as it can impact the treatment [10].

Treatment of this condition is largely based on research conducted on its precursors and relies on early management and a multi-faceted approach. As with most chronic vestibular conditions, vestibular exercises are beneficial. Medical management includes the use of SSRI or SNRI if the former is ineffective [10, 12–15]. While there is a paucity of data analyzing the benefit of these medications in PPPD, non-randomized studies have identified an improvement of symptoms in half to two thirds of patients with chronic dizziness. Further, while SSRIs have been shown to decrease symptoms of dizziness in patients with PPPD in particular, the addition of cognitive behavioral therapy (CBT) to SSRIs has been shown to both improve symptoms of dizziness when compared to the use of SSRIs alone and to decrease the amount of SSRIs required [16, 17]. While CBT seems to be useful in PPPD, the long-term sustained benefits have yet to be established [18].

Visual Vestibular Mismatch(VVM)

VVM was first described in 1995 and was referred to, at the time, as "visual vertigo" [19]. Rates of this condition are difficult to characterize. It is often associated with migraine, and these patients can develop mal de débarquement if presented with the requisite stimulation [20].

This condition refers to a sensation of dizziness, general discomfort, or nausea in the presence of complex visual stimuli. Examples of such stimulating situations include elevators or escalators, scrolling on a computer monitor, being inside a moving vehicle without a view of the surroundings, patterned carpets, checkered floors, or busy environments such as crowded malls and busy crosswalks. These individuals will often have an aversion to fluorescent lighting.

However, despite being a part of the diagnostic criteria for PPPD, when visual sensitivity is present alone, the diagnosis of VVM rather than PPPD is made. As with other functional diseases, the diagnosis of VVM is made clinically. Despite earlier reports suggesting increased sway on posturography testing, no correlation between VVM and posturography performance or caloric scores has been identified, complicating the diagnosis.

It is believed that the condition arises from overreliance on visual cues. This may be a corollary to a central re-weighting of sensory inputs. This is in contrast to the general response to disorienting stimuli, that being the dominant prioritization of vestibular input [21]. Though it is unclear why some patients develop this visual dependence while others do not [22].

Currently, the treatment of VVM is vestibular rehabilitation and desensitization to visual stimuli, which involves a graded exposure to optokinetic stimuli while the patient is initially seated, then standing, then walking [22, 23]. Pragmatic measures are often helpful, including assuming all the driving, sitting at the front of a bus, and avoiding points of visuo-vestibular conflict like a train, plane, or boats.

Concussion

Vestibular symptoms are among the most commonly reported by patients who have suffered a concussion [24–26]. While the majority of these patients will recover from their dysfunction, a subset of patients will go on to develop chronic symptoms. In fact, studies have shown that up to 50% of patients will continue to enduse symptoms of vertigo 5 years after a traumatic brain injury [27].

These patients will typically present with new-onset, difficult to characterize dizziness and imbalance following a traumatic brain injury. Other symptoms reported included light-headedness, clumsiness, and visual disorientation.

It has been postulated that these chronic vestibular deficits may be in large part due to a combination of overlooked central and peripheral vestibular diagnoses, such as BPPV or vestibular migraines, and the impaired plasticity and repair mechanisms of the brain from the trauma [28]. Other possibly overlooked vestibular disorders associated with head trauma include labyrinthine concussion, superior canal dehiscence syndrome, and post-traumatic endolymphatic hydrops [29]. Another study found 100% of patients with post-concussive dizziness to have central dysfunction, 82.9% to have cervical dysfunction, and 46.3% to have vestibular dysfunction [30]. While the pathophysiology of chronic post-concussive vestibular symptoms remains poorly understood, it is likely multifactorial.

Cervical spine rehabilitation and vestibular rehabilitation (including canalith repositioning maneuvers, vestibulo-ocular reflex (VOR), cervico-ocular reflex,, and somatosensory exercises) are an effective modality in the management of dizziness related to concussion [31–34]. In a study of 58 individuals suffering from dizziness following mild head injuries, 6–8 weeks of vestibular rehabilitation was found to improve VOR tests in 27–84% of participants [31]. In a randomized control trial assessing the benefits of cervical spine rehabilitation and vestibular rehabilitation in patients with sports-related concussions and persistent dizziness, neck pain, or headaches, patients receiving these therapies were found to have significantly decreased time to medical clearance, with 73% of patients receiving medical clearance within 8 weeks as compared to 7% of patients who received cervical spine therapy alone [35]. Early return to symptom-limited activity and reengagement in life activities following concussion may be beneficial, though the current evidence is poor [36, 37].

Vestibular Migraine

Population studies have found the prevalence of migraines to be nearly 20% [38–40]. The prevalence of migraines is even higher amongst patients with recurrent vertigo [41]. Vestibular migraines refer to migraines associated with symptoms of vertigo. This condition was officially recognized in 2012 when the Classification of Vestibular Disorders of the Bárány Society and the Migraine Classification Subcommittee of the International Headache Society established a consensus diagnostic criterion [42] (Table 13.2). Since then, awareness of this condition is increasing. In fact, 10% of patients being seen in headache clinics have been diagnosed with vestibular migraines [43]. With a 1-year prevalence of 2.7%, this condition is a common cause of dizziness, with studies showing that 12–21% of patients with dizziness have vestibular migraines [44, 45]. Nonetheless, it remains underdiagnosed with two studies discovering that only 10% of patients meeting criteria for vestibular migraines being diagnosed with such [44, 46].

Table 13.2 Diagnostic criteria of vestibular migraine and probable vestibular migraine of the Bárány Society [42]

Vestibular migraine	
(A)	At least five episodes with vestibular symptoms of moderate or severe intensity, lasting 5 min to 72 h
(B)	Current or previous history of migraine with or without aura according to the international classification of headache disorders (ICHD) (86)
(C)	One or more migraine features with at least 50% of the vestibular episodes —Headache with at least two of the following characteristics: One-sided location, pulsating quality, moderate or severe pain intensity, aggravation by routine physical activity—Photophobia and phonophobia—Visual aura
(D)	Not better accounted for by another vestibular or ICHD diagnosis
Probable vestibular migraine	
(A)	At least five episodes with vestibular symptoms of moderate or severe intensity, lasting 5 min to 72 h
(B)	Only one of the criteria B and C for vestibular migraine is fulfilled (migraine history or migraine features during the episode
(C)	Not better accounted for by another vestibular or ICHD diagnosis

This condition is more common among female patients and those with anxiety, depression, and prior head trauma [44]. Vestibular migraines can present with or without headaches. They can also present with attenuated headaches [47]. During episodes of dizziness, patients report a wide range of types of vertigo, including positional vertigo, visually induced vertigo, spontaneous vertigo, and motion-induced vertigo. Patients may also report nausea, imbalance, photophobia, phonophobia, palpitations, auras, and auditory symptoms, including tinnitus, aural fullness, and hearing loss [48]. These vestibular episodes range in duration from seconds to days however will rarely exceed 72 h [47, 49]. Patients will typically be without any signs or symptoms between episodes. While there are no specific findings on vestibular testing during episodes of acute migrainous vertigo, imbalance, spontaneous nystagmus, or positional nystagmus can be witnessed [50, 51].

The pathophysiology of vestibular migraines remains speculative and is largely based on the pathophysiology of typical migraines. As such, it is suspected that, like with typical migraines, there is a strong hereditary component to vestibular migraine [52]. Two main theories exist explaining the pathophysiology of vestibular migraines. See the chapter on headaches in this book. The ion channelopathy hypothesis postulates that defective ions cause an excess of extracellular potassium, triggering the spreading wave of depression and that these ions may also be present in the inner ear, leading to vestibular involvement. The trigemino-vascular hypersensitization theory claims that the high extracellular potassium concentration depolarizes trigeminal nerve fibers on the ventral surface of the brain, leading to the release of vasoactive neuropeptides that increase the vascular permeability and dilate cerebral and labyrinthine vessels. This increase in blood flow and permeability could in turn lead to the release of inflammatory mediators and the extravasation of plasma protein into the inner ear, triggering vestibular migraines [53, 54].

Treatments for vestibular migraines are largely based on the management of conventional migraines (see Chap. 14). In the acute vestibular phase, antiemetics and antivertigo medications are used for the nausea and vertigo. The use of non-steroidal anti-inflammatories and other rescue medication used in migraines is unlikely to be beneficial [55–57]. Prophylactic management is the current standard of treatment and includes lifestyle changes and medical management. Encouraged lifestyle modifications include avoidance of triggers, exercise, diet, and sleep hygiene [58–60]. While the evidence is weak, a recent systematic review and meta-analysis concluded that traditional pharmacological agents used in the prevention of typical migraines, such as beta blockers, anticonvulsants, calcium antagonists, tricyclic antidepressants, selective serotonin reuptake inhibitors, and serotonin–norepinephrine reuptake inhibitors, do also demonstrate improvement in symptoms and frequency of events in patients with vestibular migraines [61]. Triptan medications are useful for migraine headaches, but less so for vestibular migraine. As with typical migraines, it is recommended to select the medication based on a patient's comorbidities. Finally, while findings remain inconclusive, the use of vestibular rehabilitation may also prove beneficial [62].

Cervicogenic Dizziness

Cervicogenic dizziness is characterized by symptoms of dizziness in patients with neck pain, limited mobility, or injury. Generally, these individuals suffer from imbalance more than actual vertigo. There is controversy regarding the diagnostic entity; however, a recent study evaluating dizziness in the elderly population found 65% of their dizziness to be due to cervical spondylosis [63].

Aside from the coexistence of neck concerns and dizziness, there are no defined criteria or specific tests used for the diagnosis of cervicogenic dizziness [64]. As such, this condition remains a diagnosis of exclusion [65]. Diagnosis may include the identification of dizziness occurring with neck pain and changes in neck positioning. The onset of these symptoms may be sudden or may develop gradually. Often, patients do not experience vertigo but imbalance, and symptoms typically last minutes to hours [65]. Physical assessment should include a cervical range of motion and provocative maneuvers.

The underlying etiology of cervicogenic dizziness is debated; however, various mechanisms have been proposed: acceleration–deceleration injuries, degenerative cervical spine disorders, sympathetic disorders, and vascular disorders. Fundamentally, it is suspected that cervical mechanoreceptor function and vestibular/cervico-proprioceptive input/weighting mismatch result in symptoms.

The treatment of cervicogenic dizziness is dependent on the suspected etiology. Treatment can include physiotherapy, medical treatment (NSAID, muscle relaxants) and surgical management [66].

Conclusion

In summary, treatment of chronic, nonspecific dizziness may involve explanation, which can be therapeutic, medications, and physical therapy. The most appropriate medications are antidepressants. Perhaps 75% of patients with chronic, nonspecific dizziness respond to an SSRI [13], but SNRIs and SSRIs have similar effects. SNRIs may be more appropriate for associated pain (see neck pain and headache chapters in this book). In a young person with poor sleep, a tricyclic, such as amitriptyline, may be a good choice, providing better sleep and some pain control. If anxiety is a strong component, sometimes a low-dose benzodiazepine such as lorazepam or clonazepam can be helpful. Physical therapy is more appropriate for chronic, ongoing imbalance than for infrequent, episodic symptoms.

Functional dizziness, like its organic counterpart, remains challenging to categorize, diagnose, and manage. Overall, the evidence surrounding these conditions is being accrued but at the current time is limited. There is a significant need for research elucidating these conditions in order to guide the future development of evidence-based practice guidelines.

References

1. Mendel B, Bergenius J, Langius-Eklöf A. Dizziness: A common, troublesome symptom but often treatable. J Vestib Res Equilib Orientat. 2010;20(5):391–8.
2. Bisdorff A, Von Brevern M, Lempert T, Newman-Toker DE. Classification of vestibular symptoms: towards an international classification of vestibular disorders. J Vestib Res. 2009. Jan 1;19(1,2):1–13;19:1.
3. Neuhauser HK, Radtke A, von Brevern M, Lezius F, Feldmann M, Lempert T. Burden of dizziness and vertigo in the community. Arch Intern Med. 2008;168(19):2118–24.
4. Lin HW, Bhattacharyya N. Impact of dizziness and obesity on the prevalence of falls and fall-related injuries. Laryngoscope. 2014;124(12):2797–801.
5. Agrawal Y, Carey JP, Della Santina CC, Schubert MC, Minor LB. Disorders of balance and vestibular function in US adults: data from the National Health and nutrition examination survey, 2001-2004. Arch Intern Med. 2009;169(10):938.
6. Neuhauser HK, von Brevern M, Radtke A, Lezius F, Feldmann M, Ziese T, et al. Epidemiology of vestibular vertigo: a neurotologic survey of the general population. Neurology. 2005;65(6):898–904.
7. Dieterich M, Staab JP. Functional dizziness: from phobic postural vertigo and chronic subjective dizziness to persistent postural-perceptual dizziness. Curr Opin Neurol. 2017;30(1):107–13.
8. Staab JP, Eckhardt-Henn A, Horii A, Jacob R, Strupp M, Brandt T, et al. Diagnostic criteria for persistent postural-perceptual dizziness (PPPD): consensus document of the committee for the classification of vestibular disorders of the Bàràny society. J Vestib Res. 2017;27(4):191–208.
9. ICD-11 - Mortality and Morbidity Statistics [Internet]. [cited 2021 Jan 7]. Available from: https://icd.who.int/browse11/l-m/en#/http://id.who.int/icd/entity/2005792829.
10. Popkirov S, Staab JP, Stone J. Persistent postural-perceptual dizziness (PPPD): a common, characteristic and treatable cause of chronic dizziness. Pract Neurol. 2018;18(1):5–13.
11. Staab JP. Chronic subjective dizziness. Continuum (Minneap Minn). 2012;18(5 Neuro-otology):1118–41.
12. Staab JP, Ruckenstein MJ. Chronic dizziness and anxiety: effect of course of illness on treatment outcome. Arch Otolaryngol Head Neck Surg. 2005;131(8):675–9.
13. Staab JP, Ruckenstein MJ, Amsterdam JD. A prospective trial of sertraline for chronic subjective dizziness. Laryngoscope. 2004 Sep;114(9):1637–41.
14. Staab JP, Ruckenstein MJ, Solomon D, Shepard NT. Serotonin reuptake inhibitors for dizziness with psychiatric symptoms. Arch Otolaryngol Head Neck Surg. 2002;128(5):554.
15. Horii A, Uno A, Kitahara T, Mitani K, Masumura C, Kizawa K, et al. Effects of fluvoxamine on anxiety, depression, and subjective handicaps of chronic dizziness patients with or without neuro-otologic diseases. J Vestib Res. 2007;17(1):1–8.
16. Mahoney AEJ, Edelman S, Cremer PD. Cognitive behavior therapy for chronic subjective dizziness: longer-term gains and predictors of disability. Am J Otolaryngol. 2013;34(2):115–20.
17. Trinidade A, Goebel JA. Persistent postural-perceptual dizziness-A systematic review of the literature for the balance specialist. Otol Neurotol. 2018;39(10):1291–303.
18. Holmberg J, Karlberg M, Harlacher U, Magnusson M. One-year follow-up of cognitive behavioral therapy for phobic postural vertigo. J Neurol. 2007;254(9):1189–92.
19. Bronstein AM. Visual vertigo syndrome: clinical and posturography findings. J Neurol Neurosurg Psychiatry. 1995;59(5):472–6.
20. Beh SC, Chiang H-S, Sanderson C. The Interconnections of Mal de Débarquement Syndrome and Vestibular Migraine. Laryngoscope. 2020 Epub ahead of print.
21. Guerraz M, Yardley L, Bertholon P, Pollak L, Rudge P, Gresty MA, et al. Visual vertigo: symptom assessment, spatial orientation and postural control. Brain. 2001;124(Pt 8):1646–56.

22. Bronstein AM, Golding JF, Gresty MA. Vertigo and dizziness from environmental motion: visual vertigo, motion sickness, and drivers' disorientation. Semin Neurol. 2013;33(3):219–30.
23. Pavlou M, Lingeswaran A, Davies RA, Gresty MA, Bronstein AM. Simulator based rehabilitation in refractory dizziness. J Neurol. 2004;251(8):983–95.
24. Lau BC, Kontos AP, Collins MW, Mucha A, Lovell MR. Which on-field signs/symptoms predict protracted recovery from sport-related concussion among high school football players? Am J Sports Med. 2011;39(11):2311–8.
25. Merritt VC, Rabinowitz AR, Arnett PA. Injury-related predictors of symptom severity following sports-related concussion. J Clin Exp Neuropsychol. 2015;37(3):265–75.
26. Chorney SR, Suryadevara AC, Nicholas BD. Audiovestibular symptoms as predictors of prolonged sports-related concussion among NCAA athletes. Laryngoscope. 2017;127(12):2850–3.
27. Berman JM, Fredrickson JM. Vertigo after head injury--a five year follow-up. J Otolaryngol. 1978;7(3):237–45.
28. Arshad Q, Roberts RE, Ahmad H, Lobo R, Patel M, Ham T, et al. Patients with chronic dizziness following traumatic head injury typically have multiple diagnoses involving combined peripheral and central vestibular dysfunction. Clin Neurol Neurosurg. 2017;155:17–9.
29. Chung J, Jung HJ, Kim CS, Kim YH. A case of post-traumatic Meniere's disease. Korean J Audiol. 2014;18(1):41–4.
30. Reneker JC, Cheruvu VK, Yang J, James MA, Cook CE. Physical examination of dizziness in athletes after a concussion: A descriptive study. Musculoskelet Sci Pract. 2018;34:8–13.
31. Hoffer ME, Gottshall KR, Moore R, Balough BJ, Wester D. Characterizing and treating dizziness after mild head trauma. Otol Neurotol. 2004;25(2):135–8.
32. Alsalaheen BA, Mucha A, Morris LO, Whitney SL, Furman JM, Camiolo-Reddy CE, et al. Vestibular rehabilitation for dizziness and balance disorders after concussion. J Neurol Phys Ther. 2010;34(2):87–93.
33. Broglio SP, Collins MW, Williams RM, Mucha A, Kontos AP. Current and emerging rehabilitation for concussion: a review of the evidence. Clin Sports Med. 2015;34(2):213–31.
34. Gurley JM, Hujsak BD, Kelly JL. Vestibular rehabilitation following mild traumatic brain injury. NeuroRehabilitation. 2013;32(3):519–28.
35. Schneider KJ, Meeuwisse WH, Nettel-Aguirre A, Barlow K, Boyd L, Kang J, et al. Cervicovestibular rehabilitation in sport-related concussion: a randomised controlled trial. Br J Sports Med. 2014;48(17):1294–8.
36. DiFazio M, Silverberg ND, Kirkwood MW, Bernier R, Iverson GL. Prolonged activity restriction after concussion: are we worsening outcomes? Clin Pediatr (Phila). 2016;55(5):443–51.
37. Mucci V, Meier C, Bizzini M, Romano F, Agostino D, Ventura A, et al. Combined optokinetic treatment and vestibular rehabilitation to reduce visually induced dizziness in a professional ice hockey player after concussion: A clinical case. Front Neurol. 2019;10:1200.
38. Merikangas KR. Contributions of epidemiology to our understanding of migraine. Headache. 2013;53(2):230–46.
39. Burch RC, Loder S, Loder E, Smitherman TA. The prevalence and burden of migraine and severe headache in the United States: updated statistics from government health surveillance studies. Headache. 2015;55(1):21–34.
40. Lipton RB, Stewart WF, Diamond S, Diamond ML, Reed M. Prevalence and burden of migraine in the United States: data from the American migraine study II. Headache. 2001;41(7):646–57.
41. Cha Y-H, Lee H, Santell L, Baloh R. Association of Benign Recurrent Vertigo and Migraine in 208 patients. Cephalalgia. 2009;29(5):550–5.
42. Lempert T, Olesen J, Furman J, Waterston J, Seemungal B, Carey J, et al. Vestibular migraine: diagnostic criteria. J Vestib Res. 2012;22(4):167–72.
43. Cho S-J, Kim B-K, Kim B-S, Kim J-M, Kim S-K, Moon H-S, et al. Vestibular migraine in multicenter neurology clinics according to the appendix criteria in the third beta edition of the international classification of headache disorders. Cephalalgia. 2016;36(5):454–62.
44. Formeister EJ, Rizk HG, Kohn MA, Sharon JD. The epidemiology of vestibular migraine: A population-based survey study. Otol Neurotol. 2018;39(8):1037–44.

45. Yollu U, Uluduz DU, Yilmaz M, Yener HM, Akil F, Kuzu B, et al. Vestibular migraine screening in a migraine-diagnosed patient population, and assessment of vestibulocochlear function. Clin Otolaryngol. 2017;42(2):225–33.
46. Geser R, Straumann D. Referral and final diagnoses of patients assessed in an academic vertigo center. Front Neurol. 2012;3:169.
47. Lempert T, von Brevern M. Vestibular Migraine. Neurol Clin. 2019;37(4):695–706.
48. Neff BA, Staab JP, Eggers SD, Carlson ML, Schmitt WR, Van Abel KM, et al. Auditory and vestibular symptoms and chronic subjective dizziness in patients with Meniere's disease, vestibular migraine, and Meniere's disease with concomitant vestibular migraine. Otol Neurotol. 2012;33(7):1235–44.
49. Teggi R, Colombo B, Albera R, Asprella Libonati G, Balzanelli C, Batuecas Caletrio A, et al. Clinical features, familial history, and migraine precursors in patients with definite vestibular migraine: the VM-phenotypes projects. Headache. 2018;58(4):534–44.
50. Von Brevern M, Zeise D, Neuhauser H, Clarke AH, Lempert T. Acute migrainous vertigo: clinical and oculographic findings. Brain. 2005;128(2):365–74.
51. Polensek SH, Tusa RJ. Nystagmus during attacks of vestibular migraine: an aid in diagnosis. Audiol Neurootol. 2010;15(4):241–6.
52. Lee H, Jen JC, Cha Y-H, Nelson SF, Baloh RW. Phenotypic and genetic analysis of a large family with migraine-associated vertigo. Headache. 2008;48(10):1460–7.
53. Baloh RW. Vestibular migraine I: mechanisms, diagnosis, and clinical features. Semin Neurol. 2020;40(1):76–82.
54. Espinosa-Sanchez JM, Lopez-Escamez JA. New insights into pathophysiology of vestibular migraine. Front Neurol. 2015;6(6):12.
55. Jahn K. Vertigo and balance in children - diagnostic approach and insights from imaging. Eur J Paediatr Neurol. 2011;15(4):289–94.
56. Sargent EW. The challenge of vestibular migraine. Curr Opin Otolaryngol Head Neck Surg. 2013;21(5):473–9.
57. Neuhauser H, Radtke A, Von Brevern M, Lempert T. Zolmitriptan for treatment of migrainous vertigo: a pilot randomized placebo-controlled trial. Neurology. 2003;60(5):882–3.
58. Bisdorff AR. Management of vestibular migraine. Ther Adv Neurol Disord. 2011;4(3):183–91.
59. Liu F, Ma T, Che X, Wang Q, Yu S. The efficacy of venlafaxine, Flunarizine, and Valproic acid in the prophylaxis of vestibular migraine. Front Neurol. 2017;8:524.
60. Lee Y-Y, Yang Y-P, Huang P-I, Li W-C, Huang M-C, Kao C-L, et al. Exercise suppresses COX-2 pro-inflammatory pathway in vestibular migraine. Brain Res Bull. 2015;116:98–105.
61. Byun YJ, Levy DA, Nguyen SA, Brennan E, Rizk HG. Treatment of vestibular migraine: A systematic review and meta-analysis. Laryngoscope. 2021;131(1):186–94.
62. Alghadir AH, Anwer S. Effects of vestibular rehabilitation in the Management of a Vestibular Migraine: A review. Front Neurol. 2018;9:440.
63. Colledge NR, Barr-Hamilton RM, Lewis SJ, Sellar RJ, Wilson JA. Evaluation of investigations to diagnose the cause of dizziness in elderly people: a community based controlled study. BMJ. 1996 Sep;313(7060):788–92.
64. Knapstad MK, Nordahl SHG, Goplen FK. Clinical characteristics in patients with cervicogenic dizziness: A systematic review. Health Sci Rep. 2019;2(9):e134.
65. Wrisley DM, Sparto PJ, Whitney SL, Furman JM. Cervicogenic dizziness: a review of diagnosis and treatment. J Orthop Sports Phys Ther. 2000;30(12):755–66.
66. Devaraja K. Approach to cervicogenic dizziness: a comprehensive review of its aetiopathology and management. Eur Arch Otorhinolaryngol. 2018;275(10):2421–33.

Headaches 14

Leigh Sowerby, Boipelo Tselapedi-Sekeitto,
and Lik Hang Tommy Chan

Facial Pain

Facial pain or secondary headache can be caused by different disorders within the head and neck region. These may range from trauma, inflammatory disorders and tumours. The main focus of this chapter will be to discuss facial pain that is attributed to the nose/paranasal sinuses (previously known as sinugenic facial pain) and non-sinugenic facial pain-related disorders (see Table 14.1). Non-sinugenic facial pain is caused by disorders of the head and neck region, other than nose/paranasal sinus disorders and primary headaches [1]. These include several regions in the head and neck region such as temporomandibular joint and cranial nerves. There is an overlap of shared symptoms and aggravating factors between migraine and rhinosinusitis, and therefore patients with migraine may end up being referred to an otolaryngologist [2].

L. Sowerby
Rhinology and Anterior Skull Base Surgery, Otolaryngology - Head and Neck Surgery, University of Western Ontario, London, ON, Canada

B. Tselapedi-Sekeitto
Western University, London, ON, Canada

L. H. T. Chan (✉)
Department of Clinical Neurological Sciences, Western University (Schulich School of Medicine and Dentistry), London, ON, Canada
e-mail: tommy.chan@lhsc.on.ca

© The Author(s), under exclusive license to Springer Nature Switzerland AG 2023

B. W. Blakley, J. E. Blakley (eds.), *Functional Illness of the Head and Neck*,
https://doi.org/10.1007/978-3-031-12998-8_14

Table 14.1 The differences between sinugenic and non-sinugenic pain [2]

Features	Sinugenic pain	Non-sinugenic pain
Pain severity	Mild to moderate	Moderate to severe
Pain quality	Facial pressure and nasal congestion	Throbbing and excruciating pain
Duration	72 h or more	Less than 72 h
Site	Depends on the sinus that is involved, mostly unilateral	Maybe be generalised or localised. There is a poor correlation between location of pain and sinus anatomy
Aggravating factors	Changes in atmospheric pressure (e.g. diving, skiing and flying)	It depends on the site of inflammation. Chewing, exercise, light touch and certain food (chocolate and cheese), bright lights
Associates signs and symptoms	Anterior and post nasal drip, nasal congestion, obstruction, hyposmia and anosmia	Photophobia, phonophobia, with or without aura, nausea or vomiting.
ENT examination	Nasal congestion and thick purulent rhinorrhoea	Anterior and posterior rhinoscopy normal
Rhinoscopy	Anterior and post nasal drip Oedema of nasal cavity with or without nasal polyps	Anterior and posterior rhinoscopy normal
Paranasal CT-scan	Opacification of paranasal sinuses and occlusion of osteomeatal complex	Normal or minimal findings on paranasal CT scan

Primary Headache Disorders

Primary headache disorders are functional illnesses that are not caused by anatomic, inflammatory, infectious, or physiological abnormalities. Approximately 98% of patients who present with a headache for medical evaluation will have a type of primary headache. The two major primary headache categories are migraine and tension-type headache [3].

Migraine

Migraine is an inherited disorder of the brain in which the brain is hypersensitive to the changes in the environment as well as changes that occur within the body. Changes in sleep, stress level, activity level, hormones and any traumas or other medical conditions that the body is experiencing can be common triggers – triggers are usually partial and additive.

Many epidemiological studies have documented its high prevalence and socio-economic and personal impacts. In the Global Burden of Disease Study, migraine is the second leading cause of years lived with disability (YLDs) and accounts for more disability than all other neurologic disordered combined [4].

The diagnosis is based on clinical criteria established by the International Classification of Headache Disorders, third Edition (ICHD-3): Migraine is a recurrent headache disorder manifesting in attacks lasting 4–72 h. Typical characteristics of the headache are unilateral location, pulsating quality, moderate or severe intensity, aggravation by routine physical activity and association with nausea and/or photophobia and phonophobia [5]. Migraine is a functional disorder and is a disabling primary headache disorder. Brain imaging is usually unrevealing, but non-specific white matter lesions can be seen in the subcortical or periventricular white matter regions demonstrated on MRI of the head, reported in 12–48% of migraine patients compared with 2–11% of control subjects [6].

Migraine has two major types: migraine with and without aura. Migraine without aura is a clinical syndrome characterized by headache with specific features and associated symptoms as discussed above. Migraine with aura is primarily characterized by the transient focal neurological symptoms (visual, sensory, motor, retinal and brainstem) that usually precede or accompany the headache [5].

The understanding of the pathogenesis of migraine remains incomplete: it involves the trigeminal nerve and its axonal projections to the intracranial vessels. Nociceptive signals from the trigeminovascular system are related to areas of the brain that are responsible for the perception of pain [7]. There are signalling molecules involved in a migraine attack, such as calcitonin gene-related peptides (CGRP), which are potent vasodilators that are widely distributed in the trigeminovascular system [7] (Fig. 14.1).

CGRP ligands and receptors are widely distributed in the trigeminovascular system.

The physiological basis of the aura phase of migraine is hypothesized to be related to cortical spreading depression, a self-propagating wave of depolarization across the cerebral cortex that disrupts ionic gradients and is followed by cerebral hypoperfusion [9]. Hemodynamic changes accompanying cortical spreading depression have been documented on neuroimaging in patients who have migraine with aura, and not in patients who have migraine without aura [10].

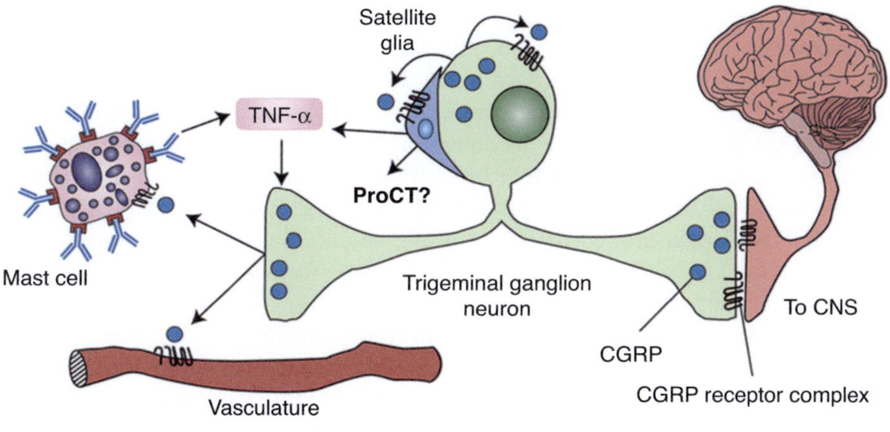

Fig. 14.1 CGRP action at peripheral receptors [8]

Misdiagnosis – 'Sinus' Headache

It is worth mentioning since migraine is a functional disorder and imaging is often unrevealing, misdiagnosis is common. A very large population-based study, entitled American Migraine Study II [11], demonstrated that many people who were diagnosed with migraine thought they had 'sinus' headache. Significantly, there were almost 20,000 study participants – only about 50% who were diagnosed with migraine knew they had migraine before the study. The most common misdiagnosis was 'sinus' headache.

True 'sinus' headache, more properly called rhinosinusitis, is a rare condition and is secondary to a viral or bacterial sinus infection characterized by thick, discoloured nasal discharge, alteration of smell, facial pain and/or fever. Symptoms should resolve within 7 days after the remission of viral symptoms or after successful treatment with antibiotics [12].

In a study of 3000 patients with 'sinus' headache, 88% of the participants were found to have migraine headache and not 'sinus headache' upon evaluation. Strict criteria from the ICHD-3 were used to tell the difference between the two headache types. In addition to their common symptoms of nasal and sinus congestion and facial pain and pressure, migraine patients had nausea, photophobia, moderate to severe headache, pulsing/throbbing pain and/or headache worsened by activity. In this study, almost 3000 patients with the complaint of 'sinus' headache were taking excessive over-the-counter and prescription decongestants, analgesics, antihistamines and nasal sprays without good relief. The lack of response supports the pain is related to migraine and not rhinosinusitis [13].

Facial Pain Secondary to Rhinosinusitis

Sinugenic facial pain is an uncommon cause of isolated facial pain. Incorrect diagnosis may lead to unnecessary medical costs [14]. Acute rhinosinusitis (ARS) or acute-on-chronic rhinosinusitis can be attributed to the cause of facial pain or headache. Chronic rhinosinusitis (CRS) alone typically does not cause significant facial pain unless there is an acute exacerbation. The site of facial pain depends on which paranasal sinus is involved. Patients commonly present with unilateral facial pain, fever and nasal symptoms (see Table 14.2). Toothache and unilateral facial pain are usually attributed to maxillary sinus infection. Frontal sinusitis may present with fever and facial pain around the eye and the supraorbital ridge. Recurrent acute sinusitis is often not sinusitis, and acute CT scans performed at the time of concern have demonstrated an absence of sinus disease [15].

The International Consensus Allergy and Rhinosinusitis (ICAR): rhinosinusitis 2021 has formulated recommendations for the management of rhinosinusitis in adults (see Table 14.3). The primary goal of performing endoscopic sinus surgery (ESS) is to optimize sinus drainage and allow for better topical therapy delivery. A long-term study of over 5 years has shown the resolution of facial pain post ESS in 47% of 51 cases [16].

Table 14.2 Diagnosis of ARS and CRS [17]

Rhinosinusitis	Duration	Symptoms	Nasal endoscopy	CT changes
ARS	Sudden onset Less than 12 weeks	Inflammation of the nose and paranasal sinuses characterised by two or more symptoms, one of which should be either nasal blockage/obstruction/ congestion or nasal discharge (anterior/posterior nasal drip): ± facial pain/ pressure ± reduction or loss of sense of smell and either	Nasal polyps and/ or mucopurulent discharge primarily from middle meatus and/or oedema/mucosal obstruction primarily in middle meatus and/or	Mucosal changes within the osteomeatal complex and/ or sinuses
CRS	More than 12 weeks			

Table 14.3 Recommendations from international consensus allergy and rhinology: rhinosinusitis 2021

	ARS	ABRS
Duration	<7 days	ARS > 7 days
INCS Fluticasone 100 μg Mometasone 200 μg Budesonide 400 μg	Recommended	Recommended
Saline irrigation	Not recommended	Recommended
Antibiotics	Not recommended	Recommended
Decongestants	Not recommended	Not recommended
Antihistamine	Not recommended	Not recommended

Medical Therapy

Corticosteroid Therapy in ARS

Corticosteroids have anti-inflammatory properties and therefore help to reduce intranasal mucosal inflammation which restores mucociliary clearance (MCC). Intranasal corticosteroid (INC) therapy has been recommended to be used as monotherapy within 7 days of ARS [18]. Although several studies [19–21] have looked at the use of oral corticosteroids in ARS, there is no conclusive evidence to support the use of oral corticosteroids in ARS. A Cochrane review meta-analysis of 1193 patients did not provide evidence to support the use of oral corticosteroids in ARS [22].

Antibiotics in ARS

Literature has shown that a watchful waiting approach may be beneficial in patients with ARS. It is recommended that antibiotics may be considered if there is no improvement after 7 days or if the patient develops worsening signs and symptoms. The choice of antibiotics is amoxicillin and clavulanate at a high dose of 4 g per day.

A systematic review has shown improvement of 88–97% in patients with acute bacterial rhinosinusitis (ABRS) in penicillin-resistant pneumococcal and beta-lactamase positive infection [23]. A Cochrane review has shown that the most common side effects such as gastrointestinal upset have been implicated in patient discontinuing antibiotic therapy. Moreover, these side effects were not debilitating, patients could still continue with their respective activities of daily living. Options after failing amoxicillin ± clavulanate or for penicillin allergy include trimethoprim-sulfamethoxazole, doxycycline or a fluoroquinolone [24].

Saline Irrigation in ARS

The use of saline irrigation as an adjunct to antibiotics has been recommended for patients with ABRS. Use of large volume (250 ml) saline nasal irrigation is a preferred method over low volume (10 ml) saline irrigation [24, 25]. Inanli et al. [26] assessed the effects of different concentrations of saline on MCC. Three groups of subjects were 10 ml 0.9% saline group, 10 ml 3% saline group and group without topical treatment. The resultant MCC time was compared amongst the groups and showed no difference. However, Gerlardy et al. showed the benefits of using 250 ml saline irrigation over 10 ml saline with improvement in rhinorrhea and postnasal drip [27].

Decongestants in ARS and ABRS

Decongestants help to reduce nasal congestion and restores patency of the sinuses. The risk of using decongestants poses a risk of the patient developing rhinitis medicamentosa if not monitored. The use of decongestants may help to reduce nasal congestion in ABRS [24].

Antihistamine in ARS and ABRS.

Braun et al. [28] in an RCT have shown an improvement in the use of loratadine in patients with allergic rhinitis. However European position paper on rhinosinusitis and nasal polyps (EPOS) 2020 guidelines and ICAR rhinitis 2021 have shown that there is no support for use of antihistamine in ARS/ABRS [24, 29].

Migraine Treatment

The foundation of migraine management is lifestyle modification. Specific strategies to create a regular and predictable schedule and environment that can be helpful for migraine. It is imperative that the patient keep a regular sleep schedule and meal schedule. Studies show routine aerobic exercise can decrease migraine frequency, severity and disability, ranging from 10% to 50% improvement [30–33].

In terms of pharmacological options, it can be divided into abortive and preventive treatments.

The most widely used abortive medications for migraine are nonsteroidal anti-inflammatory drugs (NSAIDs), which are low-cost, over-the-counter analgesic agents. Effectiveness has been best documented for acetylsalicylic acid, ibuprofen, and diclofenac with a success rate of around 20% for achieving pain freedom in 2 h [34–36] (Fig. 14.2). NSAIDs have anti-inflammatory effects via depression of prostanoid biosynthesis by inhibiting the COX enzymes and are able to prevent neurogenic inflammation [37].

Triptans are considered second-line medications. Triptans bind to 5-hydroxytryptamine (5-HT serotonin) receptors in the brain. Increasing the effects of serotonin mediates pain and mood. The downstream effect results in a reduction of CGRP. Currently, there are seven oral triptans (almotriptan, eletriptan, frovatriptan, naratriptan, rizatriptan, sumatriptan and zolmitriptan) available for clinical use. Standard dose triptans relieve headaches within 2 h in 42–76% of patients, and 2-h sustained freedom from pain was achieved for 18–50% of patients. Standard dose triptans provided sustained headache relief at 24 h in 29–50% of patients, and sustained freedom from pain in 18–33% of patients [39]. An example of treatment response with sumatriptan is illustrated in Fig. 14.3.

In practice, providers might use subcutaneous sumatriptan preparations for a patient who requires rapid onset of action. For patients with nausea and vomiting, rizatriptan or zolmitriptan are good alternatives. Rizatriptan, almotriptan and eletriptan have the advantage of the fastest onset. Almotriptan, frovatriptan and naratriptan have the advantage of having a favourable side effect profile. Frovatriptan and naratriptan offer advantages if the patient has problems with recurrence and if the headaches have a slow onset. Both might also have advantages in prevention and/or migraine with a prodrome [40]. Refer to Table 14.4 for the pharmacokinetics of the triptans.

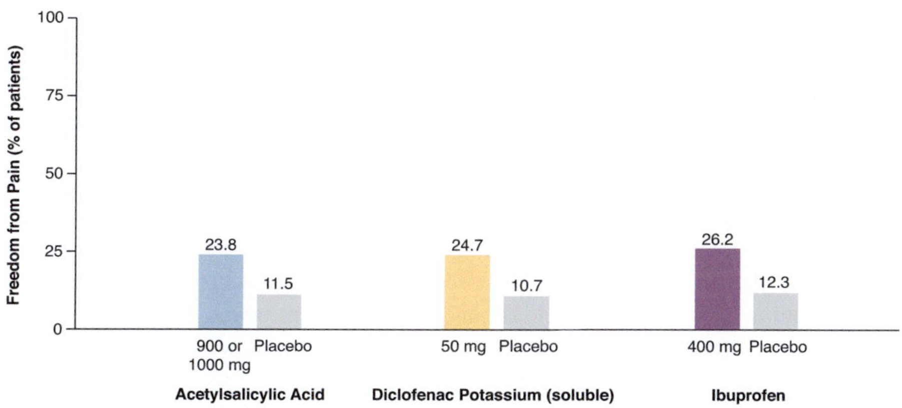

Fig. 14.2 Freedom from migraine pain (% of patients) from acetylsalicylic acid, diclofenac potassium (soluble) and ibuprofen [38]: all three analgesics demonstrated pain freedom in greater than 20% of patients in each respective studies [34]

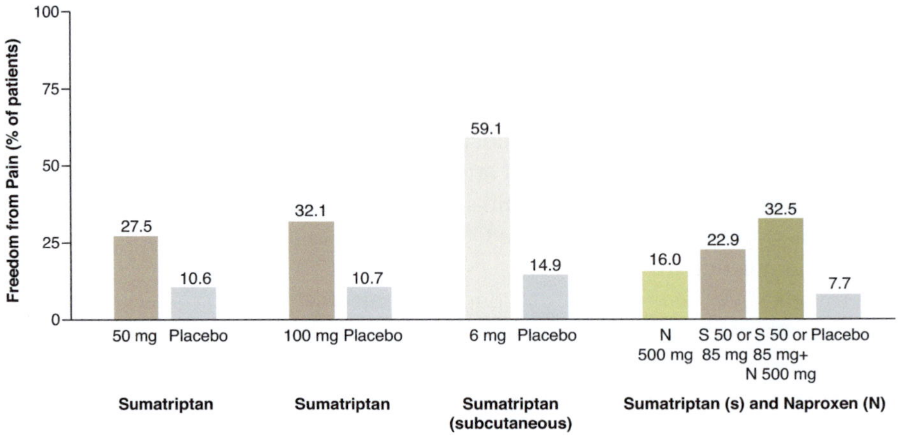

Fig. 14.3 Freedom from migraine pain (% of patients) from sumatriptan [38]

Table 14.4 Pharmacokinetics of the triptans [41]

Drug	Route	Onset	T_{max} (h)	$T_{1/2}$ (h)	Bioavailability
Sumatriptan	SQ	10–15 min	0.17	2	97%
	Intranasal	15–20 min	1.5	2	17%
	Oral	30–90 min	1.5	2	15%
Naratriptan	Oral	1–3 h	2	5.5	70%
Rizatriptan	Oral	0.5–2 h	1	2	45%
Zolmitriptan	Oral	1 h	1.5	2–3 h	40%
Almotriptan	Oral	1–3 h	2.5	3	70%
Frovatriptan	Oral	2–4 h	3	26 h	20–30%

NSAID-triptan combinations, dihydroergotamine, non-opioid combination analgesics (acetaminophen, ASA and caffeine) and several anti-emetics (metoclopramide, domperidone and prochlorperazine) are additional evidence-based options for migraine treatment. Opioid-containing combination analgesics may be helpful in specific patients but should not be used routinely [42]. Consensus guidelines advise against the use of opioids and barbiturates in the treatment of migraine, because of adverse effects and the risk of dependency and medication overuse headache [42].

New abortive migraine treatments are becoming available: small-molecule CGRP receptor antagonists, called gepants and the 5-HT1F receptor agonists, called ditans. The ditans act specifically on the 5 HT1F receptor as opposed to the traditional triptans which act on 5HT 1B and 1D receptors, hence the ditans can be administered in patients with comorbid or history of cardiovascular diseases [43].

Long-term management, such as preventive treatment may be required. The aim is to reduce the frequency, duration and/or severity of migraine attacks. The most widely used drug classes are antihypertensive agents (e.g. beta-blockers and candesartan), antidepressant agents (e.g. amitriptyline) and anticonvulsant agents (e.g. topiramate and sodium valproate) [44]. For chronic migraine (greater than 15 headache days a month for more than 3 months, at least 8 migraine days and 5 migraine attacks) [5], the evidence-based effectiveness of topiramate and onabotulinumtoxinA (Botox) has been documented [45, 46]. New mechanism-based preventive therapies have recently been introduced, targeting the CGRP ligands or receptors. These include four injectable monoclonal antibodies (eptinezumab, erenumab, fremanezumab, and galcanezumab), which all have documented effectiveness in randomized trials for the preventive treatment of episodic and chronic migraine [47–53].

Tension-Type Headache

Tension-type headache is the most common type of primary headache disorder, with a lifetime prevalence in the general population ranging in different studies between 30% and 78% and it has a high socio-economic impact [4].

Tension-type headaches usually last from 30 min to 7 days. It is often a bilateral pain described as 'a band around the head' or vice-like. The pain is generally mild to moderate and is not worse with routine physical activity, which means that most people with tension-type headache continue their normal daily activities despite having their headache. A tension-type headache is not accompanied by nausea or vomiting. It may be accompanied by photophobia or phonophobia, but not both [5, 54].

The infrequent episodic tension-type headache usually has very little impact on the individual and, in most instances, requires no attention from the medical profession in contrast to frequent episodic tension-type headache which can be associated with disability [55]. Chronic tension-type headache (greater than 15 headache days a month for more than 3 months) is associated with decreased quality of life and high disability [56].

The exact mechanisms of tension-type headache are not known. Peripheral pain mechanisms are most likely to play a role in infrequent episodic tension-type headache and frequent episodic tension-type headache [46], whereas central pain mechanisms play an important role in chronic tension-type headache similarly in chronic migraine [56]. Increased pericranial tenderness can be seen in patients with any type of tension-type headache [57, 58].

Treatment.

Simple analgesics, such as NSAIDs or aspirin, are treatment options for infrequent episodic tension-type headaches. The use of combination therapies containing either butalbital or opioids for the treatment of tension-type headache is generally not recommended because of the risk of tolerance, dependency, toxicity, and the development of medication overuse headache [59]. If tension-type headaches are frequent, long-lasting, or associated with a significant amount of disability, then preventive treatment is recommended. Amitriptyline has shown to be effective in both episodic and chronic tension-type headaches [55, 60, 61] and non-pharmacological treatments, such as biofeedback, relaxation, cognitive-behavioural therapy, acupuncture, massage therapy and/or physical therapy have shown to be beneficial in the management of tension-type headaches [62–67].

Diagnostic Dilemma

The diagnostic difficulty most often encountered among the primary headache disorders is in discriminating between tension-type headache and mild forms of migraine. Stricter diagnostic criteria have been suggested for tension-type headache in hope of excluding probable migraine that phenotypically resembles tension-type headache [5, 68]. There is a debate that tension-type headache and migraine are on the same disease spectrum and not completely distinct [69, 70].

Facial Pain

Functional facial pain can involve the trigeminal nerve, which is responsible for pain and sensation of the face through three main branches, ophthalmic: maxillary, and mandibular nerves. Trigeminal neuralgia (TN) is one of the most common causes of facial pain [71]. It is reported that 150,000 people are diagnosed with TN every year and it is most common in people over the age of 50 with a preponderance for females [72].

TN is a disorder characterized by recurrent unilateral, brief electric shock-like pains, abrupt in onset, affecting one or more divisions of the trigeminal nerve and triggered by innocuous stimuli [5, 73]. It may develop without an apparent cause (idiopathic) or as a result of a secondary cause such as demyelination, space-occupying lesion, infection, inflammation, neoplasm, etc. [74]. Classical TN is one of the most common types of TN suggestive of a vascular loop is in proximity to the trigeminal nerve identified on imaging [75].

Idiopathic TN is managed symptomatically. Anticonvulsant medications such as carbamazepine and oxcarbazepine are first-line treatments [76]. Other medications include gabapentin, baclofen, amitriptyline, nortriptyline, pregabalin, phenytoin, valproic acid, clonazepam, lamotrigine and topiramate [77].

If medications are ineffective in treating TN, several surgical procedures may help control the pain including microvascular decompression for classical TN [78] or lesioning procedures for idiopathic TN (percutaneous radiofrequency rhizotomy, percutaneous balloon compression, percutaneous glycerol rhizotomy and stereotactic radiosurgery) [77, 79–82]. If a secondary cause is identified, addressing the underlying cause is the treatment of choice.

Other cranial nerves and branches of the cranial nerves can be affected in a similar fashion as TN, including the glossopharyngeal nerve and nervus intermedius of the facial nerve [83, 84]. Treatment is similar to TN depending on the aetiology [84, 85]. The diagnostic criteria for these conditions can be found in Sect. 13 of the ICHD-3 [5].

Other Headaches and Red Flags.

Other primary headache disorders to consider include the trigeminal autonomic cephalalgias (TACs), primary cough headache, primary exercise headache and primary headache associated with sexual activity.

TACs are characterized by unilateral head pain associated with ipsilateral cranial autonomic features such as lacrimation, conjunctival injection and rhinorrhea [5]. A brain MRI is required to exclude intracranial pathologies, such as cavernous sinus and pituitary lesions [86]. Examples of TACs include cluster headache, paroxysmal hemicrania, short-lasting unilateral neuralgiform headache attacks with conjunctival injection and tearing (SUNCT), short-lasting unilateral neuralgiform headache attacks with cranial autonomic symptoms (SUNA) and hemicrania continua [87]. The diagnostic criteria of these TACs are based on the frequency and duration of the headaches [88]. Acute treatments for cluster headache include triptans and oxygen [89, 90]. Treatments of prevention for cluster headache include verapamil [91], lithium [92] and galcanezumab [93]. Treatment for paroxysmal hemicrania and hemicrania continua respond completely to therapeutic doses of indomethacin [94]. SUNCT and SUNA may be responsive to lamotrigine or intravenous lidocaine [95].

Primary cough headache is a headache precipitated by coughing or other Valsalva (straining) manoeuvre and headache last between 1 s and 2 h [96]. Brain imaging is required to rule out a space-occupying lesion, especially in the posterior fossa [97]. Primary exercise headache is a headache precipitated by any form of exercise and the headache lasts for less than 48 h [98]. Primary headache associated with sexual activity is a headache precipitated by sexual activity. It often lasts from 1 min to 24 h with severe intensity and up to 72 h with mild intensity [99]. Brain imaging with vessel imaging is required to rule out vascular aetiology in both primary exercise headache and primary headache associated with sexual activity [100]. Indomethacin has been used to manage these primary headache disorders with some effectiveness [101].

Other rare primary disorders not discussed here are listed in the ICHD-3, including primary stabbing headache, nummular headache, hypnic headache and new daily persistent headache [5].

Contact Point Headache (Sluder's Neuralgia)

This is facial pain due to a contact point between two structures within nasal cavity, such as a nasal septal deviation or spur, a concha bullosa or medialized/hypertrophied middle turbinate. This phenomenon is also referred to as Sluder's neuralgia or sphenopalatine ganglion neuralgia [2, 102]. The International Headache Society has recognized it as a diagnosis with the following criteria: (A) Intermittent pain in the periorbital, temporozygomatic or medial canthal region, (B) Endoscopy and/or CT evidence of contact points without acute sinusitis, (C) Evidence that the pain can be attributed to mucosal contact based on worsening with dependent positioning or on abolition of pain with local anaesthetic and (D) Pain resolves in 7 days following surgical removal of contact point [5].

The first-line treatment is a trial of nasal decongestants or local anaesthetic which should provide temporary relief of the symptoms. Surgical intervention maybe offered in the form of septoplasty or excision of concha bullosa. However, this is debatable, especially in cases where the mucosal contact point does not result in nasal obstruction [1]. Most evidence for surgical therapy is level IV, with 11–67% being pain-free after the procedure. A systematic review found there is insufficient evidence to support the removal of contact points in the management of facial pain and suggest an initial 6-week trial of amitriptyline [103].

Facial Pain and the Temporomandibular Joint

Facial pain can be directly related to pain arising from the temporomandibular joint (TMJ). Patients present with a history of facial pain that is caused by movement of the jaw, and chewing. On examination, application of pressure to the TMJ exacerbates the pain. Medical treatment involves the use of anti-inflammatories, analgesia, local warm compression to the TMJ or bite appliances. Second-line treatment may involve botox injections or be surgical and a referral to a dentist or oromaxillofacial surgeon is advised. The resolution of facial pain improves as the underlying TMJ disorder resolves [5].

Red Flags

Red flags can be elicited from a detailed headache history and exam. A commonly used published mnemonic is SNOOP (Table 14.5) [104]. If these features are identified, a secondary cause should be investigated. With regards to the choice of imaging, MRI is preferred over CT scan for most cases due to increased sensitivity, particularly for lesions in the posterior fossa, neoplasms, cervicomedullary lesions, pituitary lesions, intracranial hypertension/hypotension and vascular disease [6]. However in the acute setting, such as the emergency department, a CT scan could be performed first, especially for ruling out a gross lesion and haemorrhage including subarachnoid haemorrhage [6, 105].

Table 14.5 SNOOP mnemonics [104, 106]

	Stands for	Example	Differential diagnosis
S	Systemic symptoms	Fever, weight loss and fatigue	Infection (meningitis and encephalitis), giant cell arteritis, metastases and leptomeningeal carcinomatous
	Secondary risk factors	Malignancy, immunosuppression and HIV	
N	Neurologic symptoms/ signs	Focal neurologic deficits, altered consciousness and confusion	Mass lesion, stroke and hydrocephalus
O	Onset	Thunderclap and abrupt	Most common include: Subarachnoid haemorrhage, reversible cerebral vasoconstriction syndrome, pituitary apoplexy, cerebral venous sinus thrombosis and vasculitis
O	Older (especially >50 years)	New onset and progressive headache	Mass lesion and giant cell arteritis
P	Positional	Change lying versus sitting	Intracranial hypotension
P	Prior/ progressive	Different in quality from baseline	Mass lesion
P	Papilledema	Visual obscurations	Idiopathic intracranial hypertension
P	Precipitated by	Valsalva, coughing and sneezing	Posterior fossa lesion

References

1. Altin F, Haci C, Alimoglu Y, Yilmaz S. Is septoplasty effective rhinogenic headache in patients with isolated contact point between inferior turbinate and septal spur? Am J Otolaryngol - Head Neck Med Surg. 2019;40(3):364–7.
2. De Corso E, Kar M, Cantone E, Lucidi D, Settimi S, Mele D, et al. Facial pain: sinus or not? Acta Otorhinolaryngol Ital. 2018;38(6):485.
3. Lipton RB, Bigal ME, Steiner TJ, Silberstein SD, Olesen J. Classification of primary headaches. Neurology. 2004;63(3):427–35.
4. Stovner LJ, Nichols E, Steiner TJ, Abd-Allah F, Abdelalim A, Al-Raddadi RM, et al. Global, regional, and national burden of migraine and tension-type headache, 1990–2016: a systematic analysis for the global burden of disease study 2016. Lancet Neurol. 2018;17(11):954.
5. Headache Classification Committee of the International Headache Society (IHS). The International Classification of Headache Disorders, 3rd edition. Cephalalgia. 2018;38(1):1–211.
6. Evans RW, Rozen TD, Adelman JU. Neuroimaging and other diagnostic testing in headache. Wolff's headache and other head. Pain. 2001:27–49.
7. Ashina M, Hansen JM, Do TP, Melo-Carrillo A, Burstein R, Moskowitz MA. Migraine and the trigeminovascular system—40 years and counting. Lancet Neurol. 2019;18(8):795–804.
8. Raddant AC, Russo AF. Calcitonin gene-related peptide in migraine: intersection of peripheral inflammation and central modulation. Expert Rev Mol Med. 2011;13:e36.
9. Dalkara T, Nozari A, Moskowitz MA. Migraine aura pathophysiology: the role of blood vessels and microembolisation. Lancet Neurol. 2010;9(3):309–17.

10. Sanchez del Rio M, Bakker D, Wu O, Agosti R, Mitsikostas D, Østergaard L, et al. Perfusion weighted imaging during Migraine: spontaneous visual Aura and Headache. Cephalalgia. 1999;19(8):701–7.
11. Lipton RB, Diamond S, Reed M, Diamond ML, Stewart WF. Migraine diagnosis and treatment: results from the American Migraine study II. Headache. 2001;41(7):638–45. https://doi.org/10.1046/j.1526-4610.2001.041007638.x.
12. Novak VJMM. Pathogenesis and treatment of migraine and neurovascular headaches with rhinogenic trigger. Head Neck. 1992;14:467–72.
13. Schreiber CP, Hutchinson S, Webster CJ, Ames M, Richardson MS, Powers C. Prevalence of migraine in patients with a history of self-reported or physician-diagnosed "sinus" headache. Arch Intern Med. 2004;164(16):1769–72. https://doi.org/10.1001/archinte.164.16.1769.
14. Cady RK, Dodick DW, Levine HL, Schreiber CP, Eross EJ, Setzen M, et al. Sinus headache: a neurology, otolaryngology, allergy, and primary care consensus on diagnosis and treatment. Mayo Clin Proc. 2005;80(7):908–16.
15. Amedee RG. Acute radiology rarely confirms sinus disease in suspected recurrent acute rhinosinusitis. Am J Rhinol Allergy. 2017;31:420.
16. Lerman SF, Rudich Z, Brill S, Shalev H, Shahar G. Longitudinal associations between depression, anxiety, pain, and pain-related disability in chronic pain patients. Psychosom Med. 2015;77(3):333–41.
17. Fokkens WJ, Lund VJ, Hopkins C, Hellings PW, Kern R, Reitsma S, et al. Classification, definitions and terminology allergy. Eur Position Pap Rhinosinusitis Nasal Polyps. 2020:31–2.
18. Meltzer E, Bachert C, Staudinger H. Treating acute rhinosinusitis: comparing efficacy and safety of mometasone furoate nasal spray, amoxicillin, and placebo. J Allergy Clin Immunol [Internet]. 2005;116(6):1289–95. Available from: https://linkinghub.elsevier.com/retrieve/pii/S0091674905019342
19. Pierre Gehanno CB. Short therapy with amoxicillin-clavulanate and corticosteroids in acute sinusitis: results of a multicentre study in adults. Scand J Infect Dis [Internet]. 2000;32(6):679–84. Available from: http://www.tandfonline.com/doi/full/10.1080/003655400459621
20. Garbutt JM, Goldstein M, Gellman E, Shannon W, Littenberg B. A randomized, placebo-controlled trial of antimicrobial treatment for children with clinically diagnosed acute sinusitis. Pediatrics [Internet]. 2001;107(4):619–25. Available from: http://pediatrics.aappublications.org/lookup/doi/10.1542/peds.107.4.619
21. Ratau NP, Snyman JR, Swanepoel C. Short-course, low-dose oral betamethasone as an adjunct in the treatment of acute infective sinusitis. Clin Drug Investig [Internet]. 2004;24(10):577–82. Available from: http://link.springer.com/10.2165/00044011-200424100-00003
22. Zalmanovici Trestioreanu A, Yaphe J. Intranasal steroids for acute sinusitis. Cochrane Database Syst Rev [Internet]. 2013 Dec 2; Available from: http://doi.wiley.com/10.1002/14651858.CD005149.pub4
23. Anon JB, Berkowitz E, Breton J, Twynholm M. Efficacy/safety of amoxicillin/clavulanate in adults with bacterial rhinosinusitis. Am J Otolaryngol [Internet]. 2006;27(4):248–54. Available from: https://linkinghub.elsevier.com/retrieve/pii/S0196070905002280
24. Rhinosinusitis international Consensus Statement on Allergy and Rhinology. 2021; Available from: https://onlinelibrary.wiley.com/doi/pdf/10.1002/alr.22741
25. Rosenfeld RM, Piccirillo JF, Chandrasekhar SS, Brook I, Ashok Kumar K, Kramper M, et al. Clinical Practice Guideline (Update): Adult Sinusitis. Otolaryngol Neck Surg [Internet]. 2015;152(2_suppl):S1–39. Available from: http://journals.sagepub.com/doi/10.1177/0194599815572097
26. Inanli S, Oztürk O, Al MK, et. The effects of topical agents of fluticasone propionate, Oxymetazoline, and 3% and 0.9% sodium chloride solutions on Mucociliary clearance in the therapy of acute bacterial rhinosinusitis in vivo. Laryngoscope [Internet]. 2002;112(2):320–5. Available from: http://doi.wiley.com/10.1097/00005537-200202000-00022

27. Hayward G, Heneghan C, Perera R, Thompson M. Intranasal corticosteroids in Management of Acute Sinusitis: a systematic review and meta-analysis. Ann Fam Med [Internet]. 2012;10(3):241–9. Available from: http://www.annfammed.org/cgi/doi/10.1370/afm.1338
28. Braun JJ, Alabert JP, Michel FB, Quiniou M, Rat C, Cougnard J, et al. Adjunct effect of loratadine in the treatment of acute sinusitis in patients with allergic rhinitis. Allergy [Internet]. 1997;52(6):650–5. Available from: http://doi.wiley.com/10.1111/j.1398-9995.1997.tb01044.x
29. Fokkens WJ, Lund VJ, Hopkins C, Hellings PW, Kern R, Reitsma S, et al. Executive summary of EPOS 2020 including integrated care pathways. Rhinology. 2020;58(2):82–111.
30. Amin FM, Aristeidou S, Baraldi C, Czapinska-Ciepiela EK, Ariadni DD, Di Lenola D, et al. The association between migraine and physical exercise. J Headache Pain. 2018;19(1):83.
31. Krøll LS, Hammarlund CS, Linde M, Gard G, Jensen RH. The effects of aerobic exercise for persons with migraine and co-existing tension-type headache and neck pain. A randomized, controlled, clinical trial. Cephalalgia. 2018;38(12):805–16.
32. Overath CH, Darabaneanu S, Evers MC, Gerber W-D, Graf M, Keller A, et al. Does an aerobic endurance programme have an influence on information processing in migraineurs? J Headache Pain. 2014;15(1):11.
33. Elinoff V, Lynn SJ, Ochiai H, Hallquist M. The efficacy of Kiko exercises on the prevention of Migraine headaches: a pilot study. Am J Chin Med. 2009;37(03):459–70.
34. Rabbie R, Derry S, Moore RA. Ibuprofen with or without an antiemetic for acute migraine headaches in adults. Cochrane Database Syst Rev. 2013;10:4.
35. Kirthi V, Derry S, Moore RA, McQuay HJ. Aspirin with or without an antiemetic for acute migraine headaches in adults. Cochrane Database Syst Rev. 2010;4:CD008041.
36. Derry S, Moore RA. Diclofenac with or without an antiemetic for acute migraine headaches in adults. In: Moore M, editor. Cochrane database of systematic reviews. John Wiley & Sons, Ltd: Chichester; 2010.
37. Silberstein SD, Stirpe JC. COX inhibitors for the treatment of migraine. Expert Opin Pharmacother. 2014;15(13):1863–74.
38. Migraine AM. N Engl J Med. 2020;383(19):1866–76.
39. Cameron C, Kelly S, Hsieh S-C, Murphy M, Chen L, Kotb A, et al. Triptans in the acute treatment of Migraine: a systematic review and network meta-analysis. Headache J Head Face Pain. 2015;55(Suppl 4):221–35.
40. Oliver RL. Choosing the right triptan. Pract Pain Manag. 2003:15–8.
41. Jhee SS, Shiovitz T, Crawford AW, Cutler NR. Pharmacokinetics and pharmacodynamics of the Triptan antimigraine agents. Clin Pharmacokinet. 2001;40(3):189–205.
42. Becker WJ. Acute Migraine treatment in adults. Headache J Head Face Pain. 2015;55(6):778–93.
43. Kuca B, Silberstein SD, Wietecha L, Berg PH, Dozier G, Lipton RB. Lasmiditan is an effective acute treatment for migraine: a phase 3 randomized study. Neurology. 2018;91(24):e2222.
44. Silberstein SD. Preventive migraine treatment. Contin Lifelong Learn Neurol. 2015;21:973.
45. Silberstein SD, Lipton RB, Dodick DW, Freitag FG, Ramadan N, Mathew N, et al. Efficacy and safety of topiramate for the treatment of chronic Migraine: a randomized, double-blind, placebo-controlled trial. Headache J Head Face Pain. 2007 Feb;47(2):170–80.
46. Aurora S, Dodick D, Turkel C, DeGryse R, Silberstein S, Lipton R, et al. OnabotulinumtoxinA for treatment of chronic migraine: results from the double-blind, randomized, placebo-controlled phase of the PREEMPT 1 trial. Cephalalgia. 2010;30(7):804–14.
47. Goadsby PJ, Reuter U, Hallström Y, Broessner G, Bonner JH, Zhang F, et al. A controlled trial of Erenumab for episodic Migraine. N Engl J Med. 2017;377(22):2123–32.
48. Tepper S, Ashina M, Reuter U, Brandes JL, Doležil D, Silberstein S, et al. Safety and efficacy of erenumab for preventive treatment of chronic migraine: a randomised, double-blind, placebo-controlled phase 2 trial. Lancet Neurol. 2017;16(6):425–34.
49. Dodick DW, Silberstein SD, Bigal ME, Yeung PP, Goadsby PJ, Blankenbiller T, et al. Effect of Fremanezumab compared with placebo for prevention of episodic Migraine. JAMA. 2018;319(19):1999–2008.

50. Silberstein SD, Dodick DW, Bigal ME, Yeung PP, Goadsby PJ, Blankenbiller T, et al. Fremanezumab for the preventive treatment of chronic Migraine. N Engl J Med. 2017;377(22):113–22.
51. Stauffer VL, Dodick DW, Zhang Q, Carter JN, Ailani J, Conley RR. Evaluation of Galcanezumab for the prevention of episodic Migraine. JAMA Neurol. 2018;75(9):1080–8.
52. Detke HC, Goadsby PJ, Wang S, Friedman DI, Selzler KJ, Aurora SK. Galcanezumab in chronic migraine. Neurology. 2018;91(24):e2211–21.
53. Ashina M, Saper J, Cady R, Schaeffler BA, Biondi DM, Hirman J, et al. Eptinezumab in episodic migraine: a randomized, double-blind, placebo-controlled study (PROMISE-1). Cephalalgia. 2020;40(3):241–54.
54. Ashina S, Bendtsen L, Ashina M. Pathophysiology of tension-type headache. Curr Pain Headache Rep. 2005;9(6):415–22.
55. Cassie Scripter. Headache: tension-type headache. FP Essent . 2018;17–20.
56. Manzoni GC, Torelli P. Chronic migraine and chronic tension-type headache: are they the same or different? Neurol Sci. 2009;30(S1):81–4.
57. Fernández-de-las-Peñas C, Cuadrado ML, Arendt-Nielsen L, Ge H-Y, Pareja JA. Increased Pericranial tenderness, decreased pressure pain threshold, and headache clinical parameters in chronic tension-type headache patients. Clin J Pain. 2007;23(4):346.
58. Langemark M, Olesen J. Pericranial tenderness in tension headache: a blind. Controlled Study Cephalalgia. 1987;7(4):249–55.
59. Jensen R, Olesen J. Tension-type headache: an update on mechanisms and treatment. Curr Opin Neurol. 2000;13(3):285–9.
60. Bendtsen L, Jensen R. Amitriptyline reduces myofascial tenderness in patients with chronic tension-type headache. Cephalalgia. 2000;20(6):603–10.
61. Cerbo R, Barbanti P, Fabbrini G, Pascali MP, Catarci T. Amitriptyline is effective in chronic but not in episodic tension-type headache: pathogenetic implications. Headache J Head Face Pain. 1998 Jun;38(6):453–7.
62. Probyn K, Bowers H, Mistry D, Caldwell F, Underwood M, Patel S, et al. Non-pharmacological self-management for people living with migraine or tension-type headache: a systematic review including analysis of intervention components. BMJ Open. 2017;7(8):e016670.
63. Torelli P, Jensen R, Olesen J. Physiotherapy for tension-type headache: a controlled study. Cephalalgia. 2004;24(1):29–36.
64. Linde K, Allais G, Brinkhaus B, Fei Y, Mehring M, Shin B-C, et al. Acupuncture for the prevention of tension-type headache. Cochrane Database Syst Rev. 2016 Apr;19:4.
65. Cathcart S, Galatis N, Immink M, Proeve M, Petkov J. Brief mindfulness-based therapy for chronic tension-type headache: a randomized controlled pilot study. Behav Cogn Psychother. 2014;42(1):1–15.
66. Moraska AF, Stenerson L, Butryn N, Krutsch JP, Schmiege SJ, Mann JD. Myofascial trigger point-focused head and neck massage for recurrent tension-type headache. Clin J Pain. 2015 Feb;31(2):159–68.
67. Bendtsen L, Evers S, Linde M, Mitsikostas DD, Sandrini G, Schoenen J. EFNS guideline on the treatment of tension-type headache - report of an EFNS task force. Eur J Neurol. 2010 Nov;17(11):1318–25.
68. Rasmussen BK, Jensen R, Schroll M, Olesen J. Interrelations between migraine and tension-type headache in the general population. Arch Neurol. 1992;49(9):914–8.
69. Kaniecki RG. Migraine and tension-type headache: An assessment of challenges in diagnosis. Neurology. 2002;58(9, Supplement 6):S15–S20.
70. Vargas BB. Tension-type headache and migraine: two points on a continuum? Curr Pain Headache Rep. 2008;12(6):433–6.
71. Newman MDLC, Levin MDM. Trigeminal Neuralgia. In: Headache and facial pain. Oxford University Press; 2008. p. 93–7.
72. De Toledo IP, Conti Réus J, Fernandes M, Porporatti AL, Peres MA, Takaschima A, et al. Prevalence of trigeminal neuralgia. J Am Dent Assoc. 2016;147(7):570–6.e2.
73. Zakrzewska JM, Linskey ME. Trigeminal neuralgia. BMJ. 2015;350:h1238.

74. Schmidt RF, Willis W. Trigeminal neuralgia. Encycl Pain. 2007:2149–9.
75. Maarbjerg S, Wolfram F, Gozalov A, Olesen J, Bendtsen L. Significance of neurovascular contact in classical trigeminal neuralgia. Brain. 2015;138(2):311–9.
76. Jorns TP, Zakrzewska JM. Evidence-based approach to the medical management of trigeminal neuralgia. Br J Neurosurg. 2007;21(3):252–61.
77. Obermann M. Treatment options in trigeminal neuralgia. Ther Adv Neurol Disord. 2010;3(2):107–15.
78. Ovallath S. Textbook of trigeminal neuralgia. Nova Science Publishers, Incorporated; 2020. p. 225.
79. Sheehan J, Pan H-C, Stroila M, Steiner L. Gamma knife surgery for trigeminal neuralgia: outcomes and prognostic factors. J Neurosurg. 2005;102(3):434.
80. Taha JM, Tew JM. Comparison of surgical treatments for trigeminal neuralgia: reevaluation of radiofrequency Rhizotomy. Neurosurgery. 1996;38(5):865–71.
81. Skirving DJ, Dan NG. A 20-year review of percutaneous balloon compression of the trigeminal ganglion. J Neurosurg. 2001;94(6):913–7.
82. Fujimaki T, Fukushima T, Miyazaki S. Percutaneous retrogasserian glycerol injection in the management of trigeminal neuralgia: long-term follow-up results. J Neurosurg. 1990;73(2):212–6.
83. Blumenfeld A, Nikolskaya G. Glossopharyngeal neuralgia. Curr Pain Headache Rep. 2013;17(7):343.
84. Bruyn G. Nervus intermedius neuralgia (hunt). Cephalalgia. 1984;4(1):71–8.
85. Peris-Celda M, Oushy S, Perry A, Graffeo CS, Carlstrom LP, Zimmerman RS, et al. Nervus intermedius and the surgical management of geniculate neuralgia. J Neurosurg. 2019;131(2):343–51.
86. Goadsby PJ. Trigeminal Autonomic Cephalalgias. Contin Lifelong Learn Neurol. 2012;18:883–95.
87. Burish MJ, Rozen TD. Trigeminal Autonomic Cephalalgias. Neurol Clin. 2019;37(4):847–69.
88. Goadsby P, Cittadini E, Cohen A. Trigeminal autonomic Cephalalgias: paroxysmal Hemicrania, SUNCT/SUNA, and Hemicrania continua. Semin Neurol. 2010;30(02):186–91.
89. Cohen AS, Burns B, Goadsby PJ. High-flow oxygen for treatment of cluster headache. JAMA. 2009;302(22):2451–7.
90. Treatment of Acute Cluster Headache with Sumatriptan. N Engl J Med. 1991;325(5):322–6.
91. Leone M, D'Amico D, Frediani F, Moschiano F, Grazzi L, Attanasio A, et al. Verapamil in the prophylaxis of episodic cluster headache: a double-blind study versus placebo. Neurology. 2000;54(6):1382–5.
92. Ekbom K. Lithium for cluster headache: review of the literature and preliminary results of long-term treatment. Headache J Head Face Pain. 1981;21(4):132–9.
93. Dodick DW, Goadsby PJ, Lucas C, Jensen R, Bardos JN, Martinez JM, et al. Phase 3 randomized, placebo-controlled study of galcanezumab in patients with chronic cluster headache: results from 3-month double-blind treatment. Cephalalgia. 2020;40(9):935–48.
94. Antonaci F, Pareja JA, Caminero AB, Sjaastad O. Chronic Paroxysmal Hemicrania and Hemicrania Continua. Parenteral Indomethacin: The "Indotest.". Headache J Head Face Pain. 1998;38(2):122–8.
95. Williams MH, Broadley SA. SUNCT and SUNA: clinical features and medical treatment. J Clin Neurosci. 2008;15(5):526–34.
96. Schwedt TJ, Gladstone JP, Purdy RA, Dodick DW. Primary cough headache. In: Headache. Cambridge: Cambridge University Press; 2010. p. 124–6.
97. Cordenier A, De Hertogh W, De Keyser J, Versijpt J. Headache associated with cough: a review. J Headache Pain. 2013;14(42):1–7.
98. Alvarez R, Ramón C, Pascual J. Clues in the differential diagnosis of primary vs secondary cough, exercise, and sexual headaches. Headache J Head Face Pain. 2014;54(9):1560–2.
99. Schwedt TJ, Gladstone JP, Purdy RA, Dodick DW. Primary headache associated with sexual activity. In: Headache. Cambridge: Cambridge University Press; 2010. p. 120–3

100. Pascual J, González-Mandly A, Oterino A, Martín R. Primary cough headache, primary exertional headache, and primary headache associated with sexual activity. In: Handbook of clinical neurology, vol. 97. Elsevier; 2010. p. 459–68.
101. Summ O, Evers S. Mechanism of action of indomethacin in indomethacin-responsive headaches. Curr Pain Headache Rep. 2013;17(4):327.
102. Patel ZM, Kennedy DW, Setzen M, Poetker DM, Delgaudio JM. "Sinus headache": Rhinogenic headache or migraine? An evidence-based guide to diagnosis and treatment. Int Forum Allergy Rhinol. 2013;3:221–30.
103. Harrison L, Jones NS. Intranasal contact points as a cause of facial pain or headache: a systematic review. Clin Otolaryngol. 2013;38:8–22.
104. Dodick DW. Diagnosing headache: clinical clues and clinical rules. 2nd ed. Adv Stud Med. 2003;3:87–92.
105. Ducros A, Bousser M-G. Thunderclap headache. BMJ. 2013;346:e8557.
106. Micieli A, Kingston W. An approach to identifying headache patients that require neuroimaging. Front Public Heal. 2019;7:52.

Subjective Tinnitus

15

Valerie Dahm and Trung N. Le

Epidemiology and Risk Factors

The prevalence given for tinnitus [1] varies substantially and can be up to 15% [2], with 6% for mild tinnitus and 4% for severe tinnitus [3]. A large study on tinnitus epidemiology conducted with the Clinical Practice Research Datalink in Great Britain identified 109,783 adults newly diagnosed within a 16-year period [4]. Males and females were affected similarly. The authors found that 80% of individuals diagnosed with tinnitus were 40 years or older. The highest incidence rate was identified in individuals between 60 and 69 years of age. Women were slightly older at the time of diagnosis than men.

Classification

Acute Versus Chronic Tinnitus

Opinions about the cut-off between acute and chronic tinnitus are not standardized. Acute tinnitus can be defined as up to 3 months or even up to 12 months duration [5]. In general, the most common definition is that if it persists for over 6 months, it is viewed as chronic as opposed to shorter than 6 months during which is still seen as acute.

V. Dahm (✉)
Department of Otolaryngology, Sunnybrook Health Sciences Center, University of Toronto, Toronto, ON, Canada

Department of Otolaryngology, Head and Neck Surgery, Medical Unviersity of Vienna, Vienna, Austria
e-mail: valerie.dahm@meduniwien.ac.at

T. N. Le
Department of Otolaryngology Head and Neck Surgery, University of Toronto, Toronto, ON, Canada

© The Author(s), under exclusive license to Springer Nature Switzerland AG 2023

B. W. Blakley, J. E. Blakley (eds.), *Functional Illness of the Head and Neck*,
https://doi.org/10.1007/978-3-031-12998-8_15

Non-bothersome or Compensated Tinnitus

Tyler and Baker described tinnitus's effects on quality of life in 1983 [6] and since then many studies have focused on the influence of this symptom on patients [7–9]. There are several questionnaires used to assess quality of life and subjective severity of tinnitus. Details on available and useful questionnaires are discussed below. Non-bothersome or compensated tinnitus is perceived by patients, but it does not lead to secondary symptoms or affect the quality of life significantly. However, this level of burden can change over the course of time.

Bothersome or Non-compensated Tinnitus

Tinnitus that affects the quality of life significantly is called bothersome or non-compensated tinnitus. It can lead to secondary health issues. There is no correlation between the intensity and the frequency of tinnitus with the psychological disease burden [10]. Consequently, this distinction cannot be carried out with audiograms or tinnitus frequency and loudness assessment but only with a detailed history or even psychological testing.

The World Health Organization has grouped the effects of bothersome tinnitus into four broad groups: thoughts and emotions, hearing, sleeping, and concentration [11]. Secondary associated symptoms of tinnitus include the following [2, 6]:

- Insomnia.
- Depression.
- Anxiety disorders.
- Impaired understanding of speech.
- Impaired concentration, problems with both work and family life, can lead to:
- Anger.
- Frustration.
- Other emotional disturbances.
- Decrease of general health-related quality of life.

Primary Versus Secondary Tinnitus

Primary tinnitus is idiopathic or functional, which means that no pathology can be found. Sensorineural hearing loss might be accompanied by it but does not have to be present. Secondary tinnitus is thought to be associated with another underlying specific organic condition (which can be treated in some cases) and therefore might be reversible [2]. This form of tinnitus can occur in the context of middle ear diseases including chronic middle ear infections, eustachian tube dysfunction, otosclerosis, tympanosclerosis, Menières disease, or retrocochlear pathologies such as vestibular schwannomas or meningiomas [4, 12].

Presentation and Examinations

When diagnosing a patient with tinnitus, a careful history should be taken. This information is important to define which treatment options can be useful and to assess the degree of psychological burden.

- Assess medical history.
- Acute versus chronic tinnitus.
- Ototoxic medication.
- Noise exposure.
- Tinnitus quality – subjective versus objective, pulsatile versus non-pulsatile.
- Perform targeted otologic examination (including otoscopy) and other head and neck examinations to rule out associated conditions.
- Auscultation of the ear and the cervical internal carotid artery for pulsatile tinnitus.
- Audiogram with pure tone average (PTA) and word recognition score (WRS).
- Tympanogram and stapedial reflexes.
- Assessment of middle ear compliance and eustachian tube function.
- Psychological assessment.
- Distinguish between bothersome and non-bothersome tinnitus.
- Assess for symptoms of depression or anxiety.

Additional Tests

Imaging (MRI of internal auditory canal or CT scan of temporal bone) – if a history of unilateral tinnitus, pulsatile tinnitus, focal neurologic abnormalities, and asymmetric hearing loss on an audiogram [2].

Vestibular testing (nystagmography or video head impulse test) – if a history of vestibular symptoms and suspicious vestibular findings on examination.

Tinnitus Questionnaires

Tinnitus questionnaires are an important tool to identify non-auditory symptoms and disease burden as well as an appropriate comparative measure to assess the progression of condition or treatment efficacy. Until 2012, about nine questionnaires were validated and regularly used mainly for research purposes as self-reports. In 2012, Meikle et al. conducted a study with the aim of developing a new questionnaire, the Tinnitus Functional Index (TFI), which should measure severity and impact of tinnitus in a clinical setting and also include important aspects of treatment changes [13]. The authors concluded that, the TFI can be used in the clinical setting as well as to assess treatment efficacy in a research setting [13]. Jacquemin et al. conducted a study comparing the TFI with the Tinnitus

Questionnaire [14]. The authors concluded that both have high convergent validity and are both suitable as outcome measures [14]. Since the TFI is shorter and showed a slightly higher agreement with the self-reported effect in said study, the authors favor this questionnaire [14].

Theories of Tinnitus Etiology

Association of Hearing Loss and Tinnitus

Idiopathic tinnitus, bothersome or non-bothersome, acute or chronic, is often associated with hearing loss. Sensorineural hearing loss might be related to sudden hearing loss, noise trauma, presbyacusis, or ototoxic drugs [15]. Interestingly not everyone with hearing loss has tinnitus, and not everyone with tinnitus has hearing loss. One of the reasons for this might be that we are not able to detect every nuance of hearing loss with standard audiometry [16]. This effect underlines the parallel between tinnitus and phantom pain after limb amputation [17].

One of the most important arguments against tinnitus arising in the cochlea itself, which was thought to be the case previously, is that sectioning the cochlear nerve does not lead to tinnitus interruption, as shown by Jackson in 1985 [18]. This fact does not contradict the association between hearing loss and tinnitus, it merely shows that hearing loss can lead to a central phenomenon, which then leads to tinnitus. As a result, the next higher level, the auditory cortex, was suspected to be the origin of this symptom.

Association of Temporomandibular Joint Disorders and Tinnitus

Temporomandibular joint (TMJ) disorders have also been investigated in the context of tinnitus. Somatic structures such as the TMJ may interact with the auditory system [19]. The ear is innervated by various nerves including the trigeminal, facial, glossopharyngeal, and vagal nerve, which corresponds to the cranial nerves V, VII, IX, and X. The TMJ is innervated by the fifth (V) and seventh (VII) cranial nerves. These common cranial nerves have been suspected of connecting the TMJ to tinnitus [20]. A further theory is that the underlying mechanism is the effect of afferent somatosensory input from the trigeminal nerve and C2 fibers via interaction at the dorsal cochlear nucleus at the brainstem level on central auditory pathway activity [21, 22].

A systematic review and meta-analysis published in 2019 screened 224 publications and included 22 manuscripts on the association of TMJ disorders and tinnitus. The authors concluded that there was a strong association between these two issues, namely that the signs of TMJ disorders may augment the likelihood of developing tinnitus as well as tinnitus can also promote the signs of TMJ disorders [23]. They recommend investigating for possible TMJ pathologies in tinnitus patients as well as the other way around [23].

Association of Stress and Tinnitus

Stress is defined as a physical, chemical, or emotional factor that causes bodily or mental tension and may be a factor in disease causation. A stress response can be provoked by environmental influences of daily life or serious life events [24]. The individual response is influenced by a multitude of factors such as genetic, cognitive, and behavioral components [25, 26]. Tinnitus can be one of the reactions to an individual stressor but can clearly also be perceived as stressful.

Stress and tinnitus have been associated with hormonal, autonomic, and immunological dysregulations [27]. Mineral- and glucocorticoid receptors have been identified in the inner ear which prompted research in this area. Animal studies have shown that stress results in a stimulation of glucocorticoid receptors in the cochlea, as well as hormonal responses in the hypothalamic–pituitary–adrenal axis [28, 29]. Mazurek et al. analyzed studies investigating the association between hormonal, autonomic, and immunological dysregulation and tinnitus. The authors concluded that, in summary, there was some evidence of autonomic nervous system dysfunction in chronic tinnitus, but that it is unclear whether these changes are systematic and specific to tinnitus or associated with interacting systems commonly correlated with tinnitus onset, maintenance, or distress [27]. While short-term stress has been associated with excitement and increased motivation, in contrast, chronic stress can contribute to chronic illnesses, such as depression or hypertension [30, 31]. Similarly, acute short-term stress has been shown to protect the cochlea in animal studies, while long-term or chronic stress showed negative hearing effects [27]. For example, a four-hour isolation period, which was used as an acute stressor (i.e., acute stress), led to higher cortisone levels, which then protected against noise-induced hearing loss [32].

Chronic, repetitive, or long-term stress induced by a 24-hour exposure to regularly occurring aversive audiological stimuli led to a temporary auditory hypersensitivity [33]. A survey of 12,166 subjects showed that stress is almost as important as occupational noise exposure when it comes to discomfort due to tinnitus [34]. The difference between mild and severe tinnitus discomfort is more influenced by stress levels than noise exposure [34]. Said study also showed that exposure to stress and noise further increases the probability of experiencing tinnitus [34]. A further study by Hasson et al. underlined the results of the aforementioned study by demonstrating an association between hearing issues (tinnitus, hearing loss, or both) and various stress factors (burnout scores, chronic illness, poorer sleep, etc.) [35].

Tinnitus has also been found to be associated with depression and anxiety [36]. The intensity of tinnitus and level of depression showed some correlation [36]. The causality between these disorders is hard to find and can only be evaluated in longitudinal studies which are lacking. Further associations with tinnitus have been found for post-traumatic stress disorders [37]. Not only tinnitus but also conditions such as hyperacusis, Menières disease, vertigo, and dizziness have been found to occur alongside mental health difficulties and therefore an exact differentiation of all these symptoms and their association with tinnitus is not always possible [38–40].

Association Between Headaches and Tinnitus

Headaches and tinnitus are both extremely common complaints and somewhat of an enigma even to modern medicine. Several pathologies can cause both symptoms, such as carotid artery dissection [41] or traumatic head injury [42]. Since both headaches and tinnitus are so common it is hard to prove a relationship between them. Sindhusake et al. conducted a large population-based study in the west of Sydney, called the Blue Mountains Hearing Study [43]. The authors found that hearing loss had a modest association with tinnitus, but more importantly, the results showed that 6.6% of tinnitus may be related to migraine [43].

A study conducted in a tertiary care center on 193 patients with tinnitus and headaches found a significant correlation between tinnitus and headache laterality and severity [44]. The authors conclude that these results argue against a purely coincidental co-occurrence of these two symptoms and assume that there might be a common pathophysiological mechanism [44]. A prospective study on 286 individuals diagnosed with subjective, non-pulsatile tinnitus aimed at evaluating different types of headaches [45]. Almost half of the patients were diagnosed with headaches, most with tension-type headaches or migraine. These patients were significantly younger, mostly female. They also had bilateral tinnitus, vertigo, and depression more frequently as well as hearing loss less frequently. As also in the aforementioned study, headache side and tinnitus correlated well [44, 45]. More details on headaches can be found in the headache chapter of this book.

Association Between Insomnia and Tinnitus

Insomnia is a very frequently reported complaint. As sleep deprivation and disturbances have been used as torture methods, no proof is necessary that insomnia can lead to significant stress. A recently conducted review evaluated studies assessing tinnitus and insomnia [46]. They found that 10–80% of tinnitus patients suffer from insomnia. Most studies report that over 40% of tinnitus patients cannot fall asleep, have a hard time staying asleep, or wake up too early and are not able to get back to sleep. A prospective study was published by the same group. They interviewed 72 tinnitus patients, who were evaluated for a treatment program and found that 60% met strict diagnostic criteria for insomnia, while only 4% were being treated for it [47]. The authors additionally reported that the data suggest severer forms of tinnitus to be present in insomnia patients. These results were underlined by a further study published in 2019 [48]. Authors retrospectively investigated charts of 165 patients who were treated for tinnitus and had additionally answered questionnaires about sleep. They found that 50% of tinnitus patients reported poor sleep quality. Especially, a higher maximal intensity of tinnitus was associated with poor sleep quality. In contrast, patients with a lower tinnitus level had no issues with insomnia.

Therapeutic Options

Patient Counseling and Education

Counseling is an important factor when treating patients with tinnitus. Like all symptoms, tinnitus may be viewed as a negative factor, maybe even as a dangerous pathology. It is therefore important to counsel patients on the benign nature of this symptom. Hoare et al. performed a systematic review and meta-analysis of randomized controlled trials on tinnitus management and concluded that information or education for patients in form of a book or therapist-led session had a significant effect over no intervention or undirected self-help. Further, a self-help book with therapy sessions seems to provide greater help than the self-help book alone [49]. Education and counseling of tinnitus patients should include [2]:

- Brochures about tinnitus and self-help options.
- Recommending the use of self-help books.
- Suggesting sound therapy options (wearable and non-wearable devices).
- Describing counseling (cognitive behavioral therapy).
- Discussing the lack of proven benefits (e.g., pharmacological therapies).
- Discussing associated conditions (hearing loss, TMJ disorder, headaches, stress and anxiety disorder, and insomnia).
- Referral to other professionals as appropriate or needed (audiologists, otolaryngologists/otologists, psychiatrists, psychologists, neurologists, prosthetic dentists).

Hearing Aids (HAs) in the Setting of Tinnitus and Hearing Loss

HAs improve hearing and quality of life in patients with hearing loss, but the evidence is weakly supportive for tinnitus. Hoare et al. published a Cochrane review in 2014 only identifying one randomized controlled trial comparing HA use to sound generator use. Tinnitus Handicap Inventory score showed a benefit for both interventions but no difference was found between these two alternative treatments [50]. Since 2014, only one further randomized trial could be identified that compared HA use to no HA use. Radunz et al. performed a randomized-controlled trial with three arms. These groups were HAs, HAs plus *Ginkgo biloba* and *G. biloba* alone [51]. Tinnitus Handicap Inventory as well as a visual analog scale was used at the beginning of the study and after 90 days. Results showed that there was a significant improvement of tinnitus in all three groups with no significant difference between the groups. One of the main limitations of this study is the small sample size of 11 individuals per group as well as the missing control group.

Several other trials have evaluated different HAs as well as motivational interview additionally to HAs. Henry et al. performed a randomized trial comparing three different HAs (receiver-in-the-canal HAs, HAs with a sound generator and extended-wear, deep fit HAs) [52]. Tinnitus Functional Index improved in all three groups, with a total of 55 individuals. There was no significant difference between the three groups. Yakunina et al. randomized 114 patients into three groups: HAs using wide dynamic range compression, HAs with frequency translation, and HAs with linear frequency transposition [53]. Tinnitus was evaluated at 3 months time point using the Tinnitus Handicap Inventory, which matched tinnitus loudness and visual analog scale scores. There were no differences between the three groups. Tinnitus was effectively suppressed during HA use as well as after the second trial period of 3 months without HAs. Zarenoe et al. performed a randomized trial in 50 patients with hearing loss and tinnitus [54]. All received a HA, but only half of them received an additional motivational interview. Tinnitus Handicap Inventory improved significantly in all patients, though significantly more in the group receiving the motivational interview. In summary, the use of HAs is only a recommended option in patients with tinnitus and concurrent hearing loss due to the lack of sufficient evidence in the literature.

Cognitive Behavioral Therapy

Cognitive behavioral therapy (CBT) uses relaxation, cognitive restructuring of thoughts, and exposure to exacerbating situations in order to promote habituation. CBT may benefit patients with tinnitus. A Cochrane review by Martinez–Devesa included eight randomized controlled trials with 468 participants [55]. The primary outcome measure was subjective tinnitus loudness. Secondary outcome measures were quality of life and depression scores. CBT was compared to other therapies such as yoga, education, and minimal-contact education. The authors concluded that there was no significant difference in subjective tinnitus loudness, but there was a significant difference for quality-of-life scores as well as for depression scores. A meta-analysis including 18 studies on about 700 patients investigated the effect of CBT in randomized controlled studies on between-group design studies as well as within-group design studies [56]. The authors found that CBT was effective, especially for tinnitus annoyance. Effects on tinnitus loudness were only seen temporarily. Effects on psychological factors such as depression or anxiety were seen, but not at the same extent as for tinnitus annoyance.

CBT for tinnitus is conducted for 8–24 weeks in most studies, with weekly sessions [2]. Some studies include single therapy and group therapy. CBT can be delivered in person or remotely depending on the setup. One study has evaluated the long-term effects of CBT with a 15-year follow-up [57]. Four hundred thirty-four patients were treated with CBT in 1987 as in-patients. Fifteen years later these patients as well as a group of patients on a waiting list for therapy were assessed. Results showed significantly better results for the treatment group than for the control group when evaluating using the tinnitus questionnaire and visual analog scales for specific tinnitus variables (loudness, discomfort, control of tinnitus, stress, and general mood). The results also showed that 15 years after the conclusion of treatment symptoms were stable in comparison to the time of discharge. In conclusion, CBT is a fairly effective treatment without negative side effects, it is, however, time and cost intensive.

Sound Therapy

There are many different options for devices for sound therapy. Essentially there are four groups: environmental enrichment devices, open fit HAs, sound generators, and combination tinnitus instruments.

A large randomized controlled trial including 151 participants investigated the effect of sound therapy [58]. In this study, patients were randomized to one out of three groups. Group 1 underwent tinnitus retraining therapy which consisted of tinnitus-specific educational counseling and sound therapy. Group 2 received tinnitus-specific educational counseling and a placebo sound generator – patients and audiologists were blinded. Group 3 received a standard of care aimed at reducing negative cognitive, affective, physical, and behavioral reactions to tinnitus. They were also encouraged to use environmental sound enrichment but not sound generators. While there was a significant improvement of tinnitus in all groups, there was no meaningful difference between the treatment groups.

Drugs and Tinnitus

No medications have been shown to reduce tinnitus loudness or associated burdens significantly [2]. Intratympanic steroids have been investigated for tinnitus, as they have shown some beneficial effects as salvage therapy for patients with sudden sensorineural hearing loss [59]. Topak et al. performed a randomized controlled single-blinded trial with methylprednisolone and intratympanic placebo, applied three times over 3 weeks to patients with tinnitus [60]. The mean duration of tinnitus was 70 and 90 months in the two groups. There was no significant difference in tinnitus characteristics between the two groups (pre-treatment tinnitus intensity, tinnitus laterality, and tinnitus duration). Results showed that self-rated tinnitus loudness improved in both groups with no difference between drug and placebo. The tinnitus severity index questionnaire showed no difference between the two timepoints (before and after treatment) or between the two groups.

Araujo et al. and Choi et al. conducted similar studies on dexamethasone versus placebo [61, 62]. Both studies found an improvement in both groups, without a significant difference between drug and placebo. One of the main limitations of both trials was the low number of included patients ($n = 32$ and 36, respectively). Nevertheless, no studies have shown a benefit of intratympanic steroid injections over placebo and can therefore not be recommended.

Lidocaine is a further drug that used to be administered for persistent tinnitus. Lidocaine was administered intravenously and showed positive effects on tinnitus suppression [63, 64]. Due to substantial systemic side effects, this therapy was not continued [65]. Intratympanic lidocaine was administered while trying to circumvent side effects, which were encountered when applying it systemically. Podoshin et al. conducted a trial on 52 patients, who received intratympanic lidocaine [66]. All patients suffered from vertigo (and nausea/vomiting) for 4–6 hours after the instillation of lidocaine. Nine patients reported an improvement of tinnitus. In light of these side effects as well as limited results, lidocaine cannot be recommended as a treatment for patients with tinnitus.

Amitriptyline is a tricyclic antidepressant, which inhibits the reuptake of serotonin and noradrenaline almost equally and is used as an antidepressant as well as a therapy for insomnia. Nortriptyline inhibits the reuptake of norepinephrine as well as serotonin but to a lesser extent. Indications are similar to amitriptyline. Both medications have been studied in the context of tinnitus [67]. A placebo-controlled study on 37 patients (17 patients in the control group, 20 patients in the amitriptyline intervention group) evaluated audiometric results and tinnitus loudness as well as tinnitus questionnaires [68]. The authors reported a decrease in subjective tinnitus rating of 95% in the amitriptyline group as opposed to 12% in the placebo group. No other outcome, such as influence on insomnia, was reported. A further randomized study comparing amitriptyline to biofeedback showed that 43.5% of the latter group experienced tinnitus improvement, while the medication group only reported 27.5% tinnitus reduction. Nortriptyline was investigated in a single-blind, placebo-washout, nonrandomized pilot study in patients who also had major depression [69]. Of 19 included patients, 14 had a tinnitus improvement and 12 decided to continue to take the drug after the end of the study. The same study group continued to investigate the influence of nortriptyline on tinnitus and conducted a 12-week, double-blind, randomized controlled trial [70]. Nortriptyline showed superior results to placebo for depression scores, tinnitus-related disability, and loudness. None of the above-mentioned studies investigated the effect on insomnia or anxiety. Therefore, drug therapies should not be used to treat primary tinnitus, but should aim to target tinnitus-associated conditions such as headaches, stress and anxiety disorder, and insomnia.

Herbal and Other Supplements

G. biloba is a herbal supplement commonly associated with tinnitus therapy. Although several randomized controlled trials have been conducted as well as Cochrane reviews and many meta-analyses, the evidence of *G. biloba* is still not clear. Systematic reviews conclude that there is favorable efficacy, but a firm conclusion cannot be drawn [71]. In contrast, another meta-analysis states that 21.6% of *G. biloba*-treated patients experience benefit versus 18.4 of placebo-treated patients with an odds ratio of 1.24 [72]. The authors conclude that there is no benefit for *G. biloba*. Even more recent literature reviews cannot draw a final conclusion on the efficacy of this herb [73].

The American Academy of Otolaryngology – Head and Neck Surgery advises against the recommendation of *G. biloba* [2]. One of the main reasons to advise against the use of this herb is the suspicion of a platelet inhibitory effect, which could result in bleeding [74]. *G. biloba* was found to interact with anticoagulants and antiplatelet agents, as well as with anti-arrhythmias and antibiotics. The authors conclude that there is some concern for *G. biloba* and that it should be used cautiously in patients taking anesthetics, analgesics, anticoagulants, and antiplatelet agents[74].

Melatonin is a hormone involved in the sleep-wake cycle and an over-the-counter medication available in many countries for insomnia. A randomized clinical trial compared sertraline and melatonin in 70 tinnitus patients [75]. THI and severity of tinnitus were used as outcome measures. Both groups had a significant reduction of tinnitus, with greater efficacy in the melatonin group. It is important to note that the mentioned study, like many of the other studies cited in this chapter, is missing a control arm without treatment. A randomized, prospective, double-blind, placebo-controlled crossover trial was conducted with a 30-day period of 2 mg melatonin, which was followed or preceded by a thirty-day placebo treatment [76]. In said study, there was no statistically significant difference between THI scores. There was an improvement of sleeping in the treatment period compared to placebo. In summary, there is not sufficient evidence that melatonin improves tinnitus [2]. Given the small number of adverse effects, it might be considered in patients with tinnitus and insomnia [76].

Zinc is an essential trace element and has a role in cochlear physiology and in the synapses of the auditory system [77]. A Cochrane review conducted in 2016 concluded that there is no evidence that zinc can improve symptoms of tinnitus in adults [77]. To draw this conclusion, the authors included three trials with a total of 209 participants.

A randomized trial using Korean red ginseng was conducted and included three groups with a total of 61 patients [78]. The so-called control group was treated with 160 mg/day *G. biloba* extract. The two treatment groups received 1500 mg/day or 3000 mg/day of Korean red ginseng. Outcome measures were the THI, a visual analog scale, and a general quality of life questionnaire. There was some significant improvement for the higher dose Korean red ginseng group.

Cannabis and Tinnitus

Cannabis contains over 400 different chemicals, of which 9-tetrahydrocannabinol (THC) and cannabidiol (CBD) are by far the most researched and understood ingredients. THC leads to a euphoric feeling while CBD is a non-psychoactive substance associated with anticonvulsant, anxiolytic, and sedative effects [79–81]. Qian et al. recently (2020) reported on the results of a cross-sectional analysis of nationally representative data [82]. Data were collected from 2705 adults between 20 and 69 years, who had undergone audiometric testing, filled out questionnaires about tinnitus, drug use, current, and past medical status. The authors reported that the use of marijuana at least once per month for the previous year was significantly associated with tinnitus, even when accounting for variables such as age, gender, hearing thresholds, noise exposure, depression, anxiety, smoking, salicylate use, cardiovascular disease, hypertension, and diabetes. The use of other substances such as alcohol, cocaine, methamphetamine, and heroin was not associated with tinnitus. However, hearing loss, history of work noise exposure, and anxiety were not surprisingly also associated with tinnitus. The correlation to tinnitus was stronger for these factors than for use of marijuana. It is important to keep in mind that in the said study all variables were self-reported.

The Role of no Intervention

Tinnitus is classified as primary or secondary, with the former being a symptom without a known pathology. It can be bothersome and non-bothersome, acute and chronic. If patients have primary, non-bothersome, chronic tinnitus, can these patients be advised to not undergo any form of the above-mentioned, recommended treatments? What happens to patients with primary bothersome, persistent tinnitus, who do not undergo any treatment?

Phillips et al. conducted a meta-analysis on randomized controlled trials or observational studies utilizing a no-intervention or waiting-list group [83]. Only the data on patients who did not undergo treatment were used to perform the meta-analysis.

In total, 21 studies were included with 788 participants. The study concluded that there is a statistically significant decrease in the impact of tinnitus over time, with a 2.3% change in global tinnitus scores (as evaluated by questionnaires). The authors highlight the fact that there was a substantial heterogeneity between the studies. Eight studies reported depression changes, showing no significant change over time [83]. This meta-analysis reports on a waiting list or no-intervention time period of 1–52 weeks and average of 12 weeks.

This meta-analysis can only report on data provided by studies and therefor does not offer long-term outcomes of patients in non-treatment groups. It is, however, the most extensive analysis of a large, no intervention group published, so far. The authors do conclude that this study provides evidence that tinnitus does improve over time, a result that can cautiously be used for patient counseling.

Current Research/Developments

All above-mentioned therapies more or less focus on treating the distress caused by tinnitus instead of reducing the actual (phantom) sound. As already mentioned above, hearing loss, cochlear hair cell damage, or synaptopathy are thought to lead to a restructuring of the central nervous system and consequently to tinnitus. Although outside the scope of this chapter, ongoing research is focusing on drug, gene, and cell therapy development to reverse the neurodegenerative processes and treat sensorineural hearing loss. On the other hand, the top-down central modulation hypothesis is underlined by studies using functional brain imaging to detect responsible areas.

Conclusion

In conclusion, classification of tinnitus at first presentation is essential to exclude all possible causes of secondary tinnitus by performing a thorough history and examination. It is further important to distinguish bothersome from non-bothersome tinnitus, to decide on further necessary steps for treatment. HAs, especially for patients with audiometrically detectable hearing loss, should be offered for trial. Patient counseling and education, cognitive behavioral therapy, and optional sound therapy play an important role when treating patients with tinnitus. Drug therapeutics should be aimed to target tinnitus-associated conditions such as sudden hearing loss, TMJ disorder, headaches, stress and anxiety disorder, and insomnia. Therapies using neuromodulation are currently being investigated in various fields and show promising results.

References

1. Baguley D, McFerran D, Hall D. Tinnitus. Lancet. 2013;382(9904):1600–7.
2. Tunkel DE, Bauer CA, Sun GH, Rosenfeld RM, Chandrasekhar SS, Cunningham ER Jr, et al. Clinical practice guideline: tinnitus. Otolaryngol Head Neck Surg. 2014;151(2 Suppl):S1–S40.
3. Maes IH, Cima RF, Vlaeyen JW, Anteunis LJ, Joore MA. Tinnitus: a cost study. Ear Hear. 2013;34(4):508–14.
4. Stohler NA, Reinau D, Jick SS, Bodmer D, Meier CR. A study on the epidemiology of tinnitus in the United Kingdom. Clin Epidemiol. 2019;11:855–71.
5. Nyenhuis N, Zastrutzki S, Weise C, Jager B, Kroner-Herwig B. The efficacy of minimal contact interventions for acute tinnitus: a randomised controlled study. Cogn Behav Ther. 2013;42(2):127–38.
6. Tyler RS, Baker LJ. Difficulties experienced by tinnitus sufferers. J Speech Hear Disord. 1983;48(2):150–4.
7. Kamalski DM, Hoekstra CE, van Zanten BG, Grolman W, Rovers MM. Measuring disease-specific health-related quality of life to evaluate treatment outcomes in tinnitus patients: a systematic review. Otolaryngol Head Neck Surg. 2010;143(2):181–5.
8. Cima RF, Crombez G, Vlaeyen JW. Catastrophizing and fear of tinnitus predict quality of life in patients with chronic tinnitus. Ear Hear. 2011;32(5):634–41.
9. Lasisi AO, Gureje O. Prevalence of insomnia and impact on quality of life among community elderly subjects with tinnitus. Ann Otol Rhinol Laryngol. 2011;120(4):226–30.
10. Folmer RL, Griest SE, Meikle MB, Martin WH. Tinnitus severity, loudness, and depression. Otolaryngol Head Neck Surg. 1999;121(1):48–51.
11. Tyler RS, Gogel SA, Gehringer AK. Tinnitus activities treatment. Prog Brain Res. 2007;166:425–34.
12. Dawes P, Newall J, Stockdale D, Baguley DM. Natural history of tinnitus in adults: a cross-sectional and longitudinal analysis. BMJ Open. 2020;10(12):e041290.
13. Meikle MB, Henry JA, Griest SE, Stewart BJ, Abrams HB, McArdle R, et al. The tinnitus functional index: development of a new clinical measure for chronic, intrusive tinnitus. Ear Hear. 2012;33(2):153–76.

14. Jacquemin L, Mertens G, Van de Heyning P, Vanderveken OM, Topsakal V, De Hertogh W, et al. Sensitivity to change and convergent validity of the Tinnitus functional index (TFI) and the Tinnitus questionnaire (TQ): clinical and research perspectives. Hear Res. 2019;382:107796.
15. Langguth B, Kreuzer PM, Kleinjung T, De Ridder D. Tinnitus: causes and clinical management. Lancet Neurol. 2013;12(9):920–30.
16. Weisz N, Hartmann T, Dohrmann K, Schlee W, Norena A. High-frequency tinnitus without hearing loss does not mean absence of deafferentation. Hear Res. 2006;222(1–2):108–14.
17. De Ridder D, Elgoyhen AB, Romo R, Langguth B. Phantom percepts: tinnitus and pain as persisting aversive memory networks. Proc Natl Acad Sci U S A. 2011;108(20):8075–80.
18. Jackson P. A comparison of the effects of eighth nerve section with lidocaine on tinnitus. J Laryngol Otol. 1985;99(7):663–6.
19. Levine RA, Nam EC, Oron Y, Melcher JR. Evidence for a tinnitus subgroup responsive to somatosensory based treatment modalities. Prog Brain Res. 2007;166:195–207.
20. Ramirez LM, Ballesteros LE, Sandoval GP. Topical review: temporomandibular disorders in an integral otic symptom model. Int J Audiol. 2008;47(4):215–27.
21. Roberts LE, Eggermont JJ, Caspary DM, Shore SE, Melcher JR, Kaltenbach JA. Ringing ears: the neuroscience of tinnitus. J Neurosci. 2010;30(45):14972–9.
22. Shore S, Zhou J, Koehler S. Neural mechanisms underlying somatic tinnitus. Prog Brain Res. 2007;166:107–23.
23. Omidvar S, Jafari Z. Association between Tinnitus and temporomandibular disorders: a systematic review and meta-analysis. Ann Otol Rhinol Laryngol. 2019;128(7):662–75.
24. McEwen BS. Stress, adaptation, and disease. Allostasis and allostatic load. Ann N Y Acad Sci. 1998;840:33–44.
25. Lazarus RS. The psychology of stress and coping. Issues Ment Health Nurs. 1985;7(1–4):399–418.
26. Adler NE, Boyce T, Chesney MA, Cohen S, Folkman S, Kahn RL, et al. Socioeconomic status and health. The challenge of the gradient. Am Psychol. 1994;49(1):15–24.
27. Mazurek B, Boecking B, Brueggemann P. Association between stress and Tinnitus-new aspects. Otol Neurotol. 2019;40(4):e467–e73.
28. Horner KC. The emotional ear in stress. Neurosci Biobehav Rev. 2003;27(5):437–46.
29. Canlon B, Theorell T, Hasson D. Associations between stress and hearing problems in humans. Hear Res. 2013;295:9–15.
30. de Kloet ER, Joels M, Holsboer F. Stress and the brain: from adaptation to disease. Nat Rev Neurosci. 2005;6(6):463–75.
31. Spruill TM. Chronic psychosocial stress and hypertension. Curr Hypertens Rep. 2010;12(1):10–6.
32. Meltser I, Canlon B. The expression of mitogen-activated protein kinases and brain-derived neurotrophic factor in inferior colliculi after acoustic trauma. Neurobiol Dis. 2010;40(1):325–30.
33. Mazurek B, Haupt H, Joachim R, Klapp BF, Stover T, Szczepek AJ. Stress induces transient auditory hypersensitivity in rats. Hear Res. 2010;259(1–2):55–63.
34. Baigi A, Oden A, Almlid-Larsen V, Barrenas ML, Holgers KM. Tinnitus in the general population with a focus on noise and stress: a public health study. Ear Hear. 2011;32(6):787–9.
35. Hasson D, Theorell T, Wallen MB, Leineweber C, Canlon B. Stress and prevalence of hearing problems in the Swedish working population. BMC Public Health. 2011;11:130.
36. Halford JB, Anderson SD. Anxiety and depression in tinnitus sufferers. J Psychosom Res. 1991;35(4–5):383–90.
37. Hinton DE, Chhean D, Pich V, Hofmann SG, Barlow DH. Tinnitus among Cambodian refugees: relationship to PTSD severity. J Trauma Stress. 2006;19(4):541–6.
38. Holgers KM, Erlandsson SI, Barrenas ML. Predictive factors for the severity of tinnitus. Audiology. 2000;39(5):284–91.
39. Katzenell U, Segal S. Hyperacusis: review and clinical guidelines. Otol Neurotol. 2001;22(3):321–6. discussion 6-7
40. van Cruijsen N, Dullaart RP, Wit HP, Albers FW. Analysis of cortisol and other stress-related hormones in patients with Meniere's disease. Otol Neurotol. 2005;26(6):1214–9.

41. Biousse V, D'Anglejan-Chatillon J, Massiou H, Bousser MG. Head pain in non-traumatic carotid artery dissection: a series of 65 patients. Cephalalgia. 1994;14(1):33–6.
42. Kreuzer PM, Landgrebe M, Schecklmann M, Staudinger S, Langguth B, Group TRIDS. Trauma-associated tinnitus: audiological, demographic and clinical characteristics. PLoS One. 2012;7(9):e45599.
43. Sindhusake D, Golding M, Newall P, Rubin G, Jakobsen K, Mitchell P. Risk factors for tinnitus in a population of older adults: the blue mountains hearing study. Ear Hear. 2003;24(6):501–7.
44. Langguth B, Hund V, Busch V, Jurgens TP, Lainez JM, Landgrebe M, et al. Tinnitus and Headache. Biomed Res Int. 2015;2015:797416.
45. Nowaczewska M, Wicinski M, Straburzynski M, Kazmierczak W. The prevalence of different types of headache in patients with subjective Tinnitus and its influence on Tinnitus parameters: a prospective clinical study. Brain Sci. 2020;10(11)
46. Asnis GM, Majeed K, Henderson MA, Sylvester C, Thomas M, De La Garza R. An examination of the relationship between insomnia and Tinnitus: a review and recommendations. Clin Med Insights Psychiatry. 2018;9:1–8.
47. Asnis GM, Henderson MA, Thomas M, Kiran M, De La GR. Insomnia in Tinnitus patients: a prospective study finding a significant relationship. Int Tinnitus J. 2021;24(2):65–9.
48. Koning HM. Sleep disturbances associated with Tinnitus: reduce the maximal intensity of Tinnitus. Int Tinnitus J. 2019;23(1):64–8.
49. Hoare DJ, Kowalkowski VL, Kang S, Hall DA. Systematic review and meta-analyses of randomized controlled trials examining tinnitus management. Laryngoscope. 2011;121(7):1555–64.
50. Eysel-Gosepath K, Gerhards F, Schicketanz KH, Teichmann K, Benthien M. Attention diversion in tinnitus therapy. Comparison of the effects of different treatment methods. HNO. 2004;52(5):431–9.
51. Radunz CL, Okuyama CE, Branco-Barreiro FCA, Pereira RMS, Diniz SN. Clinical randomized trial study of hearing aids effectiveness in association with *Ginkgo biloba* extract (EGb 761) on tinnitus improvement. Braz J Otorhinolaryngol. 2020;86(6):734–42.
52. Henry JA, McMillan G, Dann S, Bennett K, Griest S, Theodoroff S, et al. Tinnitus management: randomized controlled Trial comparing extended-Wear hearing aids, conventional hearing aids, and combination instruments. J Am Acad Audiol. 2017;28(6):546–61.
53. Yakunina N, Lee WH, Ryu YJ, Nam EC. Tinnitus suppression effect of hearing aids in patients with high-frequency hearing loss: a randomized double-blind controlled Trial. Otol Neurotol. 2019;40(7):865–71.
54. Zarenoe R, Soderlund LL, Andersson G, Ledin T. Motivational interviewing as an adjunct to hearing rehabilitation for patients with Tinnitus: a randomized controlled pilot Trial. J Am Acad Audiol. 2016;27(8):669–76.
55. Martinez-Devesa P, Perera R, Theodoulou M, Waddell A. Cognitive behavioural therapy for tinnitus. Cochrane Database Syst Rev. 2010;9:CD005233.
56. Andersson G, Lyttkens L. A meta-analytic review of psychological treatments for tinnitus. Br J Audiol. 1999;33(4):201–10.
57. Goebel G, Kahl M, Arnold W, Fichter M. 15-year prospective follow-up study of behavioral therapy in a large sample of inpatients with chronic tinnitus. Acta Otolaryngol Suppl. 2006;556:70–9.
58. Tinnitus Retraining Therapy Trial Research Group, Scherer RW, Formby C. Effect of Tinnitus Retraining Therapy vs standard of care on Tinnitus-related quality of life: a randomized clinical Trial. JAMA Otolaryngol Head Neck Surg. 2019;145(7):597–608.
59. Stachler RJ, Chandrasekhar SS, Archer SM, Rosenfeld RM, Schwartz SR, Barrs DM, et al. Clinical practice guideline: sudden hearing loss. Otolaryngol Head Neck Surg. 2012;146(3 Suppl):S1–35.
60. Topak M, Sahin-Yilmaz A, Ozdoganoglu T, Yilmaz HB, Ozbay M, Kulekci M. Intratympanic methylprednisolone injections for subjective tinnitus. J Laryngol Otol. 2009;123(11):1221–5.
61. Araujo MF, Oliveira CA, Bahmad FM Jr. Intratympanic dexamethasone injections as a treatment for severe, disabling tinnitus: does it work? Arch Otolaryngol Head Neck Surg. 2005;131(2):113–7.

62. Choi SJ, Lee JB, Lim HJ, In SM, Kim JY, Bae KH, et al. Intratympanic dexamethasone injection for refractory tinnitus: prospective placebo-controlled study. Laryngoscope. 2013;123(11):2817–22.
63. Trellakis S, Lautermann J, Lehnerdt G. Lidocaine: neurobiological targets and effects on the auditory system. Prog Brain Res. 2007;166:303–22.
64. Israel JM, Connelly JS, McTigue ST, Brummett RE, Brown J. Lidocaine in the treatment of tinnitus aurium. A double-blind study Arch Otolaryngol. 1982;108(8):471–3.
65. Gil-Gouveia R, Goadsby PJ. Neuropsychiatric side-effects of lidocaine: examples from the treatment of headache and a review. Cephalalgia. 2009;29(5):496–508.
66. Podoshin L, Fradis M, David YB. Treatment of tinnitus by intratympanic instillation of lignocaine (lidocaine) 2 per cent through ventilation tubes. J Laryngol Otol. 1992;106(7):603–6.
67. Langguth B, Salvi R, Elgoyhen AB. Emerging pharmacotherapy of tinnitus. Expert Opin Emerg Drugs. 2009;14(4):687–702.
68. Bayar N, Boke B, Turan E, Belgin E. Efficacy of amitriptyline in the treatment of subjective tinnitus. J Otolaryngol. 2001;30(5):300–3.
69. Sullivan MD, Dobie RA, Sakai CS, Katon WJ. Treatment of depressed tinnitus patients with nortriptyline. Ann Otol Rhinol Laryngol. 1989;98(11):867–72.
70. Sullivan M, Katon W, Russo J, Dobie R, Sakai C. A randomized trial of nortriptyline for severe chronic tinnitus. Effects on depression, disability, and tinnitus symptoms. Arch Intern Med. 1993;153(19):2251–9.
71. Ernst E, Stevinson C. *Ginkgo biloba* for tinnitus: a review. Clin Otolaryngol Allied Sci. 1999;24(3):164–7.
72. Rejali D, Sivakumar A, Balaji N. *Ginkgo biloba* does not benefit patients with tinnitus: a randomized placebo-controlled double-blind trial and meta-analysis of randomized trials. Clin Otolaryngol Allied Sci. 2004;29(3):226–31.
73. Mahmoudian-Sani MR, Hashemzadeh-Chaleshtori M, Asadi-Samani M, Yang Q. *Ginkgo biloba* in the treatment of tinnitus: an updated literature review. Int Tinnitus J. 2017;21(1):58–62.
74. Posadzki P, Watson L, Ernst E. Herb-drug interactions: an overview of systematic reviews. Br J Clin Pharmacol. 2013;75(3):603–18.
75. Abtahi SH, Hashemi SM, Mahmoodi M, Nilforoush MH. Comparison of melatonin and sertraline therapies on Tinnitus: a randomized clinical Trial. Int J Prev Med. 2017;8:61.
76. Rosenberg SI, Silverstein H, Rowan PT, Olds MJ. Effect of melatonin on tinnitus. Laryngoscope. 1998;108(3):305–10.
77. Person OC, Puga ME, da Silva EM, Torloni MR. Zinc supplementation for tinnitus. Cochrane Database Syst Rev. 2016;2016(11):CD009832.
78. Kim TS, Lee HS, Chung JW. The effect of Korean red ginseng on symptoms and quality of life in chronic Tinnitus: a randomized. Open-Label Pilot Study J Audiol Otol. 2015;19(2):85–90.
79. Costa B, Trovato AE, Comelli F, Giagnoni G, Colleoni M. The non-psychoactive cannabis constituent cannabidiol is an orally effective therapeutic agent in rat chronic inflammatory and neuropathic pain. Eur J Pharmacol. 2007;556(1–3):75–83.
80. Chagas MH, Crippa JA, Zuardi AW, Hallak JE, Machado-de-Sousa JP, Hirotsu C, et al. Effects of acute systemic administration of cannabidiol on sleep-wake cycle in rats. J Psychopharmacol. 2013;27(3):312–6.
81. Narwani V, Bourdillon A, Nalamada K, Manes RP, Hildrew DM. Does cannabis alleviate tinnitus? A review of the current literature. Laryngoscope Investig Otolaryngol. 2020;5(6):1147–55.
82. Qian ZJ, Alyono JC. An association between marijuana use and tinnitus. Am J Otolaryngol. 2020;41(1):102314.
83. Phillips JS, McFerran DJ, Hall DA, Hoare DJ. The natural history of subjective tinnitus in adults: a systematic review and meta-analysis of no-intervention periods in controlled trials. Laryngoscope. 2018;128(1):217–27.

Head and Neck Manifestations of Fibromyalgia and Chronic Fatigue Syndrome

16

Swathi S. Rayasam, Flora Yan, and Ashley D. Agan

Introduction

Fibromyalgia (FM) and chronic fatigue syndrome (CFS) are both classified as functional somatic syndromes and can be characterized by varying degrees of myofascial pain and fatigue in the absence of objective causes [1, 2]. FM primarily involves chronic multifocal pain often musculoskeletal in nature and occurs in 2–5% of the population [3], whereas CFS is characterized by extreme fatigue with a prevalence of 0.5–2.5% [4]. CFS also takes on the name of myalgic encephalitis (ME) due to the nature of clinical symptoms revolving around myalgia, fatigue, and cognitive difficulties [5].

Although considered separate entities, FM and CFS have many overlapping symptoms with pain and fatigue both present in each, as well as a myriad of other findings such as headaches, cognitive dysfunction, stiffness, tenderness, depression, and other chronic pain syndromes such as low back and jaw pain [6]. For this reason, diagnosis of the two syndromes can be difficult and may require close attention to clinical symptom characterization. Even so, patients may often have concomitant FM and CFS, with Abbi et al. revealing that 34% of patients with CFS also have FM [7]. Additionally, it is estimated that both FM and CFS demonstrate a markedly higher prevalence of two to six-fold in women over men [1, 5–7]. FM more often affects people aged 55–64, whereas CFS is most often seen in patients from 20 to 40 years of age [7, 8].

S. S. Rayasam
University of Texas Southwestern Medical Center, Dallas, TX, USA

F. Yan
Temple University, Philadelphia, PA, USA

A. D. Agan (✉)
Department of Otolaryngology-Head and Neck Surgery, University of Texas Southwestern Medical Center, Dallas, TX, USA
e-mail: ashley.agan@utsouthwestern.edu

© The Author(s), under exclusive license to Springer Nature Switzerland AG 2023

B. W. Blakley, J. E. Blakley (eds.), *Functional Illness of the Head and Neck*,
https://doi.org/10.1007/978-3-031-12998-8_16

There have been multiple proposed diagnostic criteria of FM by two different organizations, the American College of Rheumatology (ACR) and the Analgesic, Anesthetic, and Addiction Clinical Trial Translations Innovations Opportunities and Networks (ACTTION) in conjunction with the American Pain Society (APS). The first diagnostic criteria for FM were developed by the ACR in 1990, focusing on having widespread pain throughout one's entire body along with a minimum number of 11 of 18 pre-determined tender spots for at least 3 months of symptom duration [1]. However, many found the physical examination of tender spots to be impractical [9]. These initial diagnostic criteria also did not consider other symptoms such as fatigue and sleep difficulties. Subsequently, in 2010, the ACR proposed a new set of diagnostic criteria for FM, this time focusing on the use of two subjective symptom scales: the Widespread Pain Index (WPI) and the symptom severity scale (SSS) (Table 16.1) [9]. The WPI focused on characterizing areas of pain, with 19 areas being examined. The use of the WPI index shifted the focus from chronic widespread pain to multisite pain, or a count of the number of body sites with pain. The SSS tested for other clinical symptoms such as cognitive deficits, fatigue, muscle weakness, and waking up unrefreshed. These indices were then modified multiple times, with the latest proposed changes to the 2010 ACR FM

Table 16.1 Diagnostic Criteria for Fibromyalgia and Chronic Fatigue Syndrome

Fibromyalgia			
2010 ACR	2016 modification of 2010 ACR	AAPT criteria	Chronic Fatigue Syndrome by IOM
• WPI[a] >7 and SSS[b] >5 OR WPI 3–6 and SSS >9 • 3-month duration of symptoms • No other disorder to explain the plain	• Involvement of 4 of 5 body sites (left upper, right upper, left lower, right lower, axial) • WPI ≥7 and SSS ≥5 OR WPI 4–6 and SSS ≥9 • 3-month duration of symptoms	• Multisite pain including ≥6 of 9 sites (head, R/L arm, chest, abdomen, upper back and spine, lower back and spine, R/L leg) • Moderate to severe sleep problems OR fatigue • 3-month duration of symptoms	• The following three symptoms: – Impairment of ability to engage in occupational, educational, social, or personal activities accompanied by fatigue not alleviated with rest for at least 6 months – Post-exertional malaise – Unrefreshing sleep • And at least 1 of the following: – Cognitive impairment – Orthostatic intolerance

ACR American college of rheumatology, *AAPT* Analgesic, Anesthetic, and Addiction Clinical Trial Translations Innovations Opportunities and Networks –American Pain Society Pain Taxonomy, *IOM* Institute of Medicine, *L* left, *R* right, *SSS* symptom severity scale, *WPI* widespread pain index

[a]The WPI measure the number of painful body regions from a list of 19 areas (R/L jaw, neck, R/L shoulder girdle, R/L upper arm, R/L lower arm, chest, abdomen, upper back, lower back, R/L hip, R/L upper leg, R/L lower leg)

[b]The SSS measures the degree of fatigue, feeling unrefreshed after sleep, cognitive symptoms, and number of general somatic symptoms

diagnostic criteria occurring in 2016. The 2016 modifications added another criterion: pain must be present in at least four of five body regions (composed of four quadrants and the axial area) [10]. This was in order to reduce the misclassification of regional pain syndrome with FM [11].

In a similar vein, the ACTTION-APS working group formed the ACTTION-APS Pain Taxonomy (AAPT) to establish a set of diagnostic criteria apart from the ACR in order to establish a common taxonomy across all chronic pain syndromes (including FM) and also to increase ease of use and clarity of criteria in the clinical setting [12]. The APPT focused on using an evidence-based approach and listed core diagnostic criteria that included the use of multisite pain counts (≥6 from a total of 9 different sites), other clinical symptoms outside of pain (sleep problems or fatigue), and a total duration of at least 3 months (Table 16.1) [13]. In addition to this, the AAPT recognized FM to be a multifaceted and heterogeneous disease state, and defined other common features, medical co-morbidities, and psychosocial factors that may be related to FM, however not necessary for diagnosis. As no diagnostic criteria have been deemed the gold standard for FM, both the ACR and APPT criteria have been used in clinical practice.

Similar to FM, the diagnostic criteria of CFS have varied over time, with previous definitions including symptoms such as post-exertional malaise, impaired concentration or memory, unrefreshing sleep, chronic pharyngitis, tender lymphadenopathy, headaches, muscle pain, or arthritic symptoms [2]. The most recent diagnostic criteria established by the Institute of Medicine in 2015 require three main symptoms: fatigue not alleviated by rest for 6 months in duration, post-exertional malaise, and unrefreshing sleep, with at least one of the following: cognitive impairment or orthostatic intolerance [14]. Table 16.1 demonstrates an overview of the diagnostic criteria for FM and CFS.

Multiple hypotheses have postulated the etiology of CFS and FM and have attributed these disease states to central sensitization, potential genetic predisposition, immune dysregulation/chronic inflammation, post-viral sequelae, or environmental factors. Central sensitization, also known as an increased central neuronal responsiveness contributing to allodynia and hyperalgesia, has been long established as a theory regarding the chronic widespread pain seen in FM. The reason for this hyper-responsiveness may be due to the alterations in neuromodulatory compounds (e.g., substance P) or abnormalities of neurological structures fundamental to pain perception [15]. More recently, altered pain thresholds in patients with CFS may provide support for central sensitization to play a role in CFS as well [15].

A commonly considered etiology of CFS was that of viral origin. Specifically, it was previously thought that CFS arose in the setting of viral triggers such as Epstein-Barr virus (EBV), cytomegalovirus (CMV), and human herpesviruses (HHV) [16]. These viruses were thought to incite immune dysregulation even following the resolution of the viral illness itself, leading to a chronic viral infection that manifests itself in the form of CFS. In fact, viral-like illnesses may precede CFS infections in about 50–80% of cases [17]. Nevertheless, the direct viral causation of CFS has not been confirmed and remains an area of active investigation.

Whatever the etiology, many consider severity and management of FM/CFS in the context of a biopsychosocial model [2]. Specifically, it has been seen that lifestyle factors such as acute stress or lack of personal and/or professional life satisfaction can trigger flare-ups in patients with FM [1]. It is clear that both FM and CFS can be so functionally impairing that they make daily activities of living cumbersome, and a greater portion of patients with FM (31% vs. 2% in healthy controls) report some form of work disability attributed to their medical condition [18]. Likewise, patients with CFS have reported a 54% reduction in work productivity compared to those without [19].

Interestingly, in addition to the commonly associated symptoms of pain and fatigue, many patients with FM/CFS may also experience a number of otolaryngologic symptoms or co-morbidities, such as hearing loss, tinnitus, allergic rhinitis, functional voice disorders, chronic pharyngitis, as well as temporomandibular joint disorders (TMD) (see Fig. 16.1). As these symptoms are not a part of either diagnostic criteria for FM or CFS, many times they can be overlooked. Therefore, the association between FM/CFS and otolaryngologic symptoms is further characterized in this chapter to provide readers with a heightened awareness of the overlap of these conditions.

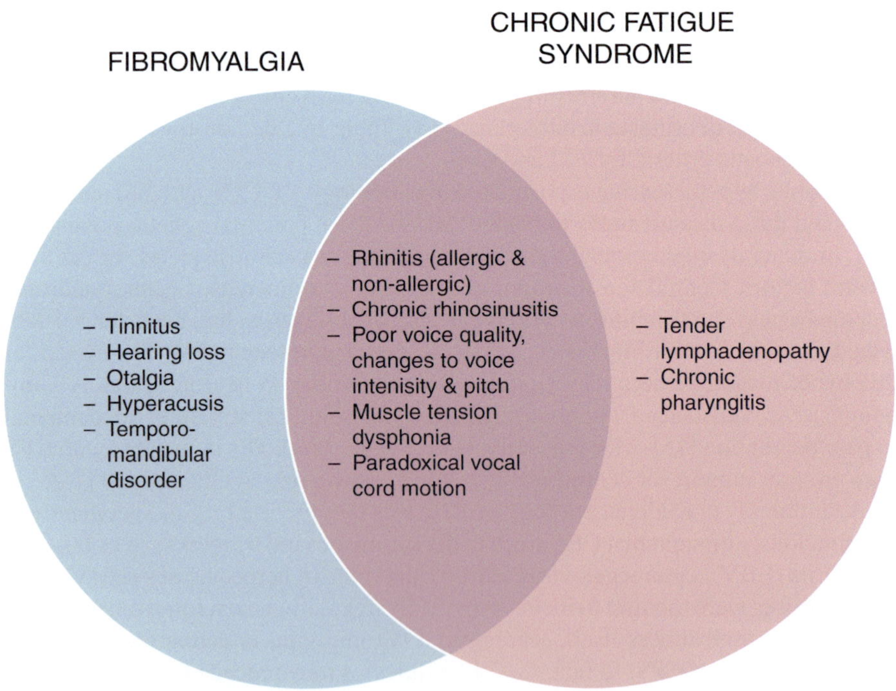

Fig. 16.1 Key otolaryngologic symptoms of fibromyalgia and chronic fatigue syndrome

Otology

FM has been associated with various otologic symptoms including hearing loss, tinnitus, otalgia, and hyperacusis. It has been hypothesized that changes in central sensitization and perception of sensory stimuli may explain the development of otologic findings after FM onset. To our knowledge, no research has found significant otologic symptoms associated with CFS, so the following section will be limited to a discussion of FM.

Many patients with FM report some degree of subjective, or self-reported, hearing loss following a diagnosis of FM. Bayazit et al. found that 12.5% of patients with FM who were enrolled in their study reported a subjective hearing loss on the Fibromyalgia Impact Questionnaire [20]. Similarly, Koca et al. shared that 45.4% of patients with FM reported "hearing problems," which was significantly higher than healthy volunteers (13.6%) [21]. Stranden et al. also reported that patients with FM are more likely to report subjective hearing loss [22]. Interestingly, they adjusted their measurement for audiometrically measured hearing loss; that is, the patients with FM reported subjective hearing loss more than the non-FM controls when matched for objective hearing threshold. However, while self-reported subjective hearing loss has a frequently reported association with fibromyalgia, the same cannot be said definitively for objectively measured hearing loss.

Objective hearing loss is commonly evaluated by electrophysiology studies, such as auditory brainstem measuring or otoacoustic emissions testing, and by audiometry, in which increases in hearing thresholds represent hearing loss. For the patients with FM who reported subjective hearing loss in Bayazit's study, no objective hearing loss was reported based on the pure-tone average and speech discrimination score components of audiometric analysis [20]. Interestingly, Koca's audiometry revealed a significant difference in hearing assessment findings between patients with FM and healthy volunteers, with patients with FM having higher hearing thresholds, and thus more hearing loss, across all frequencies (250 to 12,000 Hz) [21]. The type of hearing loss (sensorineural vs. conductive) was not specified. Notably, none of the patients in Koca's study had a history of hearing loss prior to audiometry performed during this study. Le et al. performed a large study in which patients with FM presented with a higher incidence of hearing loss than the control group [23]. Moreover, those with FM had a significantly higher risk for overall (1.46-fold), conductive (1.34-fold), sensorineural (1.46-fold), and mixed (1.56-fold) hearing loss. Patients with FM were found to have a higher risk of sensorineural hearing loss than conductive hearing loss, and among those with sensorineural hearing loss, bilateral sensory hearing loss was the most common. There is plenty of research conveying that FM patients more frequently report subjective hearing loss, but the connection between FM and objectively measured hearing loss is less clear and requires further study. Studies have not discussed treatment for hearing loss specifically in FM patients. However, hearing aids and other hearing rehabilitation devices are considered the mainstay of treatment for sensorineural hearing loss in general and should be considered in this population.

Subjective tinnitus is another otologic finding that has been associated with FM, with many patients experiencing tinnitus sometime after the onset of FM. Koca et al. shared that over half of their patients with FM (63.6%) had self-reported tinnitus when asked to select "yes" or "no" for the presence of the sensation [21]. Bayazit et al. similarly reported the presence of subjective tinnitus in their group of patients with FM (16.7%), which was a far lesser prevalence than other studies, but still more than the prevalence of tinnitus in the general American population (9.6%) [20, 24]. Iikuni et al. evaluated the time point at which patients experienced tinnitus, either before FM onset or after diagnosis of FM, and demonstrated that there was a significant increase in reported subjective tinnitus after FM onset [25]. Additionally, Cil et al. found that 74.3% of their patients with FM had self-reported tinnitus as identified using the Tinnitus Handicap Inventory (THI) [26]. This questionnaire was again administered after patients underwent a trial of pharmacologic treatment of either Pregabalin or Duloxetine. Interestingly, taking medication was found to significantly decrease subjective tinnitus as measured by the THI, but no significant difference was found between the treatment results of the two medications. These findings suggest that patients with FM may develop subjective tinnitus at a higher rate than the general population and that they may be amenable to pharmacologic treatments such as anti-convulsants, anti-depressants, and muscle relaxants [27].

Otalgia has also been seen to manifest after FM onset. Iikuni et al. evaluated whether patients experienced chronic earache in one or both ears before FM onset as well as at the time of the study [25]. The team discovered a significant increase in reported otalgia in one or both ears after FM onset in this group. Likewise, Da Silva et al. reported that significantly more patients with FM complained of bilateral earache when compared with non-FM controls despite being on a treatment regimen for FM most commonly consisting of antidepressants, physical therapy, or opioids, at the time of the study [28]. It is unknown whether FM can cause otalgia. In patients presenting with otalgia, it is important to evaluate for all possible causes including malignancies of the skull base, pharynx, and larynx. Currently, we recommend that FM patients with otalgia that cannot be attributed to any other source be treated conservatively with analgesics at the discretion of the provider.

The development of hyperacusis is a less-discussed phenomenon that may occur in patients with FM and is defined by markedly decreased tolerance for sounds at ordinary intensities. Geisser et al. used two different methods to evaluate the presence of hyperacusis in their study population of patients with FM and healthy controls [29]. First, they administered a hyperacusis questionnaire, which asked participants to answer questions about what real-life sounds are bothersome and at what volume. The questionnaire was scored to convey the degree of hearing sensitivity. Geisser's group found that patients with FM experienced a significantly higher hearing sensitivity than controls [29]. The second test that the group administered obtained loudness discomfort levels for each ear separately and then averaged the numbers to provide a single score. They found that patients with FM needed significantly lower auditory stimulation to report low, medium, and high pain intensity than healthy control subjects. Furthermore, Suhnan et al. conducted a literature review and concluded that FM patients may be more likely to develop hyperacusis as the disease progresses [30]. In terms of treatment, retraining and acoustic therapies traditionally used to alleviate hyperacusis may be worthwhile in this patient population with FM [31].

As previously mentioned, FM is a disorder in which there is an alteration in central sensitization leading to hyper-responsiveness to certain stimuli and pain signals. It is hypothesized that the otology symptoms associated with FM also stem from this phenomenon. Suhnan et al. examined global central sensitization in the context of hyperacusis and offered a few possible mechanistic explanations for this finding [30]. One idea they presented is that FM patients may experience a disturbance in pain-inhibitory mechanisms, leading to sensitization of both pain-specific and more general neurons in the spinal dorsal horn. They supported this claim by citing the weakened pain-inhibitory effect of noradrenaline in FM patients. The group concluded that otologic findings may be a result of the auditory system having connections to these very nociceptor centers in the brain due to a potential relationship between the processing of sound and bodily pressure-pain stimuli. Montoya et al. expounded on this idea by looking at pressure-pain thresholds in the hands and event-related brain potentials for patients with FM [32]. They found that these patients had abnormal processing of pain-related information as well as altered adaptation to pain stimuli. The group claimed that their findings could explain the presence of otologic symptoms in FM. Standen, Le, and Bayazit have independently offered their support in favor of this possible mechanism to explain the presence of hearing loss, tinnitus, and otalgia in patients [20, 22, 23]. Likewise, Iikuni et al. supported the idea that a central perceptual issue was behind these symptoms because they found no objective evidence of otologic changes [25]. A processing abnormality would also explain why only some patients experience these alterations.

Dizziness

Dizziness is a neuro-otological finding that may be seen in patients with FM and CFS. Koca et al. administered a Dizziness Handicap Inventory (DHI) to patients with FM to evaluate self-perceived handicapping effects of dizziness on quality of life, where a score is computed out of 100 with higher numbers representing the worse quality of life [21]. They found that the mean score was 24.6 for those with FM which was significantly higher than the control group's mean score of 11.7. Sawada et al. asked a group of patients with FM to complete a DHI and a version of the Fibromyalgia Impact Questionnaire (JFIQ) [33]. They found that

30.4% of the patients complained of dizziness, and the DHI and JFIQ scores were found to be correlated, meaning that the degree of subjective pain accompanying FM correlates with the degree of distress due to dizziness. It is hypothesized that the presence of dizziness in patients with FM can also be attributed to central sensitivity [21, 33]. Similarly, Collin et al. found that 58.2% of patients with CFS self-reported dizziness, and this information was used to sort patients into CFS phenotypes [34]. Garner et al. asked patients with CFS and healthy controls to use the Gracely Box Scale to self-rate their level of dizziness while recumbent and while standing [35]. They found that 38% of patients with CFS had recumbent dizziness and 72% of patients with CFS had standing dizziness, which was both significantly higher than healthy controls. Serotonergic medications, vestibular rehabilitation therapy, or psychotherapy may be considered for dizziness in patients with FM or CFS.

Rhinology

Both FM and CRS have been associated with a number of rhinological conditions, namely non-allergic rhinitis (NAR) and allergic rhinitis (AR) as well as chronic rhinosinusitis (CRS). In fact, the prevalence rate of FM in patients with rhinitis has ranged from 15–38% [36–38]. Additionally, when specifically examining patients with FM and/or CFS, rhinitis symptoms have been seen in 66–80% of patients [36, 39, 40]. Both positive and negative allergy skin tests resulted for these patients, making atopy a potential, however possibly not all-encompassing, a link between FM/CFS and rhinitis. In one study, nasal steroids were shown to be ineffective for the treatment of rhinitis in patients with CFS, with Kakumanu et al. revealing no significant differences in non-allergic rhinitis severity scores between use of nasal corticosteroids and saline spray as a placebo [41]. This might suggest patients with CFS may not respond to standard medical treatment for rhinitis [40]. Patients with both FM/CFS and rhinitis symptoms also appear to have a lower quality of life compared to those with rhinitis alone. Specifically, Gultana et al. demonstrated that a cohort of patients with concurrent FM and AR had significantly higher Rhinoconjunctivitis Quality of Life Questionnaire (RQLQ) and Nottingham Health Profile (NHP) scores, translating to poorer quality of life [37]. The largest differences in quality of life were seen in the following RQLQ domains: sleep, nasal problems, and emotions.

Numerous hypotheses have been investigated to explain the coexisting symptoms of NAR/AR and FM. Gultuna et al. proposed neurogenic inflammation to be a potential shared mechanism of AR and FM. It has been seen that a nasal allergen challenge, to simulate conditions of AR, results in releases of neuropeptides such as substance P and calcitonin gene-related peptides, which have also been under investigation in the pathogenesis of FM. Regarding another popular hypothesis that has been previously mentioned, many have attributed the common link between NAR/AR and FM, CFS, as well as other functional syndromes, to the role of central sensitization across these conditions.

Even more often than nasal congestion, patients with CFS may frequently experience symptoms of rhinosinusitis including facial pressure, frontal headache, and postnasal drip [40, 42]. The overall presence of sinus disease in patients with FM and CRS has not been well elucidated, however, Soler et al. did demonstrate a 9% prevalence of an FM diagnosis in a cohort of patients with medically refractory CRS versus 2–5% of FM in the general population [3, 43]. Fatigue is a commonly reported symptom in all patients with CRS [44]; Reh et al. reported that fatigue trumped congestion or nasal discharge as the most debilitating CRS symptom in 14% of patients with CRS as diagnosed by the clinical practice guidelines from the American Academy of Otolaryngology [45]. This demonstrates that fatigue may be an overlapping symptom in CRS and CFS.

In patients with CRS and FM who are refractory to medical management, surgical intervention may be appropriate. Improvement of quality of life and reduction of fatigue following endoscopic sinus surgery for CRS is comparable for patients with and without FM. Some may attribute this to result from relief of nasal obstruction, a decrease in inflammatory systemic mediators, or from a decrease in disease-associated emotional stress. Whatever the reason, Sautter et al. demonstrated that patients with FM and CRS had higher baseline fatigue visual analog scale (VAS) scores than patients with CRS alone and experienced a greater reduction of fatigue following surgery [44]. Soler et al. similarly found patients with both FM and CRS to have a poorer baseline quality of life compared to patients with CRS alone, as seen by the elevated rhinosinusitis disability index (RSDI) and chronic sinusitis survey (CSS) [43]. Patients with FM and CRS had comparable improvement in quality of life measurements as compared to patients with CRS alone following ESS. Altogether, symptoms of rhinitis and rhinosinusitis are prevalent in patients with FM and/or CFS, and can dramatically contribute to a poorer quality of life. Notwithstanding, management of rhinitis in patients with FM/CRS should follow routine treatment paradigms as those in non-FM/CRS patients.

Laryngology

Patients with FM or CFS have been seen to present with alterations to voice quality as well as a number of functional laryngological disorders. Gurbuzler et al. hypothesized that changes in voice intensity and pitch may be prevalent among patients with FM, as voice is dependent on both air expiration from the lungs as well as the vibrations from the oscillating vocal folds, and FM patients had been seen to have decreased respiratory muscle strength [46, 47]. In a cohort of 30 patients with FM, Gurbuzler et al. found significant subjective voice difference between patients with FM and the control group when comparing two administered scales: the grade, roughness, breathiness, asthenia and strain (GRBAS) scale and the Voice Handicap Index (VHI-10) [46]. The GRBAS scale is assessed by an external individual listening to and grading the quality of the patient's voice. The VHI-10 is a patient's self-assessment of how changes in their voice have affected their daily life. Specifically, patients with FM had a significantly higher VHI-10 and GRBAS scores than patients in the control group, indicating impaired perceived voice quality. Additionally, patients with FM were also found to have a shorter maximum phonation time and a decrease in voice intensity.

Functional laryngological disorders have also been associated with patients with FM and CFS and can include muscle tension dysphonia (MTD) and paradoxical vocal fold motion disorder [48]. Prevalence of these laryngological disorders among patients with FM and CFS is not well known, however, it has been investigated by Piersiala et al. in an investigation of 215 patients with a chronic pain syndrome (CPS) (including patients with FM, CFS, or irritable bowel syndrome (IBS)) versus 4034 control patients [49]. Patients with CPS were more likely to have MTD and paradoxical vocal cord motion, and less likely to have laryngeal or airway pathology such as vocal fold lesions or anatomical airway alterations like glottic or tracheal stenosis. In fact, patients with a CPS had 1.8 increased odds of having muscle tension dysphonia and 2.5 increased odds of having paradoxical vocal fold motion over control patients. Although Piersiala et al. did not examine the FM and CFS patients separately from the IBS patients, these conclusions may still be pertinent in our discussion of FM and CFS. The results of Piersiala et al. propose two major considerations in that (1) the diagnosis of FM or CFS is a risk factor for MTD development and/or (2) that FM/CFS and MTD have similar underlying pathophysiology [48, 49]. In addition to this, the prevalence of FM and CFS was studied in patients with MTD, with Craig et al. examining a group of 153 patients with MTD. It was noted that 30% had other comorbidities, including 8% with FM and 1.3% with CFS [50].

Overall, patients with FM and CFS may present with poorer voice quality and experience concomitant functional laryngological disorders such as MTD and paradoxical vocal fold motion. Notwithstanding, the degree of disorder and treatment efficacy in our patient population of interest may require further investigation.

Temporomandibular Disorders

Temporomandibular disorders (TMD), defined as any symptoms or signs associated with the temporomandibular joint, have been found to often accompany FM. Truta et al. highlighted a phenomenon referred to as masticatory FM, in which patients experience pain while using their chewing muscles, as well as tenderness to palpation in the setting of normal radiographic imaging [51]. Truta et al. also recommended that this variation of FM be treated first with antispasmodics with central analgesic properties, followed by orthotics or physical, behavioral, or pharmacologic treatment based on response. In a review of 19 studies, Ayouni et al. found a strong association between TMD and FM, demonstrating that patients with FM had around an 80% prevalence of

TMD signs/symptoms such as temporomandibular joint pain, along with tenderness to palpation along muscles of mastication [28, 52–54]. TMD prevalence was also found to be significantly higher in FM (53%) than in failed back syndrome (11%), the latter of which served as a chronic pain control group [55]. Moreover, Leblebici et al. reported that 52% of patients with TMD also had FM, and Velly et al. reported that the presence of FM predicted the persistence of clinically significant TMJ pain after 18 months, without prescribed treatment (OR 2.48, $p = 0.02$) [54, 56]. It was also concluded that in patients with FM, the pressure-pain threshold in bilateral trigeminal areas was lower than in healthy controls. The authors commented on these findings by similarly suggesting that alterations in central processing mechanisms could serve as an explanation. It is important to be aware that patients with FM may develop TMD, and vice versa.

Chronic Pharyngitis (Table 16.2)

CFS is thought to occasionally present with chronic pharyngitis or a seronegative EBV-like presentation. In fact, chronic pharyngitis as a symptom has been a previous diagnostic criterion of CFS (2). Collin et al. organized a group of CFS patients into 6 symptom-based phenotypes, of which one was sore throat/painful lymph nodes, and found that only 4.5% of the patient population was categorized as this phenotype [34]. Similarly, other studies, such as Hickie et al., have also used sore throat as part of their inclusion criteria in CFS patients, and Sullivan et al. further reported that 12% of self-reported fatigued patients without formal CFS diagnosis complained of sore throat [57, 58]. Patients with CFS of the sore throat phenotype comprised a very small percentage of all CFS patients and additionally had markedly lower fatigue scores and higher physical function scores than other patients with CFS, demonstrating that chronic pharyngitis is prevalent, but not pervasive in all patients with CFS [34, 58].

Conclusions

This chapter has outlined specific otolaryngologic symptoms that have been observed in FM and CFS. The notable prevalence of these symptoms suggests that clinicians should not only monitor patients with FM and/or CFS for the development of head and neck symptoms but also should increase their diagnostic index of suspicion for FM and CFS in healthy patients who have a new development of these symptoms. Future directions should focus on revealing the mechanisms responsible for the otolaryngologic findings in these two functional disorders. Investigation of these pathophysiologic pathways will allow for the development of targeted management or treatment regimes.

Table 16.2 Overview of literature regarding FM/CFS and ENT-related clinical symptoms

Study (year)	ENT-related disease	Design	Population (n)	Outcome	Conclusions
Gurbuzler (2013)	Dysphonia	Prospective cohort	FM (31) versus controls (31)	Grade, roughness, breathiness, asthenia, and strain (GRBAS) voice scale; VHI-10; laryngostroboscopy, acoustic analysis, maximum phonation time	Patients with FM had poorer perceived voice quality over controls, with a VHI-10 score of 7.9 vs. 1.3 ($p < 0.001$) and a GRBAS scale of 2.5 vs. 0.6 ($p < 0.001$).
Piersiala (2020)	Muscle tension dysphonia, paradoxical vocal cord paralysis	Retrospective cohort	Patients with a CPS (215) versus controls (4034)	Prevalence and odds ratios of different voice and functional voice disorders, laryngeal pathology, and airway/swallowing problems	Patients with CPS were more likely to present with muscle tension dysphonia (OR 1.9, 95% CI) or paradoxical vocal cord paralysis (OR 2.5, 95% CI) and less likely to present with laryngeal pathology (OR 0.77, 95% CI) or airway problems (OR 0.47, 95% CI)
Craig (2015)	Laryngology	Retrospective cohort	Patients with muscle tension dysphonia (153)	Changes in VHI scores following differing treatment options (voice therapy alone or with physical therapy, physical therapy alone, no treatment); prevalence of comorbidities including FM and CFS.	30% of patients with MTD had a comorbid condition including 8% with FM and 1.3% with CFS. Presence of comorbidities had no effect on baseline VHI scores or VHI improvement following treatment.
Gultana (2019)	Rhinitis	Retrospective cohort	Patients with AR (105)	Prevalence of FM and impact on quality of life using RQLQ and NHP scores	Prevalence rate of FM in patients with AR was 32%. Patients with both FM and AR have decreased RQLQ and NHP scores.
Tsiakiris (2017)	Rhinitis	Retrospective cohort	Patients with AR (298), allergic asthma (164) versus controls (2876)	Prevalence of functional somatic syndromes (FM, irritable bowel syndrome, migraine) expressed using OR	Prevalence rate of FM in patients with AR was 15%. Patients with AR had an adjusted OR of 3.5 (95% CI 2.0–6.4) over controls of having FM.

Cleveland (1992)	Rhinitis	Prospective cohort	Patients with rhinitis (allergic and non-allergic) (48)	Prevalence of symptoms of rhinitis including congestion, rhinorrhea, postnasal drip. Prevalence of FM per 1990 ACR criteria.	Prevalence rate of FM in patients with rhinitis was 38%.
Michaud (2006)	Sinus-related symptoms	Retrospective cohort	Patients with rheumatic arthritis (7243), osteoarthritis (1667), and FM (447)	Rate of physician visits for sinus problems in last 6 months from time of study, lifetime and rates of over the counter and prescription sinus medications	Prevalence rate of sinus problems in patients with FM in the last 6 months or at any time point was 25% and 63%, respectively. Of patients with FM, 37% and 35% used OTC or prescription sinus medication respectively.
Sautter (2008)	CRS	Prospective cohort	Patients with CRS (272)	Changes in fatigue following endoscopic sinus surgery evaluated using a 10-point VAS	Prevalence rate of FM in patients with CRS was 5%. Following ESS, patients with CRS and FM showed greater reductions in fatigue than patients with CRS alone.
Soler (2008)	CRS	Prospective cohort, case–control analysis	Patients with CRS (283)	Changes in QOL scores following endoscopic sinus surgery including the RSDI and CSS	Prevalence rate of FM in patients with CRS was 9%. Following ESS, patients with CRS with FM showed comparable rates of improvement in QOL compared to patients with CRS without FM.
Bayazit (2002)	Hearing loss, tinnitus	Prospective cross-sectional	Patients with FM (25)	Subjective hearing loss using FM impact questionnaire; subjective tinnitus using patient's history and standard otolaryngologic examination including audiologic assessment.	12.5% of FM patients reported subjective hearing loss with normal objective otolaryngologic examinations. 16.7% of FM patients reported subjective tinnitus.
Koca (2018)	Hearing loss, tinnitus	Prospective cross-sectional	Patients with FM (45) versus controls (45)	Subjective hearing problems and tinnitus using questionnaire; audiogram and tympanogram for objective hearing loss.	Self-reported hearing problems ($P < 0.001$) and tinnitus ($P < 0.001$) were significantly higher in FM group than controls. Significant difference found between two groups in audiometry at frequencies 250–12,000 Hz.

(continued)

Table 16.2 (continued)

Study (year)	ENT-related disease	Design	Population (n)	Outcome	Conclusions
Le (2020)	Hearing loss	Retrospective cohort	Patients with FM (55169) versus controls (110338)	Prevalence of general and hearing loss subtypes	FM group had a higher incidence of hearing loss than the control group (4.03 vs. 2.33 per 1000 person-years). FM patients had 1.46-fold higher risk for hearing loss. Diabetes, hypertension, and Meniere's disease increase risk of objective hearing loss in FM patients.
Standen (2016)	Hearing loss	Retrospective cross-sectional	Patients with subjective hearing loss (44494)	Prevalence of FM.	Prevalence of FM in patients with hearing loss was 3.3%. Those with FM had increased probability of reporting subjective hearing loss compared to non-FM controls matched for objective hearing loss level (OR 5.2 for women and 4.4 for men).
Cil (2020)	Tinnitus	Randomized control trial	Patients with FM (101)	Prevalence of self-reported tinnitus; subjective level of tinnitus before and after treatment with pregabalin or duloxetine using tinnitus handicap inventory.	Prevalence of tinnitus was 74% in patients with FM. Tinnitus level after treatment was significantly lower than before ($P < 0.001$). No significant difference between pregabalin and duloxetine in a change in tinnitus level.
Iikuni (2013)	Tinnitus, otalgia	Retrospective cohort	Patients with FM (21)	Prevalence of recalled and self-reported tinnitus and otalgia before and after FM onset.	Prevalence of tinnitus and otalgia in patients with FM was 78% and 40%, respectively. Significant post-FM increase in tinnitus and otalgia ($P < 0.001$; $P < 0.001$).
Da Silva (2012)	Otalgia	Prospective cross-sectional	Patients with FM (26) versus controls (26).	Evaluation of orofacial pain.	Significantly more patients with FM reported earache compared to controls ($P = 0.038$).
Geisser (2008)	Hyperacusis	Prospective cross-sectional	Patients with FM (31) versus controls (29)	Prevalence and level of hyperacusis based on hyperacusis questionnaire.	Patients with FM experienced higher hearing sensitivity than controls and required significantly lower auditory stimulation to report a level of pain intensity.

Suhnan (2017)	Hyperacusis, central sensitization	Literature review	Patients with hyperacusis (10 papers)	Prevalence of hyperacusis in FM patients; pathophysiology of hyperacusis.	Patients with FM more likely to develop hyperacusis as disease progresses. FM patients may experience disturbance in pain-inhibitory mechanisms, leading to otologic findings.
Montoya (2005)	Central sensitization	Prospective cross-sectional	Patients with FM (12) versus controls (12)	Pressure-pain thresholds and event-related brain potentials in FM patients.	Patients with FM had abnormal pain processing and abnormal adaptation to pain stimuli compared to controls, which could lead to otologic findings.
Ayouni (2019)	TMD	Systemic review	Patients with FM and TMD (19 papers)	Prevalence of TMD in patients with FM.	Patients with FM have high prevalence of TMD or orofacial involvement. For these patients, pressure-pain threshold in trigeminal areas was lower than controls.
Collin (2016)	Sore throat	Prospective cross-sectional	Patients with CFS (8433)	Prevalence of symptom-based sore throat/painful lymph node phenotype of CFS.	4.5% of CFS patients presented with a sore throat/painful lymph node phenotype.

AR Allergic rhinitis, *CFS* chronic fatigue syndrome, *CPS* chronic pain syndromes, *CRS* chronic rhinosinusitis, *CSS* chronic sinusitis survey, *FM* fibromyalgia, *NHP* Nottingham health profile, *ENT* otolaryngology, *RQLQ* rhinoconjunctivitis quality of life questionnaires, *RSDI* rhinosinusitis disability index, *VHI* voice handicap index, *TMD* temporomandibular disorder, *QOL* quality of life

References

1. Clauw DJ. Fibromyalgia: an overview. Am J Med. 2009;122(12 Suppl):S3–s13.
2. Yancey JR, Thomas SM. Chronic fatigue syndrome: diagnosis and treatment. Am Fam Physician. 2012;86(8):741–6.
3. Weir PT, Harlan GA, Nkoy FL, Jones SS, Hegmann KT, Gren LH, et al. The incidence of fibromyalgia and its associated comorbidities: a population-based retrospective cohort study based on international classification of diseases, 9th revision codes. J Clin Rheumatol. 2006;12(3):124–8.
4. Physicians WGotRACo. Chronic fatigue syndrome. Clinical practice guidelines--2002. Med J Aust. 2002;176(S9):S17–55.
5. Capelli E, Zola R, Lorusso L, Venturini L, Sardi F, Ricevuti G. Chronic fatigue syndrome/ Myalgic encephalomyelitis: an update. Int J Immunopathol Pharmacol. 2010;23(4):981–9.
6. McCarberg BH. Clinical overview of fibromyalgia. Am J Ther. 2012;19(5):357–68.
7. Abbi B, Natelson BH. Is chronic fatigue syndrome the same illness as fibromyalgia: evaluating the 'single syndrome' hypothesis. QJM. 2013;106(1):3–9.
8. Avellaneda Fernández A, Pérez Martín A, Izquierdo Martínez M, Arruti Bustillo M, Barbado Hernández FJ, de la Cruz LJ, et al. Chronic fatigue syndrome: aetiology, diagnosis and treatment. BMC Psychiat. 2009;9(Suppl 1):S1–S11.
9. Wolfe F, Clauw DJ, Fitzcharles MA, Goldenberg DL, Katz RS, Mease P, et al. The American College of Rheumatology preliminary diagnostic criteria for fibromyalgia and measurement of symptom severity. Arthritis Care Res. 2010;62(5):600–10.
10. Wolfe F, Clauw DJ, Fitzcharles MA, Goldenberg DL, Häuser W, Katz RL, et al. 2016 revisions to the 2010/2011 fibromyalgia diagnostic criteria. Semin Arthritis Rheum. 2016;46(3):319–29.
11. Galvez-Sánchez CM, Reyes Del Paso GA. Diagnostic criteria for fibromyalgia: critical review and future perspectives. J Clin Med. 2020;9(4):1219.
12. Fillingim RB, Bruehl S, Dworkin RH, Dworkin SF, Loeser JD, Turk DC, et al. The ACTTION-American pain society pain taxonomy (AAPT): an evidence-based and multidimensional approach to classifying chronic pain conditions. J Pain. 2014;15(3):241–9.
13. Arnold LM, Bennett RM, Crofford LJ, Dean LE, Clauw DJ, Goldenberg DL, et al. AAPT Diagnostic Criteria for Fibromyalgia. J Pain. 2019;20(6):611–28.
14. Committee on the Diagnostic Criteria for Myalgic Encephalomyelitis/Chronic Fatigue S, Board on the Health of Select P, Institute of M. The National Academies Collection: Reports funded by National Institutes of Health. Beyond Myalgic Encephalomyelitis/Chronic Fatigue Syndrome: Redefining an Illness. Washington (DC): National Academies Press (US). Copyright 2015 by the National Academy of Sciences. All rights reserved; 2015.
15. Meeus M, Nijs J. Central sensitization: a biopsychosocial explanation for chronic widespread pain in patients with fibromyalgia and chronic fatigue syndrome. Clin Rheumatol. 2007;26(4):465–73.
16. Rasa S, Nora-Krukle Z, Henning N, Eliassen E, Shikova E, Harrer T, et al. Chronic viral infections in myalgic encephalomyelitis/chronic fatigue syndrome (ME/CFS). J Transl Med. 2018;16(1):268.
17. Cortes Rivera M, Mastronardi C, Silva-Aldana CT, Arcos-Burgos M, Lidbury BA. Myalgic encephalomyelitis/chronic fatigue syndrome: a comprehensive review. Diagnostics (Basel). 2019;9(3):91.
18. Annemans L, Le Lay K, Taïeb C. Societal and patient burden of fibromyalgia syndrome. PharmacoEconomics. 2009;27(7):547–59.
19. Reynolds KJ, Vernon SD, Bouchery E, Reeves WC. The economic impact of chronic fatigue syndrome. Cost Effective Resour Alloc. 2004;2(1):4.
20. Bayazit YA, Gürsoy S, Ozer E, Karakurum G, Madenci E. Neurotologic manifestations of the fibromyalgia syndrome. J Neurol Sci. 2002;196(1–2):77–80.
21. Koca TT, Seyithanoglu M, Sagiroglu S, Berk E, Dagli H. Frequency of audiological complaints in patients with fibromyalgia syndrome and its relationship with oxidative stress. Niger J Clin Pract. 2018;21(10):1271–7.

22. Stranden M, Solvin H, Fors EA, Getz L, Helvik A-S. Are persons with fibromyalgia or other musculoskeletal pain more likely to report hearing loss? A HUNT study. BMC Musculoskelet Disord. 2016;17(1):477.
23. Le TP, Tzeng YL, Muo CH, Ting H, Sung FC, Lee SD, et al. Risk of hearing loss in patients with fibromyalgia: a nationwide population-based retrospective cohort study. PLoS One. 2020;15(9):e0238502.
24. Bhatt JM, Lin HW, Bhattacharyya N. Prevalence, severity, exposures, and treatment patterns of tinnitus in the United States. JAMA Otolaryngol Head Neck Surg. 2016;142(10):959–65.
25. Iikuni F, Nomura Y, Goto F, Murakami M, Shigihara S, Ikeda M. Why do patients with fibromyalgia complain of ear-related symptoms? Ear-related symptoms and otological findings in patients with fibromyalgia. Clin Rheumatol. 2013;32(10):1437–41.
26. Cil Ö, Zateri C, Güçlü O, Oymak S, Tezcan E. The effect of fibromyalgia treatment on tinnitus. Am J Otolaryngol. 2020;41(3):102390.
27. Beebe Palumbo D, Joos K, De Ridder D, Vanneste S. The management and outcomes of pharmacological treatments for tinnitus. Curr Neuropharmacol. 2015;13(5):692–700.
28. da Silva LA, Kazyiama HH, de Siqueira JT, Teixeira MJ, de Siqueira SR. High prevalence of orofacial complaints in patients with fibromyalgia: a case-control study. Oral Surg Oral Med Oral Pathol Oral Radiol. 2012;114(5):e29–34.
29. Geisser ME, Glass JM, Rajcevska LD, Clauw DJ, Williams DA, Kileny PR, et al. A psychophysical study of auditory and pressure sensitivity in patients with fibromyalgia and healthy controls. J Pain. 2008;9(5):417–22.
30. Suhnan AP, Finch PM, Drummond PD. Hyperacusis in chronic pain: neural interactions between the auditory and nociceptive systems. Int J Audiol. 2017;56(11):801–9.
31. Jastreboff PJ, Jastreboff MM. Tinnitus retraining therapy for patients with tinnitus and decreased sound tolerance. Otolaryngol Clin N Am. 2003;36(2):321–36.
32. Montoya P, Pauli P, Batra A, Wiedemann G. Altered processing of pain-related information in patients with fibromyalgia. Eur J Pain. 2005;9(3):293–303.
33. Sawada F, Nomura Y, Goto F, Murakami M, Jike M, Toi T, et al. Relationship of physical distress to dizziness in patients with fibromyalgia. Acta Otolaryngol. 2016;136(1):56–61.
34. Collin SM, Nikolaus S, Heron J, Knoop H, White PD, Crawley E. Chronic fatigue syndrome (CFS) symptom-based phenotypes in two clinical cohorts of adult patients in the UK and the Netherlands. J Psychosom Res. 2016;81:14–23.
35. Garner R, Baraniuk JN. Orthostatic intolerance in chronic fatigue syndrome. J Transl Med. 2019;17(1):185.
36. Cleveland CH Jr, Fisher RH, Brestel EP, Esinhart JD, Metzger WJ. Chronic rhinitis: an underrecognized association with fibromyalgia. Allergy Proc. 1992;13(5):263–7.
37. Gultuna S, Tezel N, Ozalp Ates FS. Fibromyalgia in the patients with allergic rhinitis: its prevalence and impact on the quality of life. Am J Rhinol Allergy. 2019;33(6):716–22.
38. Tsiakiris G, Neely G, Lind N, Nordin S. Comorbidity in allergic asthma and allergic rhinitis: functional somatic syndromes. Psychol Health Med. 2017;22(10):1163–8.
39. Baraniuk JN, Clauw D, Yuta A, Ali M, Gaumond E, Upadhyayula N, et al. Nasal secretion analysis in allergic rhinitis, cystic fibrosis, and nonallergic fibromyalgia/chronic fatigue syndrome subjects. Am J Rhinol. 1998;12(6):435–40.
40. Baraniuk JN, Merck SJ. The nonallergic rhinitis of chronic fatigue syndrome. In: Pawankar R, Holgate ST, Rosenwasser LJ, editors. Allergy Frontiers: clinical manifestations. Tokyo: Springer; 2009. p. 81–97.
41. Kakumanu SS, Mende CN, Lehman EB, Hughes K, Craig TJ. Effect of topical nasal corticosteroids on patients with chronic fatigue syndrome and rhinitis. J Am Osteopath Assoc. 2003;103(9):423–7.
42. Chester AC. Symptoms of rhinosinusitis in patients with unexplained chronic fatigue or bodily pain: a pilot study. Arch Intern Med. 2003;163(15):1832–6.
43. Soler ZM, Mace J, Smith TL. Fibromyalgia and chronic rhinosinusitis: outcomes after endoscopic sinus surgery. Am J Rhinol. 2008;22(4):427–32.
44. Sautter NB, Mace J, Chester AC, Smith TL. The effects of endoscopic sinus surgery on level of fatigue in patients with chronic rhinosinusitis. Am J Rhinol. 2008;22(4):420–6.

45. Reh DD, Mace J, Robinson JL, Smith TL. Impact of age on presentation of chronic rhinosinusitis and outcomes of endoscopic sinus surgery. Am J Rhinol. 2007;21(2):207–13.
46. Gurbuzler L, Inanir A, Yelken K, Koc S, Eyibilen A, Uysal IO. Voice disorder in patients with fibromyalgia. Auris Nasus Larynx. 2013;40(6):554–7.
47. Sahin G, Ulubaş B, Calikoğlu M, Erdoğan C. Handgrip strength, pulmonary function tests, and pulmonary muscle strength in fibromyalgia syndrome: is there any relationship? South Med J. 2004;97(1):25–9.
48. Misono S, Dietrich M, Piccirillo JF. The puzzle of medically unexplained symptoms—a holistic view of the patient with laryngeal symptoms. JAMA Otolaryngol Head Neck Surg. 2020;146(6):550–1.
49. Piersiala K, Akst LM, Hillel AT, Best SR. Chronic pain syndromes and their laryngeal manifestations. JAMA Otolaryngol Head Neck Surg. 2020;146(6):543–9.
50. Craig J, Tomlinson C, Stevens K, Kotagal K, Fornadley J, Jacobson B, et al. Combining voice therapy and physical therapy: a novel approach to treating muscle tension dysphonia. J Commun Disord. 2015;58:169–78.
51. Truta MP, Santucci ET. Head and neck fibromyalgia and temporomandibular arthralgia. Otolaryngol Clin N Am. 1989;22(6):1159–71.
52. Ayouni I, Chebbi R, Hela Z, Dhidah M. Comorbidity between fibromyalgia and temporomandibular disorders: a systematic review. Oral Surg Oral Med Oral Pathol Oral Radiol. 2019;128(1):33–42.
53. Pimentel MJ, Gui MS, Martins de Aquino LM, Rizzatti-Barbosa CM. Features of temporomandibular disorders in fibromyalgia syndrome. Cranio. 2013;31(1):40–5.
54. Leblebici B, Pektaş ZO, Ortancil O, Hürcan EC, Bagis S, Akman MN. Coexistence of fibromyalgia, temporomandibular disorder, and masticatory myofascial pain syndromes. Rheumatol Int. 2007;27(6):541–4.
55. Balasubramaniam R, de Leeuw R, Zhu H, Nickerson RB, Okeson JP, Carlson CR. Prevalence of temporomandibular disorders in fibromyalgia and failed back syndrome patients: a blinded prospective comparison study. Oral Surg Oral Med Oral Pathol Oral Radiol Endod. 2007;104(2):204–16.
56. Velly AM, Look JO, Schiffman E, Lenton PA, Kang W, Messner RP, et al. The effect of fibromyalgia and widespread pain on the clinically significant temporomandibular muscle and joint pain disorders--a prospective 18-month cohort study. J Pain. 2010;11(11):1155–64.
57. Hickie I, Davenport T, Vernon SD, Nisenbaum R, Reeves WC, Hadzi-Pavlovic D, et al. Are chronic fatigue and chronic fatigue syndrome valid clinical entities across countries and health-care settings? Aust N Z J Psychiatry. 2009;43(1):25–35.
58. Sullivan PF, Pedersen NL, Jacks A, Evengård B. Chronic fatigue in a population sample: definitions and heterogeneity. Psychol Med. 2005;35(9):1337–48.

Sleep and Functional Illness

17

Reena Dhanda Patil

Introduction

Good quality sleep is increasingly recognized as paramount to one's health and well-being. The medical community has evolved its thinking about sleep over the past decades to understand it as a dynamic state that is critically important to an individual's psychological and physiological health. In particular, the specialty of otolaryngology has traveled far in its understanding of sleep medicine as it pertains to the burgeoning field of sleep surgery. Otolaryngologists regularly encounter the two most common sleep disorders, obstructive sleep apnea, and insomnia, in patients who are unable to tolerate positive airway pressure (PAP) treatment and are seeking alternative surgical therapy. Functional illnesses such as chronic fatigue syndrome (CFS) and fibromyalgia (FM), which often include sleep-related complaints among their diagnostic criteria, are similarly common in patients seeking care for sleep disorders such as OSA [1, 2]. The subtleties of these conditions as well as contributions from mood disorders can certainly impact sleep and the otolaryngologist's ability to offer successful treatment with sleep surgery. It is of great relevance to any provider who wishes to treat patients with sleep disorders to understand the complexities and nuances of sleep, which touch many aspects of a person's ability to function optimally during the daytime.

R. D. Patil (✉)
Department of Otolaryngology-Head and Neck Surgery, University of Cincinnati College of Medicine, Cincinnati, OH, USA

Cincinnati VA Medical Center, Cincinnati, OH, USA

© The Author(s), under exclusive license to Springer Nature Switzerland AG 2023

B. W. Blakley, J. E. Blakley (eds.), *Functional Illness of the Head and Neck*,
https://doi.org/10.1007/978-3-031-12998-8_17

Sleep and Health: A Psychoneuroimmunologic Perspective

It is helpful to briefly review the ways in which sleep affects one's bodily health in a holistic sense. Sleep can be defined as a reversible state of decreased responsiveness to stimuli within one's environment [3]. Sleep influences two major neurobiological systems, the hypothalamic–pituitary–adrenal (HPA) axis and the sympathetic nervous system (SNS), which are responsible for the regulation of both innate and adaptive immunity as well as inflammation [4]. Both sleep deprivation and excessive sleep are related to the ability to fight common infectious processes such as pneumonia and the common cold [5, 6]. In addition, short sleep duration and fragmentation reported by insomniacs are more likely to have higher levels of inflammatory markers such as catecholamines and their metabolites in urine samples than those not reporting these sleep deficits [7]. Dysfunctional sleep may mediate and potentiate inflammation that contributes to hypertension, diabetes, cardiovascular disease, cancer, and increased mortality as well as less well-defined functional illnesses such as CFS and FM. Not only is poor sleep duration associated with physical disease, but the inflammatory state resulting from poor sleep may also play a role in mood disorders such as depression [4]. Prolonged insomnia lasting up to a year has been found to be associated with a 14-fold increased risk for depression in the following year [8]. Depression in turn may provide subtle changes in one's perception of illness that can contribute to the manifestations of common functional illnesses.

Relationship of Sleep to Fatigue

What Is Fatigue?

Fatigue is an exceedingly common complaint experienced by the general population. Nonpathologic fatigue is universally experienced and described as short term (less than 3 months) with an easily identifiable cause, such as an acute febrile illness, endocrine pathology, or recovery from trauma or surgery. In contrast, pathologic fatigue is often associated with chronic illnesses such as cancer, multiple sclerosis and depression and has a longer duration [9]. One study found that chronic fatigue (lasting more than 6 months) was present in 2.7–4.2% of patients in a community-based study in a large US city [10]. In particular, fatigue is a subjective experience that can lead to physiological and psychological impairments including poor strength, tiredness, difficulty concentrating as well as decreased morale and mood [11, 12]. It can be difficult in practice to elucidate fatigue because of its multifactorial nature including physical and psychological factors as well as sociocultural and environmental influences [12]. Excessive fatigue is characteristic of patients presenting with chronic insomnia, which is the most common sleep disorder presenting in the primary health care setting [11]. Primary insomnia, labeled as such when it is not due to another sleep, medical, psychosocial or substance abuse disorder, can be more difficult to treat given the lack of an obvious underlying cause.

Chronic Fatigue Syndrome and Sleep

When addressing fatigue in the context of treatment for sleep disorders, it is helpful for the primary care provider, sleep medicine physician and otolaryngologist to understand chronic fatigue syndrome (CFS). CFS is one of a number of mind–body illnesses that is controversial and not well understood with regard to its etiology [13]. It is widespread with an estimated one to two million Americans suffering from this illness, more commonly women, and poses substantial economic costs related to lost productivity and unemployment in the United States [13, 14]. CFS is defined by at least 6 months of "persistent, relapsing fatigue associated with substantial impairments". In addition, four out of eight additional symptoms must be present for diagnosis, one of which is unrefreshing sleep [13]. Many CFS patients are assessed as having poor sleep hygiene and insomnia and can benefit from sleep-focused treatment including cognitive behavioral therapy for insomnia (CBT-i) and exercise therapy. Sleep hygiene should address the "wired but tired" state of mind in patients with CFS. Sleep scheduling, limiting daytime napping, and wind-down activities at night should be encouraged to improve sleep quality [13].

Relationship of Sleep to Pain

Effect of Pain on Sleep

Whether acute or chronic, pain that is severe enough to negatively affect sleep can have physiological and emotional effects on an individual's health, which can then play into the complex factors affecting coexistent functional illness. From a polysomnographic standpoint, the effect of pain on quality and architecture of sleep is related to increased arousals as well as the decreased duration of slow-wave sleep, the most restful phase of sleep [3]. Overall decreased sleep efficiency is also common in patients with widespread musculoskeletal pain and headaches (HA) [3]. In addition, sleep disturbances related to periodic limb movements have been found more often in patients with chronic pain when compared to controls [15].

FM and Sleep

FM, a functional illness that is similar to CFS with the addition of chronic widespread pain as its primary feature, also presents diagnostic and treatment challenges to both primary care and specialist providers. FM is a common musculoskeletal pain syndrome that was first described per rheumatologic criteria in 1990 [16]. It continues to be controversial, having been described by some as the "medicalization of misery" [17]. Its prevalence is estimated at 2% worldwide, and it is reportedly experienced by three to six million people in the United States [13, 18]. FM is defined by 3 or more months of generalized body pain and tenderness, with many specific tender points described by patients [16]. Debilitation in FM is multifactorial, characterized not only by pain but also by nonrefreshing sleep, fatigue, functional impairment, low energy, and depression among other symptoms. Sleep disturbances affect more than 90% of patients with FM [18]. Like CFS, FM causes significant economic strain on society and the healthcare system due to lost productivity and healthcare utilization [18].

A number of investigators have examined objective sleep data and found that certain patients with FM have fragmented sleep, decreased slow wave sleep, and low sleep efficiency [18]. With regard to these sleep disturbances, they have traditionally been thought to be a result of sleeplessness caused by chronic pain and depression in FM. On the other hand, sleep dysfunction in itself has been found to result in hyperalgesia and a decreased pain threshold [18, 19]. As a result of such findings, researchers postulate a bidirectional relationship between sleep dysfunction and FM that merits further study given that appropriate, early treatment of sleep disorders such as insomnia and OSA may significantly improve symptoms referable to FM [18]. In addition, careful management of pain symptoms in FM with pharmacology and other modalities such as acupuncture and massage may ameliorate the poor sleep experienced by the majority of FM patients.

Sleep and HA

HA are intrinsically related to sleep in that poor sleep can trigger HA, particularly migraines, while chronic migraines and tension-type HA can certainly cause sleep disturbance [3]. Patients with chronic migraines often also experience insomnia, resulting in complaints related to poor sleep time, sleepiness, and unrefreshing sleep [20]. It is important to recognize the link between poor sleep and HA in functional illness given the overlap of these two complaints in common disorders such as CFS and FM [21, 22]. Interestingly, one study showed that FM comorbidity was present in 36% of patients suffering from primary HA, with high levels of tenderness at trigger points, poor sleep adequacy, and severe fatigue when compared to those without FM [21]. HA was also more frequent in CFS patients, with 84% experiencing migraine HA and 81% tension-type HA, and sleep severity scores were significantly worse compared to healthy controls [22].

Patients often present to a primary care provider, sleep medicine specialist, or otolaryngologist with HA contributing to poor sleep, while in fact those HA may be related to the lack of sleep seen in undiagnosed OSA. Providers should have a low threshold to perform polysomnogram (PSG) in patients with suspected OSA and HA among other complaints. In patients found to have concomitant OSA and HA, effective treatment of OSA with PAP has been shown to improve HA [23]. Despite these promising results, patients with OSA and HA undergoing surgical treatment for sleep apnea should be counseled that while successful surgery may improve HA symptoms, the ongoing relationship of an individual's HA to functional illness, chronic pain, fatigue, medication effects, and other disorders will require continued management in the postoperative period.

Surgical Treatment for OSA in the Context of Functional Illness

As the prevalence of OSA reaches 9–38% in the United States, patients with OSA are increasingly referred to an otolaryngology practice for the consideration of sleep surgery [24]. Despite growing attention to OSA and its impact on an individual's cardiovascular and mental health, quality of life, and motor vehicle safety, this disorder remains undiagnosed in a majority of men and women [25]. One factor leading to underdiagnosis may be related to past diagnostic criteria for OSA which emphasized excessive daytime sleepiness (EDS) to ascertain if OSA was present but did not focus on other common symptoms such as "fatigue," "tiredness," or "lack of energy" [26]. Only recently has the American Academy of Sleep Medicine revised its criteria to include fatigue and insomnia as part of the symptomatology of OSA [27]. In practice, a common and complex phenotype of a patient with OSA presents with multiple and often vague complaints of sleepiness, fatigue, and/or low energy. To complicate matters further, OSA can be comorbid with and potentiate other sleep and health conditions, including functional disorders such as primary insomnia, CFS, and FM [1, 2]. Fatigue and chronic pain in these disorders may worsen sleep fragmentation and hypersomnolence already present in OSA, making it difficult to pinpoint the cause of a patient's complaints as only due to the objective presence of apneas and hypopneas.

To accurately understand sleep disorders in the preoperative setting, the otolaryngologist must obtain a comprehensive history, recognizing the interchangeability of the terms fatigue, tiredness, and sleepiness. It is also important to understand that these complaints can coexist in many pathophysiological states, including OSA, especially when comorbid with conditions such as insomnia and depression [11]. A review of sleep aid medications is important given their effects on sleep stages and possible effects on daytime hypersomnolence (see Table 17.1). The otolaryngologist can utilize simple questionnaires, such as the Insomnia Severity Index, Epworth Sleepiness Scale (ESS), and Functional Outcomes of Sleep Questionnaire to not only recognize the nature and severity of the patient's EDS and fatigue complaints but also to counsel patients on realistic expectations of the benefits of sleep surgery. The practitioner should also probe a patient's history to determine if the presence of a functional illness such as CFS and FM may be contributing to the perception of deficits caused by OSA. Recognition of symptoms that point to diagnosed or undiagnosed functional illness may lead to fruitful consultations with primary care, rheumatology, and/or mental health services to address underlying conditions with a variety of modalities prior to pursuing the irreversible option of surgical treatment for OSA. In addition, patients must be counseled that although EDS may be objectively eliminated after surgical treatment of OSA, residual sleepiness and fatigue can remain and be refractory to treatment.

Chronic pain also remains highly relevant to the otolaryngologist's practice when evaluating patients referred for sleep surgery. Patients with FM and their providers should be cognizant of the relationship between poor sleep quality and the experience of pain and how it affects PAP tolerance. Given the highly reported

Table 17.1 Commonly used sleep aid medications and their effects [28, 29]

Class of medication	Example(s)	Mechanism of action	Comments
Sedative-hypnotics			
Benzodiazepines	Temazepam, triazolam	GABA receptor agonist	Excellent sleep induction, risk of addiction and tolerance, withdrawal effects including REM rebound, respiratory depression
Benzodiazepine-like agents	Zolpidem, eszoplicone	GABA receptor agonist	Excellent efficacy, minimal side effects, low abuse potential
Antihistamines	Diphenhydramine	Histamine-1 receptor antagonist	Varyingly effective, side effects of daytime sleepiness, cognitive impairment
Barbiturates	Methaqualone, glutethimide	GABA receptor agonist	Historical interest, high risk of addiction, tolerance, and overdose
Ethanol	Liquor, wine, beer	GABA receptor agonist	Widely used, chronic use causes tolerance, dependence, and diminished sleep efficiency/quality
Sedating antidepressants			
Tricyclic antidepressants	Amitriptyline, imipramine	Serotonin and norepinephrine reuptake inhibitor	Anticholinergic effects, daytime hangover, danger with overdose
Tetracyclic antidepressants	Mirtazipine	Alpha-2-adrenergic receptor antagonist	Dry mouth, weight gain, constipation
Serotonin antagonist and reuptake inhibitor	Trazodone	Serotonin receptor antagonist	Nausea, vomiting, diarrhea, daytime sleepiness, dizziness
Circadian rhythm synchronizer			
Pineal hormone	Melatonin	Intracellular effect on suprachiasmatic nucleus	Adjusts body's internal clock and sleep-wake cycles, useful for shift-work disorder and jet lag; can cause headaches, dizziness, depression, drowsiness

GABA gamma aminobutyric acid

prevalence of FM, it is possible that patients presenting for treatment of OSA also have comorbid FM. In these cases, the surgeon should thoroughly discuss with the patient how wakefulness from nocturnal pain poses treatment challenges with regard to adherence to patient-initiated surgical treatments such as hypoglossal nerve stimulator (HNS), similar to PAP. Importantly, any patient with chronic pain may also be at risk for opioid abuse which can complicate the post-surgical course. Opioid abuse has been found to increase nocturnal hypoxemia and central sleep apnea, which can hamper the surgeon's success in treating patients referred for obstructive sleep apnea [3, 30]. The important role of poor sleep in potentiating pain and vice versa suggests the need to develop multidisciplinary treatments, including pain management services, to improve sleep quality in this complex patient population. Ideally, pain control should be optimized preoperatively, utilizing pharmacologic treatments such as anti-inflammatory and psychotropic medications as well as alternative treatments such as acupuncture and hypnotherapy [19].

Choice of Sleep Surgery in Patients with Functional Illness

Sleep surgery as a field began in the 1980s in the United States with the introduction of the uvulopalatopharyngoplasty (UPPP) by Fujita [31]. Other static surgical procedures, including expansion pharyngoplasty, hyoid suspension, midline partial glossectomy, and tongue base suspension have been developed over the years with varying levels of success. More recently, dynamic therapies are available to patients, most notably the HNS, which has shown promising results in improving the severity of sleep apnea and sleepiness measures [32]. From the author's experience, it is important to tailor the choice of sleep surgery not only to a patient's anatomy but also to their self-motivation and involvement in their own care. In particular, patients undergoing surgery for OSA with sleep issues related to functional disorders will need thorough, individualized counseling as to the nature of the procedure and how it will affect them postoperatively. For example, an OSA patient with comorbid severe insomnia and/or chronic pain in CFS and FM may have worsened sleep fragmentation and sleep time than a patient with OSA only at baseline. If this patient underwent HNS, they would likely require special attention to device settings tailored to their sleep cycle and habits to prevent poor adherence to HNS. On the other hand, static surgical procedures such as UPPP and hyoid suspension may not provide the same objective surgical success as recent results from HNS [32], but will provide patients with a constant result after healing is complete without the need for nightly activation of a device [33]. Whichever procedure is selected, an open and knowledgeable discussion with the patient should take place, taking into account their individual profile with regard to fatigue, insomnia, pain, and mental health issues.

Residual Sleepiness and Fatigue After Treatment of OSA

Otolaryngologists should understand how residual EDS and fatigue, which are well documented in the PAP literature, may affect the perceived success of surgery for OSA. Residual EDS remains a common problem that has been estimated to occur in 5–55% of those using PAP for OSA, with a prevalence of 10–12% remaining even after excluding poor PAP users [34, 35]. Patients with residual EDS after appropriate treatment of OSA with PAP were found to have impaired daytime functioning, more fatigue, and overall worse health than patients without residual EDS [34]. This subjective sense of a poorer quality of life and sleep is also common in patients with functional illnesses and may be a result of the comorbidity of these conditions with OSA.

When evaluating residual EDS after what is considered successful sleep surgery, it is important to confirm the objective efficacy of surgery by tests such as full night PSG, perhaps with a home sleep test, to optimize patient comfort and sleep time. Residual sleepiness can also be confirmed utilizing a multiple sleep latency test as well as a subjective test such as the ESS. If residual EDS exists after successful surgical treatment, the otolaryngologist may need to refer the patient for a thorough evaluation to rule out other causes of sleepiness, including conditions such as narcolepsy, mood disorders, multiple sclerosis, and neurologic disorders [34]. Adverse effects of residual sleepiness after seemingly successful surgery for OSA must be addressed with the patient, as these patients may still be at risk for detrimental cardiovascular health outcomes as well as an increased risk for home, work, or traffic accidents [35].

Treatment of EDS and fatigue that persist after objectively successful treatment of OSA is challenging. Prevention by early recognition of patients at risk for persistent sleepiness or fatigue starts by identifying patients with significant insomnia, chronic pain, mental health disorders, and functional illnesses such as CFS or FM before surgery. This can aid in counseling patients as to preoperative pharmacologic and psychosocial interventions that may provide a better chance for subjective success after surgery. For example, patients with comorbid depression and insomnia may benefit from sedating antidepressants such as mirtazapine and trazodone rather than the commonly used classes of serotonin and norepinephrine reuptake inhibitors and activating tricyclic antidepressants which have been shown to impair sleep through dysregulation of rapid eye movement (REM) sleep and onset of restless leg syndrome [36]. Close follow-up as to the effects of these medications with mental health professionals is required as sedating antidepressants can also cause a "hangover effect" of increased daytime somnolence.

Postoperatively, residual EDS and fatigue attributable to insomnia can be treated with sleep aid medications and CBT-i to improve a patient's perception of sleep quality and restfulness. Daytime symptoms of tiredness and low energy can be addressed with pharmacologic therapy. In the United States, wake stimulants such as modafinil have been found to be effective in promoting wakefulness through the ascending arousal pathway beginning in the hypothalamus [34]. Mental health providers can also utilize therapy and psychotropic medications to optimize conditions such as depression, anxiety, and post-traumatic stress that often coexist with functional disorders. Otolaryngologists must consider themselves as part of a team caring for these patients and recruit their colleagues in behavioral health, primary care, pain management, rheumatology, and sleep medicine to provide the best chance for objective and subjective success with surgery for sleep apnea.

Summary

Over the past several decades, the medical community has increasingly recognized that sleep is a complex, dynamic state that is critically important to an individual's psychological and physiological health. Sleep disturbances related to functional illness are widespread throughout the general population; in particular, patients experiencing conditions such as CFS and FM often complain of symptoms such as insomnia, daytime sleepiness, and tiredness. Primary care providers and sleep medicine specialists also commonly encounter patients with OSA and may consider referral to otolaryngology for surgery as treatment options become more extensive and individualized. Referring providers and otolaryngologists must understand how sleep complaints related to functional illnesses may act in concert with OSA when considering sleep surgery. The best chance for the sleep surgeon to develop a productive relationship with a patient and provide relief for their symptoms resides with a careful history that allows for accurate preoperative assessment of functional illness symptoms and realistic expectations for postoperative outcomes with regard to sleepiness and fatigue. Most importantly, the otolaryngologist must function as part of a multidisciplinary team to ensure that patients' functional illnesses are appropriately managed to optimize decision making for surgery and postoperative surgical success.

References

1. Mariman A, Delesie L, Tobback E, Hanoulle I, Sermijn E, Vermeir P, Pevernagie D, Vogelaers D. Undiagnosed and comorbid disorders in patients with presumed chronic fatigue syndrome. J Psychosom Res. 2013;75:491–6.
2. Marvisi M, Balzarini L, Mancini C, Ramponi S, Marvisi C. Fibromyalgia is frequent in obstructive sleep apnea and responds to CPAP therapy. Eur J Intern Med. 2015;26:49–50.
3. Ferini-Strambi L, Galbiati A, Combi R. Sleep disorder-related headaches. Neurol Sci. 2019;40:107–13.
4. Irwin MR. Why sleep is important for health: a psychoneuroimmunology perspective. Annu Rev Psychol. 2015;66:143–72.
5. Patel SR, Malhotra A, Gao X, Hu FB, Neuman MI, Fawzi WW. A prospective study of sleep duration and pneumonia risk in women. Sleep. 2012;35:97–101.
6. Cohen S, Doyle WJ, Alper CM, Janicki-Deverts D, Turner RB. Sleep Habits and Susceptibility to the Common Cold. Arch Intern Med. 2009;169:62.
7. Vgontzas AN, Fernandez-Mendoza J, Liao D, Bixler EO. Insomnia with objective short sleep duration: the most biologically severe phenotype of the disorder. Sleep Med Rev. 2013;17:241–54.
8. Lee E, Cho HJ, Olmstead R, Levin MJ, Oxman MN, Irwin MR. Persistent sleep disturbance: a risk factor for recurrent depression in community-dwelling older adults. Sleep. 2013;36:1685–91.
9. Jason LA, Evans M, Brown M, Porter N. What is fatigue? Pathological and nonpathological fatigue. PM R. 2010;2:327–31.
10. Jason LA, Jordan KM, Richman JA, et al. A community-based study of prolonged fatigue and chronic fatigue. J Health Psychol. 1999;4:9–26.
11. Kim SA, Koo BB, Kim DE, Hwangbo Y, Yang KI. Factors affecting fatigue severity in patients with obstructive sleep apnea. Clin Respir J. 2017;11:1045–51.
12. Bardwell WA, Moore P, Ancoli-Israel S, Dimsdale JE. Fatigue in obstructive sleep apnea: driven by depressive symptoms instead of apnea severity? Am J Psychiatry. 2003;160:350–5.
13. Friedberg F. Chronic fatigue syndrome, fibromyalgia, and related illnesses: a clinical model of assessment and intervention. J Clin Psychol. 2010;66(6):641–65.
14. Yancey JR, Thomas SM. Chronic fatigue syndrome: diagnosis and treatment. Am Fam Physician. 2012;86:741–6.
15. Rains JC, Penzien DB. Sleep and chronic pain: challenges to the alpha-EEG sleep pattern as a pain specific sleep anomaly. J Psychosom Res. 2003;54:77–83.
16. Wolfe F, Smythe HA, Yunus MB. The American College of Rheumatology 1990 criteria for the classification of fibromyalgia. Arthritis Rheum. 1990;33(2):160–72.
17. Hadler NM. "Fibromyalgia" and the medicalization of misery. J Rheumatol. 2003;30:1668–70.
18. Choy EHS. The role of sleep in pain and fibromyalgia. Nat Rev Rheumatol. 2015;11:513–20.
19. Moldofsky H. Fibromyalgia, sleep disorder and chronic fatigue syndrome. CIBA Found Symp. 1993;173:262–71.
20. Ong JC, Park M. Chronic headaches and insomnia: working toward a biobehavioral model. Cephalalgia. 2012;32:1059–70.

21. de Tommaso M, Sardaro M, Serpino C, Costantini F, Vecchio E, Prudenzano MP, Lamberti P, Livrea P. Fibromyalgia comorbidity in primary headaches. Cephalalgia. 2009;29:453–64.
22. Ravindran MK, Zheng Y, Timbol C, Merck SJ, Baraniuk JN. Migraine headaches in chronic fatigue syndrome (CFS): comparison of two prospective cross-sectional studies. BMC Neurol. 2011;11:30.
23. Johnson KG, Ziemba AM, Garb JL. Improvement in headaches with continuous positive airway pressure for obstructive sleep apnea: a retrospective analysis. Headache. 2013;53:333–43.
24. Senaratna CV, Perret JL, Lodge CJ, Lowe AJ, Campbell BE, Matheson MC, Hamilton GS, Dharmage SC. Prevalence of obstructive sleep apnea in the general population: a systematic review. Sleep Med Rev. 2017;34:70–81.
25. Chervin RD. Sleepiness, fatigue, tiredness, and lack of energy in obstructive sleep apnea. Chest. 2000;118:372–9.
26. American Sleep Disorders Association. The international classification of sleep disorders. Psychol Med. 2001;21(4):1079.
27. American Academy of Sleep Medicine. International classification of sleep disorders. Diagnostic and coding manual. Westchester, IL: American Academy of Sleep Medicine; 2005. p. 51–5.
28. Pagel JF, Parnes BL. Medications for the treatment of sleep disorders: an overview. Prim care companion. J Clin Psychiatry. 2001;3:118–25.
29. do Amaral FG, Cipolla-Neto J. A brief review about melatonin, a pineal hormone. Arch Endocrinol Metab. 2018;62:472–9.
30. Farney RJ, Walker JM, Cloward TV, Rhondeau S. Sleep-disordered breathing associated with long-term opioid therapy. Chest. 2003;123:632–9.
31. Fujita S, Conway W, Zorick F, Roth T. Surgical correction of anatomic abnormalities in obstructive sleep apnea syndrome: uvulopalatopharyngoplasty. Otolaryngol Head Neck Surg. 1981;89:923–34.
32. Woodson BT, Strohl KP, Soose RJ, et al. Upper airway stimulation for obstructive sleep apnea: 5-year outcomes. Otolaryngol Head Neck Surg. 2018;159:194–202.
33. Robinson S, Chia M, Carney AS, Chawla S, Harris P, Esterman A. Upper airway reconstructive surgery long-term quality-of-life outcomes compared with CPAP for adult obstructive sleep apnea. Otolaryngol Head Neck Surg. 2009;141:257–63.
34. Chapman JL, Serinel Y, Marshall NS, Grunstein RR. Residual daytime sleepiness in obstructive sleep apnea after continuous positive airway pressure optimization: causes and management. Sleep Med Clin. 2016;11:353–63.
35. Launois SH, Tamisier R, Lévy P, Pépin J-L. On treatment but still sleepy: cause and management of residual sleepiness in obstructive sleep apnea. Curr Opin Pulm Med. 2013;19:601–8.
36. Adam W, Aleksandra W, Małgorzata W, Wojciech J. Effects of antidepressants on sleep. Curr Psychiatry Rep. 2017;19:11920–017.

18 Functional Disorders of the Larynx: Muscle Tension Dysphonia, Paradoxical Vocal Cord Dysfunction, and Globus Pharyngeus

Brendan D. McNeely and Amanda Hu

Introduction

The larynx is located in the neck, a vulnerable part of the body. A complex interrelationship between voluntary and reflexive motor output of the true vocal cords controls laryngeal function. The larynx has three main functions: voice, respiration, and airway protection [1]. Functional disorders of the larynx can affect these three functions. In this chapter, we highlight three representative functional disorders; muscle tension dysphonia which can cause hoarseness, paradoxical vocal fold dysfunction which can cause dyspnea, and globus pharyngeus which can cause the sensation of a lump in the throat, but not true dysphagia.

This chapter will focus on the diagnosis and treatment of functional disorders of the larynx. Diagnosis of such functional disorders requires careful consideration as they can be mistaken for other respiratory or esophageal diagnoses. The treatment of functional disorders of the larynx is often multidisciplinary and involves collaboration with speech-language pathologists. Lastly, some functional disorders of the larynx have been correlated with specific psychometric traits and psychiatric disorders, which may contribute to symptomatology.

B. D. McNeely · A. Hu (✉)
Division of Otolaryngology - Head and Neck Surgery, Department of Surgery, University of British Columbia, Vancouver, BC, Canada

© The Author(s), under exclusive license to Springer Nature Switzerland AG 2023

B. W. Blakley, J. E. Blakley (eds.), *Functional Illness of the Head and Neck*,
https://doi.org/10.1007/978-3-031-12998-8_18

Muscle Tension Dysphonia

Clinical Features

Muscle tension dysphonia (MTD) is a condition of vocal impairment characterized by improper tension in the laryngeal and paralaryngeal muscles [2–6]. The term MTD was introduced in 1983 by Morrison et al. and can be divided into two forms: primary and secondary [5]. Primary MTD describes dysphonia due to abnormal laryngeal muscle activation without organic vocal cord pathology [3]. Alternatively, in secondary MTD, dysphonia is precipitated by an underlying organic condition. MTD has also been called as muscle misuse dysphonia however, MTD is currently the preferred term as it allows for etiological factors to be described and thus may aid to focus treatment options [3].

Clinically, patients with MTD often present with variable dysphonia and rapid changes in voice [6]. The onset of dysphonia may coincide with changes in environmental temperature, airborne irritants, or viral infections [4]. In MTD, persistent forceful vocal cord closure can produce a strained voice, quiet voice, or no voice at all, leading to chronic muscle soreness and vocal cord nodules or polyps [4].

Epidemiology

There is limited data surrounding MTD prevalence. In general, functional dysphonia has been seen in all age groups greater than 15 years old, wherein 73% of functional dysphonia is found in people between 15 and 44 years of age [7]. Primary MTD is believed to occur more commonly in women, particularly those who are middle-aged; however, any patient population may be affected [8]. Primary MTD is frequently seen at voice centers and may account for 10–40% of all clinical presentations [9, 10].

Pathophysiology

Extrinsic laryngeal musculature including suprahyoid and infrahyoid muscles maintain the larynx in a stable position so that the smaller intrinsic muscles can coordinate vocal fold abduction and adduction [1]. In patients with MTD, the extrinsic laryngeal musculature is held in an elevated level of contraction at rest and during phonation such that vocal cord function is disturbed [11, 12].

Several factors may cause elevated tension in the extrinsic laryngeal musculature that is responsible for MTD. Primary MTD is generally believed to arise due to the misuse of the voluntary muscles related to phonation including oral, perioral, and respiratory muscles [6, 13, 14]. The improper use or overuse of these muscles can progress into eventual voice decompensation and is common among those who have careers with high voice demands. A subset of patients with primary MTD may be linked to certain personality traits including introversion, social anxiety, depression, neuroticism, constraint, and stress reactivity [15–17].

Secondary MTD, also known as organic MTD, may result as compensation for an underlying organic disease, such as laryngopharyngeal reflux, aging or hormonal changes, and upper respiratory infections. Hyperfunction of the thyrohyoid and cricopharyngeal muscles, as a protective mechanism against regurgitated gastric acid in the larynx, can lead to MTD [18–20]. A previous study has shown that 78% of patients with secondary MTD have abnormal reflux testing [21]. In a similar fashion, laryngeal muscle tension can change in an effort to compensate for hormone-related changes in laryngeal mucosa thickness. Either an increase or decrease in mucosal thickness can impair vocal cord adduction leading to subsequent laryngeal muscular strain, false vocal cord hyperfunction, and ultimately MTD [22–24]. MTD following acute viral laryngitis has also been described by Koufman et al., who report that laryngeal inflammation can cause abnormal false vocal cord function [14]. Subsequent false vocal cord compensation may become habituated and thereby result in chronic abnormal laryngeal posturing.

Diagnosis and Workup

The diagnosis of MTD is based upon a history of vocal misuse, psychological, and laryngoscopic evaluations [25]. A careful history of patients with dysphonia would include any changes in phonation and any aggravating factors. Clinical assessment that includes a poorly controlled breath stream and an abnormally low-pitched phonation often raises the suspicion of MTD [4, 19].

Hyperactive laryngeal musculature may be compensating for inappropriate vocal fold function in MTD. Consequently, visualization of the larynx and palpation of neck muscles are important first steps in the diagnosis. Visualization of the true vocal cords and supraglottic region can be challenging in patients with MTD as supraglottic compression can obstruct the laryngscopic view [4]. However, this supraglottic compression can raise the suspicion of an MTD diagnosis. Moreover, palpable tightness in the extrinsic laryngeal musculature, observed laryngeal rise, and decreased thyrohyoid space during rest or phonation also raise the suspicion of an MTD diagnosis [18].

Treatment

Muscle tension dysphonia can be caused by a number of interacting factors that must be considered to provide improvement of patients' symptoms. In general, education on good vocal hygiene is recommended for all patients with dysphonia. Vocal hygiene has been described in three subgroups: environmental, vocal use, and individual behavioral advice [3, 13, 26, 27]. Specifically, it is advised that patients with MTD should avoid yelling or whispering, should avoid speaking in dry and dusty environments, should avoid fumes or allergens, should not clear their throat when speaking, and should limit the number of hours they speak in a day [3]. Behavioral accommodations include reducing alcohol and caffeine use, avoiding smoking, and maintaining regular sleeping patterns [3]. In addition, profession-specific voice accommodations such as microphones may be required.

Voice therapy is often the principal, direct treatment for primary MTD and can generate remarkable improvements in phonation at medium and long-term follow-up [26, 28–30]. During voice therapy, speech-language therapists work with patients to improve their laryngeal posture, breathing mechanics, and articulation. Direct interventional techniques for MTD include laryngeal manipulation, the yawn-sign method and optimal pitch establishment with biofeedback [26]. Additionally, circumlaryngeal manual therapy (CMT), where mechanical pressure is placed over specific sites of the larynx prone to muscular stiffness and cramping, has been shown to have broad symptom and voice improvements in patients with MTD [31–33]. Twenty-four out of 25 patients (96%) showed an improved symptom burden although 68% of those had a mild recurrence of MTD following therapy [33]. CMT presents clinicians and patients with an alternative therapy should good voice hygiene not provide the patient with symptom relief. Together, patient-specific voice hygiene and voice therapy are the mainstays of treatment for nonorganic MTD. It is important to note that primary MTD may cause organic changes such as vocal cord lesions which may require alternative intervention.

In patients with organic or secondary MTD, common medical treatments exist to treat the underlying conditions such as laryngopharyngeal reflux, sinusitis, and upper respiratory tract infection that can cause MTD. For example, laryngopharyngeal reflux can be treated with lifestyle and dietary modifications and stomach acid-reducing medications [34]. Alternatively, surgery is rarely used to treat MTD [3].

Summary

Muscle tension dysphonia is defined by sustained and inappropriate contraction in the extrinsic muscles of the larynx that presents as disrupted phonation. Primary MTD may present without organic cause due to improper use or overuse, which can subsequently lead to structural changes in the larynx. Alternatively, medical conditions such as laryngopharyngeal reflux, hormonal dysregulation, and upper respiratory infections can result in laryngeal compensation resulting in secondary MTD. Treatment of MTD is focused on rehabilitating laryngeal muscle use and promoting good vocal hygiene. Primary MTD often requires voice therapy, whereas secondary MTD may require medical intervention to restore proper phonation; however, due to the fluid pathophysiology of MTD, treatment should be specific to each patient with MTD.

Paradoxical Vocal Cord Dysfunction

Clinical Features

Paradoxical vocal cord dysfunction (PVCD) describes the inappropriate and episodic closure of otherwise normally functioning vocal cords during inspiration or expiration, resulting in dyspnea [35, 36]. Typically, PVCD presents acutely and can range from mild discomfort to severe respiratory distress with stridor [37]. Patients may also have a dry cough, aphonia, neck and subcostal indrawing, and, in its most severe form, a sensation of choking [38–40]. Some of the most common triggers have been reported as environmental exposures, intense exercise, stress, phonation, and upper respiratory infections, all of which are not mutually exclusive [36]. Patients with PVCD are often misdiagnosed with asthma and may have adverse effects from concomitant medical therapy [35]. Altogether, PVCD is often distressing for patients and common misdiagnosis necessitates a greater awareness of this condition.

Epidemiology

The incidence of PVCD is not well studied as it is often misdiagnosed as an asthma exacerbation and can occur in combination with asthma. Of note, a review of 1536 patients with PVCD found a broad range of patient age (0.2–82 years), in which 65% were over 19 years of age and a 3:1 female preponderance. Despite its predominance in females, PVCD has also been well documented in males [41]. In adolescents and young adults, PVCD incidence has been reported to occur in up to 27% of the population [42]. Lastly, one study demonstrated that PVCD is not more prevalent among those with a medical condition, as had been previously assumed [43].

Pathophysiology

Similar to other functional disorders of the larynx, the pathophysiology of PVCD is unclear. Both organic and non-organic causes have been identified as precipitating factors of PVCD with the most common inducing agents being irritants, exercise, and emotional stress [36]. In PVCD, such precipitating factors may cause inappropriate vocal cord closure due to laryngeal hyper-responsiveness to a normal stimulus in the larynx [44, 45]. Moreover, gastroesophageal reflux disease (GERD) is speculated to play a role in predisposing patients to PVCD [37, 39]. Lastly, psychogenic factors including emotional stress, competitive sports, and depression may cause an attack of PVCD to be more likely to occur [37].

Diagnosis and Workup

A careful clinical history and physical exam are essential to the diagnosis of PVCD. Three main criteria are generally used to establish a diagnosis of PVCD: (1) stridor and/or dyspnea, (2) laryngoscopic observation of vocal cord adduction, and (3) truncated inspiration measured on spirometry [37]. The "gold standard" for diagnosing PVCD is direct visualization of paradoxical vocal cord movement during inspiration by flexible laryngoscopy. Previous reports show diagnostic laryngoscopy findings in 100% of symptomatic patients with PVCD and 60% of asymptomatic patients with PVCD [46]. In addition, laryngoscopic evaluation in patients with PVCD will often reveal erythematous and inflamed mucosa of the larynx [37, 47].

There are substantial overlaps in the symptoms of asthma and PVCD; however, the onset and recovery period are important differentiators between diagnoses. In PVCD, onset and recovery periods are approximately <5 and 5–10 min, respectively, whereas asthma has a longer onset and recovery period of approximately >10 and 15–60 min, respectively [37]. PVCD alone does not have any characteristic radiographic findings and chest X-rays are often normal [48]. During a PVCD attack, spirometry may show a truncated inspiratory flow loop with variable reproducibility in subsequent respiratory cycles, whereas asthma is characterized by normal inspiratory curves [47, 49]. In addition, PVCD symptoms do not typically resolve with asthma medications and do not have improvement to the flow-volume loops on spirometry. Agents such as histamine, methacholine, and exercise have been used to induce PVCD attacks for clinical observation; however, it is unclear whether such agents can truly recreate patient symptoms [36, 50]. Importantly, PVCD and other respiratory conditions may coexist and thus an alternative diagnosis does not necessarily rule out the possibility of concomitant PVCD.

Treatment

Acute management of patients with a current attack of PVCD requires careful understanding from the healthcare provider. While reassurance alone has been shown to be effective in resolving the acute airway symptoms of PVCD [35, 36], speech-language pathology interventions such as using specific respiratory patterns may be helpful [51]. Techniques used by speech-language pathologists are targeted at maintaining an adequate airway opening during respiration [52]. Such direct techniques include instructing patients to nasal sniff, pant, or breathe with pursed lips, although the evidence is only anecdotal [51]. Heliox (a mixture of helium and oxygen) administration [53] and sedation with anti-anxiety medications are rarely required [54]. Lastly, botulism toxin injections have been used in rare instance to paralyze vocal cords in an abducted position and should only be considered when intubation or tracheostomy are the only remaining options [55, 56].

In the chronic setting, speech therapy is often regarded as the principal treatment of PVCD. Direct speech-language therapy techniques teach patients with PVCD to maintain a laryngeal opening during respiration while suppressing irritating behaviors of the larynx (coughing and throat clearing) [57]. Moreover, indirect speech therapy techniques are also used by patients and healthcare providers to identify specific triggers that precede PVCD attacks so that careful avoidance may prevent future attacks [36, 58]. Similarly, it is important for patients to follow overall healthy voice hygiene. Psychotherapy and hypnosis continue to be used in the treatment of PVCD despite no clear therapeutic evidence [36]. It is believed that such techniques promote emotional and physical relaxation to prevent the onset of PVCD attacks. Medications for reflux are also recommended to prevent laryngospasm. Other treatments such as inhaled anticholinergics and positive airway pressure have been reported in some patients but lack evidence [36, 59].

Summary

In summary, PVCD presents as dyspnea due to partial or full vocal cord adduction during respiration. Acute attacks of PVCD can be instigated by environmental triggers, exercise, stress, and upper respiratory infections. This functional disorder of the larynx can be differentiated from other respiratory disorders due to its rapid onset and resolution. Flexible laryngoscopic evaluation remains the gold standard for direct diagnosis of PVCD, particularly during an acute attack. While careful reassurance is often sufficient to treat acute PVCD, indirect and direct speech therapy may prevent the recurrence of PVCD attacks.

Globus Pharyngeus

Clinical Features

Globus pharyngeus is a functional disorder of the larynx characterized by a persistent or intermittent sensation of a lump or foreign body in the throat [60, 61]. The functional symptom of globus is most commonly episodic and located midline between the thyroid cartilage and the sternal notch [60, 62]. Patients may also report throat tightness or itchiness with associated mucus accumulation or particulate retention. Despite the sensation of dysphagia, globus pharyngeus does not impair the passage of an oral bolus. In general, there is no associated odynophagia and the sensation of discomfort may be improved with eating and swallowing [61, 63]. To confirm a diagnosis of globus pharyngeus, other organic causes must be excluded [61].

Epidemiology

The characteristic sensation of a lump in the throat is notably prevalent in the general population, where previous studies report globus pharyngeus to occur in 8.1–46% of otherwise healthy individuals [64–66]. This functional disorder affects men and women equally; however, in the past, women have been more likely to seek healthcare for the above symptom [64]. In practice, globus pharyngeus can account for 4% of all patient encounters at Otolaryngology clinics with a peak onset between 36 and 51 years of age [65]. Globus pharyngeus symptoms often persist; in 75% of patients' symptoms last more than 3 years and as many as 50% of patients can have symptoms lasting up to 7 years [67].

Pathophysiology

The current understanding of the pathogenesis of globus pharyngeus is limited. Upper esophageal motor dysfunction, reflux disorders, psychologic abnormalities, and visceral hypersensitivity have all been implicated in the pathophysiology of this disorder [61, 63, 68].

Gastric reflux into the esophagus has been suggested to produce the symptom of globus pharyngeus by low pH exposure at the distal esophagus, albeit without consensus [69–75]. Symptoms may also consist of pharyngeal irritation, reflex contraction of the UES, and altered sensation in the neck. Esophageal endoscopy has revealed peptic esophagitis and hiatal hernia in 5–38% and 6–52% of patients with globus pharyngeus, respectively [71]. Despite these findings, the relationship between globus pharyngeus and gastric reflux may simply be correlational as both are prevalent among the general population and have an indistinct temporal relationship.

Patients with globus pharyngeus report higher self-assessed measures of neuroticism, introversion, anxiety, and depression, thus making them more likely to be diagnosed with an affective disorder [76–78]. Among 104 participants with globus pharyngeus, 53% had features of anxiety disorder and 41% had borderline or true depression [79]. Acute stress may also precipitate episodes of globus pharyngeus, particularly in urban versus rural patients [80].

The current theory dominating the etiology of idiopathic globus pharyngeus is visceral hypersensitivity. One study found hypersensitivity to mechanical balloon distension but not electrical stimulation in the esophagus of patients with globus pharyngeus relative to controls [81]. Visceral hypersensitivity may be present with concomitant and contributing gastric reflux or mucosal changes. Overall, there is no singular etiology for globus pharyngeus and patients may have differing or multiple co-existing pathologies contributing to their symptoms.

Diagnosis

The diagnosis of globus pharyngeus is made by eliciting a compatible clinical history, particularly distinguishing esophageal dysphagia and upper airway symptoms. Moreover, the diagnosis of globus pharyngeus does not include additional red flag features such as a sore throat, odynophagia, or unintentional weight loss [61]. Among standardized questionnaires, a subscale within the Glasgow Edinburgh

Table 18.1 Rome IV criteria for globus pharyngeus. All criteria must be fulfilled for the last 3 months with initial symptom onset at a minimum of 6 months prior to diagnosis

Rome IV criteria for globus pharyngeus
1. Persistent or intermittent, non-painful sensation of a lump or foreign body in the throat with no structural lesion identified on physical examination, laryngoscopy, or endoscopy
2. Occurrence of globus sensation between meals
3. Absence of dysphagia or odynophagia
4. Absence of a gastric inlet patch in the proximal esophagus
5. Absence of evidence that gastroesophageal reflux/eosinophilic esophagitis is causing symptoms
6. Absence of major esophageal motor disorders

Throat Scale was found to objectively characterize globus pharyngeus with high sensitivity [82].

Idiopathic globus pharyngeus is diagnosed when the sensation of a foreign body in the throat is present with the concomitant exclusion of identifiable cause according to the Rome IV criteria (Table 18.1) [60]. The Rome Foundation has published guidelines for the diagnosis of functional disorders, including irritable bowel syndrome, cyclic vomiting syndrome, and globus [83]. Identifiable causes for the aforementioned symptom can include a structural lesion, GERD, eosinophilic esophagitis, or a major esophageal motor dysfunction. Laryngoscopic evaluation can be used as a first step to rule out any structural lesion of the upper airway. When red flag symptoms are present, an upper gastrointestinal endoscopy can be ordered to rule out esophageal disorders including eosinophilic esophagitis [71, 84]. Without the direct visualization of structural causes, it is important to investigate GERD as a potential mechanism leading to the patient's symptoms. Due to its prevalence, GERD is often an assumed component of the patient's presentation. A trial of proton pump inhibitors (PPI) can be used to manage symptoms but does not delineate between a diagnosis of GERD or globus pharyngeus [60, 61, 71]. Recent evidence suggests that pH monitoring could detect abnormal acid reflux related to GERD thereby justifying medication [85, 86]. Videofluoroscopy has limited diagnostic use for globus pharyngeus because hyoid bone displacement, pharyngeal transit time, pharyngeal constriction ratio, and maximum width of esophageal opening during bolus propulsion did not differ between healthy patients and patients with globus pharyngeus [87–89]. In contrast, esophageal manometry and barium swallow testing serve an important role to rule out any major esophageal motor disorder, such as achalasia [90]. While all patients with globus sensation should receive a laryngoscopic evaluation, more extensive investigations including pH monitoring and esophageal manometry should be conducted on a patient-specific basis taking into account each individual's symptoms.

Treatment

The single most effective treatment of globus pharyngeus has yet to be defined. This may be in part due to the nonspecific etiology of the disease, however, patients should be reassured that it is a benign disease. In fact, up to half of globus pharyngeus patients can have symptom resolution with careful reassurance alone when compared to patients receiving antidepressant medications for their symptoms [91, 92]. Importantly, such conservative management does not entail any medication-specific risks.

Speech-language therapy can be a conservative method of treating globus pharyngeus [63, 68]. Khalil et al. showed globus symptom improvement in a randomized cohort of 36 participants by using exercises to relieve pharyngolaryngeal tension such as yawning, a "giggling" posture, and liquid swallowing when compared to reassurance alone [93]. In patients with persistent symptoms and the absence of any laryngeal mucosa abnormalities, the initial management is often a PPI trial for 6–8 weeks, most commonly omeprazole 20 mg twice daily [68]. Alternatively, current evidence demonstrates a role for ablative therapy on any heterotopic gastric inlet patches by gastroenterology [94, 95].

When alternative therapies fail, neuromodulators may be used in the management of idiopathic globus pharyngeus with good results, although the evidence remains conflicted [60]. One randomized controlled trial showed that amitriptyline improved symptoms in 76% of patients with globus pharyngeus, whereas pantoprazole had a response in only 36% of patients [96]. Selective serotonin reuptake inhibitors have also been successful in treating globus symptoms and is suggested to be due in part to their management of visceral hypersensitivity or anxiety disorders [97].

Summary

Globus pharyngeus is characterized by the sensation of a lump or tightness in the throat that is not due to an underlying structural lesion, GERD, or esophageal motor disorder. The symptoms are often intermittent but may persist for years. Due to an uncertain underlying etiology, no singular management protocol is established. Some therapies that have demonstrated improvement include a trial of PPI, neuromodulator treatment, and most recently heterotrophic gastric islet patch ablation. All patients with symptoms of globus pharyngeus should undergo a thorough laryngeal work up including a laryngoscopic visualization of the upper airway and possibly esophageal investigations to rule out any potentially more sinister diagnoses. In most instances of true globus pharyngeus, patients are reassured that it is a benign disorder.

References

1. Sasaki CT, Issacson G. Functional anatomy of the larynx. Otolaryngol Clin N Am. 1988;21(4):595.
2. Beslie GM, Morrison MD. Anatomic correlation for muscle tension dysphonia. J Otolaryngol. 1983;12(5):319–21.
3. Van Houtte E, Van Lierde K, Claeys S. Pathophysiology and treatment of muscle tension dysphonia: a review of the current knowledge. J Voice. 2011;25(2):202–7.

4. Gardner GM, Benninger MS. Other neuromuscular causes of dysphonia and trauma. In: Otolaryngoloy: a color handbook. Boca Raton, FL: CRC Press; 2016. p. 189–200.
5. Morrison MD, Rammage LA, Beslie GM, Pullan CB, Nichol H. Muscular tension dysphonia. J Otolaryngol. 1983;12(5):302–6.
6. Morrison MD, Rammage LA. Muscle misuse voice disorders: description and classification. Acta Otolaryngol. 1993;113(3):428–34.
7. Van Houtte E, Van Lierde K, D'Haeseleer E, Claeys S. The prevalence of laryngeal pathology in a treatment-seeking population with dysphonia. Laryngoscope. 2010;120(2):306–12.
8. Roy N. Functional dysphonia. Curr Opin Otolaryngol Head Neck Surg. 2003;11:144–8.
9. Bridger MW, Epstein R. Functional voice disorders: a review of 109 patients. J Laryngol Otol. 1983;97(12):1145.
10. Sama A, Carding PN, Price S, Kelly P, Wilson JA. The clinical features of functional dysphonia. Laryngoscope. 2001;111(3):458–63.
11. Hočevar-Boltežar I, Janko M, Žargi M. Role of surface EMG in diagnostics and treatment of muscle tension dysphonia. Acta Otolaryngol. 1998;118(5):739–43.
12. Redenbaugh MA, Reich AR. Surface EMG and related measures in normal and vocally hyperfunctional speakers. J Speech Hear Disord. 1989;54(1):68.
13. Koufman JA, Blalock PD. Functional voice disorders. Otollaryngol Clin North Am. 1991;1(24):1059–73.
14. Koufman JA, Blalock PD. Classification and approach to patients with functional voice disorders. Ann Otol Rhinol Laryngol. 1982;91:372–7.
15. Roy N, Bless DM, Heisey D. Personality and voice disorders: a superfactor trait analysis. J Speech Lang Hear Res. 2000;43:749–68.
16. Roy N, McGrory JJ, Tasko SM, Bless DM, Heisey D, Ford CN. Psychological correlates of functional dysphonia: an investigation using the Minnesota multiphasic personality inventory. J Voice. 1997;11(4):443–51.
17. Van Mersbergen M, Patrick C, Glaze L. Functional dysphonia during mental imagery: testing the trait theory of voice disorders. J Speech Lang Hear Res. 2008;51(6):1405–23.
18. Angsuwarangsee T, Morrison MD. Extrinsic laryngeal muscular tension in patients with voice disorders. J Voice. 2002;16(3):333–43.
19. Altman KW, Atkinson C, Lazarus C. Current and emerging concepts in muscle tension dysphonia: a 30-month review. J Voice. 2005;19(2):261–7.
20. McGarey PO, Barone NA, Freeman M, Daniero JJ. Comorbid dysphagia and dyspnea in muscle tension dysphonia: a global laryngeal musculoskeletal problem. OTO Open. 2018;2(3):2473974X1879567.
21. Koufman JA, Amin MR, Panetti M. Prevalence of reflux in 113 consecutive patients with laryngeal and voice disorders. Otolaryngol Head Neck Surg. 2000;123(4):385–8.
22. Abitbol J, Abitbol P, Abitbol B. Sex hormones and the female voice. J Voice. 1999;13(3):424–46.
23. D'Haeseleer E, Depypere H, Claeys S, Van Borsel J, Van Lierde K. The menopause and the female larynx, clinical aspects and therapeutic options: a literature review. Maturitas. 2009;64(1):27–32.
24. Bielamowicz S. Aging voice or vocal fold paresis. Arch Otolaryngol Neck Surg. 2004;130(9):1114.
25. Morrison MD, Nichol H, Rammage LA. Diagnostic criteria in functional dysphonia. Laryngoscope. 1986;96(1):1.
26. Ruotsalainen J, Sellman J, Lehto L, Verbeek J. Systematic review of the treatment of functional dysphonia and prevention of voice disorders. Otolaryngol Head Neck Surg. 2008;138(5):557–65.
27. Smith ME, Houtz DR. Muscle tension dysphonia and puberphonia. Multidisciplinary management of pediatric voice and swallowing disorders. Cham: Springer; 2020. p. 239–44.
28. Mackenzie K, Millar A, Wilson JA, Sellars C, Deary IJ. Is voice therapy an effective treatment for dysphonia? A randomised controlled trial. BMJ. 2001;323(7314):658.

29. Carding PN, Horsley IA, Docherty GJ. A study of the effectiveness of voice therapy in the treatment of 45 patients with nonorganic dysphonia. J Voice. 1999;13(1):72–104.
30. Ruotsalainen JH, Sellman J, Lehto L, Jauhiainen M, Verbeek JH. Interventions for treating functional dysphonia in adults. Cochrane Database Syst Rev. 2007;(3):CD006373.
31. Roy N, Leeper HA. Effects of the manual laryngeal musculoskeletal tension reduction technique as a treatment for functional voice disorders: perceptual and acoustic measures. J Voice. 1993;7(3):242–9.
32. Roy N, Ford CN, Bless DM. Muscle tension dysphonia and spasmodic dysphonia: the role of manual laryngeal tension reduction in diagnosis and management. Ann Otol Rhinol Laryngol. 1996;105(11):851–6.
33. Roy N, Bless DM, Heisey D, Ford CN. Manual circumlaryngeal therapy for functional dysphonia: an evaluation of short- and long-term treatment outcomes. J Voice. 1997;11(3):321–31.
34. Ali MES. Laryngopharyngeal reflux: diagnosis and treatment of a controversial disease. Curr Opin Allergy Clin Immunol. 2008;8(1):28–33.
35. Ibrahim WH, Gheriani HA, Almohamed AA, Raza T. Paradoxical vocal cord motion disorder: past, present and future. Postgrad Med J. 2007;83(977):164–72.
36. Halvorsen T, Walsted ES, Bucca C, Bush A, Cantarella G, Friedrich G, et al. Inducible laryngeal obstruction: an official joint European Respiratory Society and European Laryngological Society statement. Eur Respir J. 2017;50(3):1602221.
37. Morris MJ, Christopher KL. Diagnostic criteria for the classification of vocal cord dysfunction. Chest. 2010;138(5):1213–23.
38. Lee J, Denton E, Hoy R, Tay TR, Bondarenko J, Hore-Lacy F, et al. Paradoxical vocal fold motion in difficult asthma is associated with dysfunctional breathing and preserved lung function. J Allergy Clin Immunol Pract. 2020;8(7):2256–62.
39. Koufman JA, Block C. Differential diagnosis of paradoxical vocal fold movement. Am J Speech Lang Pathol. 2008;17(4):327.
40. Marcinow AM, Thompson J, Chiang T, Forrest LA, Desilva BW. Paradoxical vocal fold motion disorder in the elite athlete: experience at a large division i university. Laryngoscope. 2014;124(6):1425–30.
41. Forrest LA, Husein T, Husein O. Paradoxical vocal cord motion: classification and treatment. Laryngoscope. 2012;122(4):844–53.
42. Seear M, Wensley D, West N. How accurate is the diagnosis of exercise induced asthma among Vancouver schoolchildren? Arch Dis Child. 2005;90(9):898–902.
43. Pasternak K, Thibeault SL. Factors affecting initiation of voice therapy for paradoxical vocal fold motion disorder. J Voice. 2020;34(4):559–66.
44. Bucca C. Are asthma-like symptoms due to bronchial or extrathoracic airway dysfunction? Lancet. 1995;345(8978):791–5.
45. Ayres JG, Gabbott PLA. Vocal cord dysfunction and laryngeal hyperresponsiveness: a function of altered autonomic balance? Br Med J. 2002;57(4):284.
46. Newman KB, Mason UG, Schmaling KB. Clinical features of vocal cord dysfunction. Am J Respir Crit Care Med. 1995;152(4):1382.
47. Christopher KL, Eckert RC, Blager FB, Raney RA, Souhrada JF. Vocal-cord dysfunction presenting as asthma. N Engl J Med. 1983;308(26):1566.
48. Brugman SM, Simons SM. Vocal cord dysfunction: don't mistake it for asthma. Phys Sportsmed. 1998;26(5):63–85.
49. Morris MJ, Deal LE, Bean DR, Grbach VX, Morgan JA. Vocal cord dysfunction in patients with exertional dyspnea. Chest. 1999;116(6):1676–82.
50. Guss J, Mirza N. Methacholine challenge testing in the diagnosis of paradoxical vocal fold motion. Laryngoscope. 2006;116(9):1558–61.
51. Pitchenik AE. Functional laryngeal obstruction relieved by panting. Chest. 1991;100(5):1465–7.
52. Patel RR, Venediktov R, Schooling T, Wang B. Evidence-based systematic review: effects of speech-language pathology treatment for individuals with paradoxical vocal fold motion. Am J Speech Lang Hear Res. 2015;24(2):1–14.

53. Weir M. Vocal cord dysfunction mimics asthma and may respond to heliox. Clin Pediatr (Phila). 2002;41(1):37–41.
54. Morris MJ, Allan PF, Perkins PJ. Vocal cord dysfunction: etiologies and treatment. Clin Pulm Med. 2006;13(2):73–86.
55. Woisard V, Liu X, Bes MCA, Simonetta-Moreau M. Botulinum toxin injection in laryngeal dyspnea. Eur Arch Otorhinolaryngol. 2017;274(2):909–17.
56. deSilva B, Crenshaw D, Matrka L, Forrest LA. Vocal fold botulinum toxin injection for refractory paradoxical vocal fold motion disorder. Laryngoscope. 2019;129(4):808–11.
57. Christopher KL, Morris MJ. Vocal cord dysfunction, paradoxic vocal fold motion, or laryngomalacia? Our understanding requires an interdisciplinary approach. Otolaryngol Clin N Am. 2010;43(1):43–66.
58. Rameau A, Foltz RS, Wagner K, Zur KB. Multidisciplinary approach to vocal cord dysfunction diagnosis and treatment in one session: a single institutional outcome study. Int J Pediatr Otorhinolaryngol. 2012;76(1):31–5.
59. Heiser JM, Kahn ML, Schmidt TA. Functional airway obstruction presenting as stridor: a case report and literature review. J Emerg Med. 1990;8(3):285–9.
60. Aziz Q, Fass R, Gyawali CP, Miwa H, Pandolfino JE, Zerbib F. Esophageal disorders. Gastroenterology. 2016;150(6):1368–79.
61. Zerbib F, Rommel N, Pandolfino J, Gyawali CP. ESNM/ANMS review. Diagnosis and management of globus sensation: a clinical challenge. Neurogastroenterol Motil. 2020;32(9):1–8.
62. Ortiz AS, Lawton A, Rives E, Gutierrez G, Dion GR. Correlating videofluoroscopic swallow study findings with subjective globus location. Laryngoscope. 2019;129(2):335–8.
63. Lee BE, Kim GH. Globus pharyngeus: a review of its etiology, diagnosis and treatment. World J Gastroenterol. 2012;18(20):2462–71.
64. Tang B, Da CH, Xie HL, Chen DY, Jiang SM, Jia L. Epidemiology of globus symptoms and associated psychological factors in China. J Dig Dis. 2016;17(5):319–24.
65. Moloy PJ, Charter R. The Globus Symptom. Arch Otolaryngol. 1982;108(11):740.
66. Josefsson A, Palsson O, Simrén M, Sperber AD, Törnblom H, Whitehead W. Oesophageal symptoms are common and associated with other functional gastrointestinal disorders (FGIDs) in an English-speaking Western population. United Eur Gastroenterol J. 2018;6(10):1461–9.
67. Timon C, O'Dwyer T, Cagney D, Walsh M. Globus pharyngeus: long-term follow-up and prognostic factors. Ann Otol Rhinol Laryngol. 1991;100:351–4.
68. Järvenpää P, Arkkila P, Aaltonen LM. Globus pharyngeus: a review of etiology, diagnostics, and treatment. Eur Arch Otorhinolaryngol. 2018;275(8):1945–53.
69. Vakil NB, Kahrilas PJ, Dodds WJ, Vanagunas A. Absence of an upper esophageal sphincter response to acid reflux. Am J Gastroenterol. 1989;84(6):606–10.
70. Thompson WG, Heaton KW. Heartburn and globus in apparently healthy people. Can Med Assoc J. 1982;126(1):46–8.
71. Selleslagh M, Van Oudenhove L, Pauwels A, Tack J, Rommel N. The complexity of globus: a multidisciplinary perspective. Nat Rev Gastroenterol Hepatol. 2014;11(4):220–33.
72. Van Daele DJ. Esophageal manometry, pH testing, endoscopy, and videofluoroscopy in patients with globus sensation. Laryngoscope. 2020;130(9):2120–5.
73. Norder Grusell E, Mjörnheim AC, Finizia C, Ruth M, Bergquist H. The diagnostic value of GerdQ in subjects with atypical symptoms of gastro-esophageal reflux disease. Scand J Gastroenterol. 2018;53(10–11):1165–70.
74. Hill J, Stuart RC, Fung HK, Ng EKW, Cheung FM, Chung SCS, et al. Gastroesophageal reflux, motility disorders, and psychological profiles in the etiology of globus pharyngis. Laryngoscope. 1997;107(10):1373–7.
75. Tokashiki R, Yamaguchi H, Nakamura K, Suzuki M. Globus sensation caused by gastro epophageal reflux disease. Auris Nasus Larynx. 2002;29(4):347–51.
76. Cook IJ, Dent J, Collins SM. Upper esophageal sphincter tone and reactivity to stress in patients with a history of globus sensation. Dig Dis Sci. 1989;34(5):672–6.

77. Deary IJ, Smart A, Wilson JA. Depression and "hassles" in globus pharyngis. Br J Psychiatry. 1992;161(JULY):115–7.
78. Wilson JA, Deary IJ, Maran AGD. Is globus hystericus? Br J Psychiatry. 1988;153(Sep.):335–9.
79. Khan M, Saha M, Mamun M, Salam K, Chowdhury M, Hasque M, et al. Upper GIT endoscopic evaluation and psychological state assessment of patients with globus sensation. Mymensingh Med J. 2019;28(2):405–9.
80. Tang B, Wang X, Chen C, Deng X, Ouyang X, Jia L, et al. The differences in epidemiological and psychological features of globus symptoms between urban and rural Guangzhou, China: a cross-sectional study. Medicine. 2018;97(43):16–8.
81. Chen CL, Szczesniak MM, Cook IJ. Evidence for oesophageal visceral hypersensitivity and aberrant symptom referral in patients with globus. Neurogastroenterol Motil. 2009;21(11):1142–8.
82. Wilson JA, Harris MB, Deary IJ. Globus pharyngis: development assessment scale. J Psychosom Res. 1995;39(2):203–13.
83. The Rome Foundation. Rome IV Diagnostic Criteria. Rome IV Book.
84. Sanyaolu LN, Jemah A, Stew B, Ingrams DR. The role of transnasal oesophagoscopy in the management of globus pharyngeus and non-progressive dysphagia. Ann R Coll Surg Engl. 2016;98(1):49–52.
85. Gawron AJ, Rothe J, Fought AJ, Fareeduddin A, Toto E, Boris L, et al. Many patients continue using proton pump inhibitors after negative results from tests for reflux disease. Clin Gastroenterol Hepatol. 2012;10(6):620–5.
86. Yadlapati R, Ciolino JD, Craft J, Roman S, Pandolfino JE. Trajectory assessment is useful when day-to-day esophageal acid exposure varies in prolonged wireless pH monitoring. Dis Esophagus. 2019;32(3):1–7.
87. Dworkin JP, Dowdall JR, Kubik M, Thottam PJ, Folbe A. The role of the modified barium swallow study and esophagram in patients with globus sensation. Dysphagia. 2015;30(5):506–10.
88. Järvenpää P, Ilmarinen T, Geneid A, Pietarinen P, Kinnari TJ, Rihkanen H, et al. Work-up of globus: assessing the benefits of neck ultrasound and videofluorography. Eur Arch Otorhinolaryngol. 2017;274(2):931–7.
89. Li J, Zhang J, Guo P, Tian S, Li K. Dynamic swallowing study for globus patients. World J Otorhinolaryngol Head Neck Surg. 2016;2(4):198–202.
90. Kahrilas PJ, Bredenoord AJ, Fox M, Gyawali CP, Roman S, Smout AJPM, et al. The Chicago Classification of esophageal motility disorders, v3.0. Neurogastroenterol Motil. 2015;27(2):160–74.
91. Cybulska EVAM. Globus Hystericus—a somatic symptom of depression ? The role of electroconvulsive therapy and antidepressants. Psychosom Med. 1997;69(10):67–9.
92. Brown SR, Schwartz JM, Summergrad P, Jenike MA. Globus hystericus syndrome responsive to antidepressants. Am J Psychiatry. 1986;143(7):917–8.
93. Khalil HS, Bridger MW, Hilton-Pierce VJ. The use of speech therapy in the treatment of globus pharyngeus patients. A randomised controlled trial. Rev Laryngol Otol Rhinol (Bord). 2002;124(4):187–90.
94. Kristo I, Rieder E, Paireder M, Schwameis K, Jomrich G, Dolak W, et al. Radiofrequency ablation in patients with large cervical heterotopic gastric mucosa and globus sensation: closing the treatment gap. Dig Endosc. 2018;30(2):212–8.
95. Klare P, Meining A, Von Delius S, Wolf P, Konukiewitz B, Schmid RM, et al. Argon plasma coagulation of gastric inlet patches for the treatment of globus sensation: it is an effective therapy in the long term. Digestion. 2013;88(3):165–71.
96. Weijenborg PW, de Schepper HS, Smout AJPM, Bredenoord AJ. Effects of antidepressants in patients with functional esophageal disorders or gastroesophageal reflux disease: a systematic review. Clin Gastroenterol Hepatol. 2015;13(2):251–259.e1.
97. Zhou W-C, Jia L, Chen D-Y, Liu Y, Liu J, Jiang S-M, et al. The effects of paroxetine and amitriptyline on the upper esophageal sphincter (UES) pressure and its natural history in globus pharyngeus. Dig Liver Dis. 2017;49(7):757–63.

A Psychological Approach to Functional Illness

19

Anna Marie A. Carlson and Gregg A. Tkachuk

A History of Psychological Conceptualization of Functional Illness

The biomedical model, introduced into medical thinking by Descartes in the seventeenth century, assumes a dualistic view in which somatic symptoms are considered either somatogenic (i.e., the result of physical pathology), or in the case where no medical cause can be ascertained, psychogenic (i.e., psychological in origin). Traditional medicine has adopted this dichotomous, Cartesian mind–body dualistic view. Psychogenic views of unexplained physical symptoms have been inculcated since the formulation of psychodynamic theory and have been criticized as overly stigmatizing patients and providing too narrow an explanation, particularly for chronic medical conditions where no cure is available. Nonetheless, this view remains pervasive both within and outside of the health care system.

The Biopsychosocial Perspective

Human beings differ in their expression of physical symptoms, their propensity to seek medical care, and their responses to medical treatments. Melzack was instrumental in expanding the dualistic mind- or body framework in his study of chronic pain. The Gate-Control Theory [1, 2] encouraged consideration of the psychological factors in the pain experience through interaction with modulation of ascending

A. M. A. Carlson (✉)
Department of Clinical Health Psychology, University of Manitoba, Brandon, MB, Canada
e-mail: annamarie.carlson@umanitoba.ca

G. A. Tkachuk
Department of Clinical Health Psychology, University of Manitoba, Winnipeg, MB, Canada

© The Author(s), under exclusive license to Springer Nature Switzerland AG 2023

B. W. Blakley, J. E. Blakley (eds.), *Functional Illness of the Head and Neck*,
https://doi.org/10.1007/978-3-031-12998-8_19

and descending pathways in the central nervous system. In 1999 [3], Melzack reported on the Neuromatrix Theory of pain, which combined gate-control theory with an expanded view of the brain's neural network combined with the body's natural adaptations to stress. This theory has continued to be widely supported and offers an explanation for a number of chronic pain conditions such as fibromyalgia, and migraine.

Similarly, Engel [4] proposed a biopsychosocial perspective to explain both the disease process and the subjective experience that a disease is present, including how an individual and the individual's wider social network perceive and adapt to physical symptoms and disability. The hallmark of the biopsychosocial model is a complex, dynamic, and reciprocal interaction of biological, psychological, and social variables.

Functional Somatic Syndromes

Based on the earlier work of Kellner [5–7] the term *functional somatic syndrome* (FSS) was first introduced by Barsky and Borus [8] to describe categories of bodily symptoms frequently encountered in many areas of medical practice that have no well-defined structural organic pathology. Nonetheless, the presence of functional somatic symptoms results in considerable distress and disability, rendering patients and medical practitioners alike susceptible to frustration due to a lack of effective treatments. Common bodily symptoms include pain, dizziness, heart palpitations, gastrointestinal distress, weakness, and generalized fatigue of varying levels of severity. Some patients present with a single persistent symptom, or set of symptoms from the same organ system, while others describe multiple symptoms relating to several organ systems. Accompanying features may, but do not necessarily, include high health anxiety, bodily checking behaviors, high rates of anxiety and/or depression, and personality disorders. As a result, quality of life tends to be lower, disability rates higher, and long-term outcomes poorer in those with multiple, and more severe, bodily symptoms [9].

There is a high comorbidity between functional somatic symptoms and psychological disorders. For example, Kleykamp et al. (2021) [10] reported that over half of individuals with fibromyalgia experienced depression in their lifetime. Carta et al. [11] reported a significant risk of lifetime prevalence of mood disorders (65%), post-traumatic stress disorder (PTSD) (8.4%), and panic disorder (28.2%) in individuals with fibromyalgia, and referenced the possibility of vulnerability to chronic stress. Janssens et al. (2015) [12] reported that mood and anxiety disorders are more prevalent in individuals with FSS, however, the authors found most persons with FSS do not have mood or anxiety disorders. Adding to the disease burden of individuals with FSS, there is also consideration of comorbidity with other functional disorders (39–76%) [10].

Etiology of FSS

It is beyond the scope of this chapter to review all available etiological models of FSS. The factors most notably included for consideration in traditional models include predisposing, perpetuating, and precipitating factors as well as the dynamic and reciprocal interplay among these factors in explaining the experience of bodily distress [9, 13, 14].

Predisposing factors include genetics, early experience with illness, vicarious learning of familial illness behavior, cultural views of illness, a history of adverse childhood experiences including physical or sexual trauma, neuroticism (i.e., heightened reactivity to stressors, tendency toward experiencing negative affect such as anxiety or depression), and a general predisposition to experience distress related to bodily symptoms or health anxiety.

Perpetuating factors include central nervous system sensitization to previously encountered stressful stimuli and positive and negative feedback loops involving the hypothalamus–pituitary–adrenal (HPA) axis in the regulation of cortisol and release of inflammatory cytokines. Features of attention, perception, focus, health-related attributions, illness-related beliefs, and behavioral responses to illness such as avoidance and deconditioning have also been implicated. The latter of these components are typically targeted for change in behavioral treatment approaches.

Precipitating factors are events that are hypothesized to trigger the start of the self-perpetuating cycle. These are essentially major life events or persistent daily stressors that confront the sympathetic nervous system such as illness, accidents, injuries, significant losses, work, family, or relationship stressors, and perceived threats to one's well-being. Maladaptive coping responses to these events can potentially lead to a chronic or prolonged state of activation that is maintained by cognitive factors (i.e., perseverative worry, rumination, or catastrophizing) and experiential (i.e., cognitive, emotional, and behavioral) avoidance that can also be a focus of psychological treatment.

As mentioned earlier, another important feature of etiological models is the dynamic interplay among these factors in explaining the experience of bodily distress. This can be characterized as an autopoietic process of symptom generation and perpetuation [13]. As an example, consider an individual with a predisposition to experience bodily distress who is subjected to an adverse childhood experience or observes a parent responding with high anxiety to a relatively minor illness. These early life events could sensitize the central nervous system to lower the threshold for symptom detection. A precipitating stressor later in life such as a minor injury or relatively common viral illness, loss of a loved one or important relationship triggers the experience or expectation of physical symptoms, which are catastrophically misinterpreted as signifying danger or serious disease, and a significant emotional response that has previously been paired with physical symptoms through classical conditioning. A maladaptive coping response such as frequent bodily checking behavior or seeking frequent reassurance from medical providers and significant others temporarily reduces anxiety but reinforces the further need for such reassurance seeking whenever similar symptoms inevitably resurface. The individual also seeks to avoid important life activities that may provoke physical symptoms, and this avoidance is maintained by operant conditioning. Over time, physical deconditioning and increased disability and depression are the results. This further sensitizes the individual by lowering the threshold for symptom detection and accompanying emotional distress. The individual becomes stuck in the perpetual cycle of symptom maintenance, anxiety, and despair [9].

More recent etiological models attempt to expand upon the traditional models to address how symptom perception is initiated and why symptom-related distress is maintained despite reassurance from physicians. One influential model is based on the idea that the central nervous system is a predictive coding machine whereby disorders of interoception can occur when peripheral sensory inputs do not match the centrally based (i.e., central nervous system) predictions [15]. It proposes a mechanism whereby FSS patients may construct the perception of bodily symptoms in the absence of peripheral physiological sensations. In this view, somatic symptoms are essentially considered to be "somatovisceral illusions" or memories of previous sensations. Another relatively recent model addresses the question of why symptom-related distress persists despite medical reassurance and negative test results [16]. It proposes that, while patients with FSS may be initially relieved by medical reassurance, they later negatively reappraise the information presented by the physician and thus, reinvoke the original concern. They further suggest that this process eventually renders FSS patients "immune" to medical reassurance.

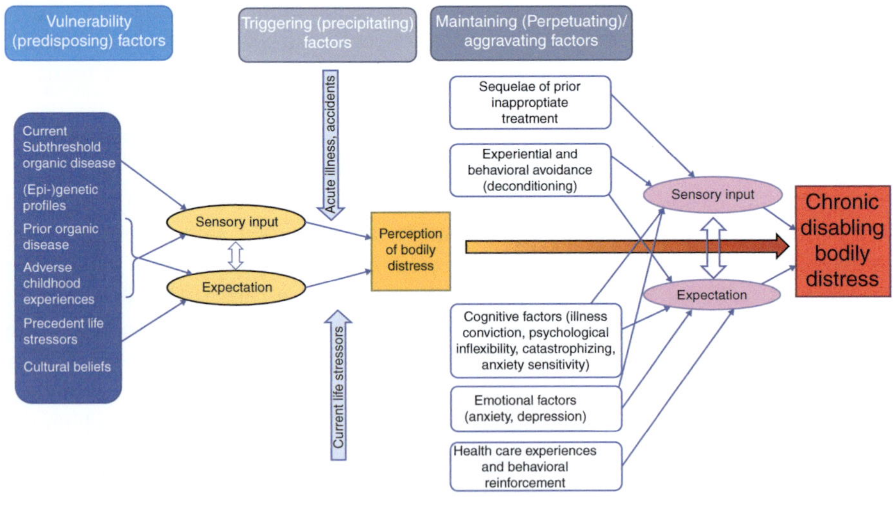

Fig. 19.1 Schematic model of the etiology of bodily distress. Note: The distinction between vulnerability/triggering and perpetuating/aggravating factors is to some extent artificial as most factors influence on both sides. Adapted from Henningsen et al. [9]. Reproduced with permission from S. Karger AG, Basel

Within a comprehensive framework that includes both the traditional and contemporary models, some etiological factors will preferentially act either via centrally or peripherally acting routes, but most can influence both routes (see upper and lower parts of Fig. 19.1, called "sensory input" and "expectation").

Psychological Assessment of Functional Illness

As previously outlined, FSS symptoms may be influenced by a number of autopoietic biopsychosocial factors and as such the assessment will focus on these factors. The purpose of the assessment is to gather information about the physical symptoms (see Table 19.1), level of distress and dysfunction caused by the symptoms, psychological functioning and psychological comorbidities, social situation, general background and upbringing, early life experiences with health and physical symptoms, and coping skills [17]. The intention in this phase is to have information to facilitate differential diagnosis, create a conceptualization of the biopsychosocial factors influencing the physical symptoms, begin forming a therapeutic alliance, and be able to start direct treatment planning [18].

Table 19.1 Targets of assessment in psychological interview

• Physical symptom assessment
• Description of symptoms
• Description of symptom onset and progression
• Frequency, severity, duration of symptoms
• Triggers/patterns of symptoms
• Perception of cause
• Medical investigations and results
• Understanding and level of acceptance of functional diagnosis
• Previous treatments (helpful and unhelpful) – medications for symptoms (prescription and nonprescription), patterns of use – allied health, and alternative treatments
• Dysfunction/limitations/distress linked to the interpretation of the physical symptoms and/or by the symptoms themselves
• Strategies employed to cope with/influence symptoms
• Goals for symptom reduction (e.g., total absence, 50% improvement, and improved function)
General medical history
• Diagnoses, other functional, and otherwise
• Limits to function as result of other medical conditions
• Medications
• Hospitalizations, surgeries, notable procedures
• History of head injury
• Relationships with/attitudes towards health care providers
• Significant frustrations with receiving health care, diagnostics, etc.
Lifestyle assessment
• Sample daily schedule
• Sleep

(continued)

Table 19.1 (continued)

• Exercise
• Appetite
• Recreational substances including caffeine, alcohol, and nicotine, and substance abuse history
Psychological symptoms and personality functioning
• Current mood
• Symptoms of depression
• Symptoms of anxiety – How does a person typically experience stress? Body symptoms? – Symptoms of generalized anxiety disorder (GAD) and Panic disorder – obsessive-compulsive disorder (OCD), Social Anxiety, Specific phobia
• Trauma history – Early childhood, assault, accidents, medical procedures – Symptoms of PTSD
• Suicidal/homicidal ideation – Plan, intent, means, history of same – Current safety
• Psychological/psychiatric including treatment history
• Life stressors
• Changes in symptoms/stressors/mood in timeline with functional symptoms
Social history
• Family of origin
• Family history – Medical, mental health, and substance use – Family's understanding of/stigma toward health medical and mental health concerns
• Current living situation
• Support systems/significant relationships
• Current source of income, financial hardship
• Developmental and social history
• Experience with illness, physical symptoms (if not obtained in medical history)
• Education history
• Work history
• Hobbies/recreational life
Treatment indicators
• Goals of treatment such as "miracle cure", and/or reduction of medication, symptoms, distress, dysfunction, etc.
• Relative resistance/acceptance to mind-body connection (biopsychosocial model of treatment)
• Motivation for treatment—willing to take active steps for change
• Secondary gain
• Function/reinforcement of symptoms in environment
• Active psychosis, untreated bipolar disorder
• Adequate physical health
Behavioral observations
• Pain/symptom behavior (grimacing, wincing, rubbing, and bracing)
• Use of assistive devices (i.e., walking aid, earplugs, and neck brace)
• Level of openness in sharing personal details, sense of insight into mind-body connection
• Cognitive status
• Mood – range of affect – stated mood with observable mood

Patients seen in this setting are likely to be hesitant to see the role psychology may play and are concerned the referral implies that their symptoms are "all in their head"—suggesting a feigning or imagination of the symptoms, or that a potentially serious condition is being ignored by a referral to psychology. These patients typically will report high distress from their symptoms and are keen on finding a medical "fix". Assessment may begin with inquiring as to the patient's understanding of the referral and thoughts about meeting with a psychologist [18].

As such, it is typically prudent to initially focus the psychological assessment on the physical symptoms before moving into a more traditional psychological and lifestyle evaluation. This information is typically gathered through clinical interview, self-report symptom questionnaires and/or symptom diaries of varying length and symptom focus. The most widely used patient self-report scales to assess for severe health anxiety/somatization include the Whitely Index [19], Illness Attitudes Scales [20], and Health Anxiety Inventory [21] and these measures have been shown to have good psychometric properties [22]. Self-report scales are also available to assess psychological constructs that may be associated with higher symptom intensity and disability such as anxiety sensitivity [23] and pain catastrophizing [24]. Behavioral observations of the patient are also typically included in the assessment.

Psychological assessment is often a dynamic process and typically continues over the course of treatment. Over time, patients become more invested in understanding their own triggers and tend to remember more about circumstances that corresponded to symptom onset as they become aware of physical and emotional experiences during the course of therapy [18].

As reviewed previously, individuals with functional illness are likely to have a comorbid psychological diagnosis such as an anxiety or depressive disorder. A number of other DSM-5 diagnoses may be indicated specifically in relation to the functional symptoms. The key differentials are related to the timing of symptom onset, the context in which the symptoms occur, and distress related specifically to

Table 19.2 DSM-5 diagnostic considerations for functional symptoms

Adjustment disorder • when physical symptoms came first and changes in mood and anxiety are related to the stress of having the physical symptom(s)
Trauma-related disorder • if physical symptoms began within the context of post-traumatic distress
Other anxiety disorder • if symptoms are transient and/or only occur in the context of other anxiety disorder (i.e., tinnitus during social interactions for someone with social anxiety disorder)
Depressive disorder • full criteria for disorder needs to be met to diagnose instead of adjustment disorder even if a change in mood seems connected to the symptoms • if a physical symptom is consistent with somatic symptoms of depression

(continued)

Table 19.2 (continued)

Conversion disorder (functional neurological disorder) • voluntary motor or sensory symptoms inconsistent with known medical condition, cannot be accounted for by another mental or medical disorder, and are distressing, impairing, or subject to medical investigation • coded with and without the psychological stressor. Criteria for PTSD should not be met
Illness anxiety disorder • physical symptoms are mild at best but the individual is concerned about acquiring an illness • typically strong checking and avoidance patterns related to the physical symptoms
Somatic symptom disorder • physical symptoms are present, often in more than one physical domain • symptoms cause significant distress and limitations characterized by concern regarding the seriousness of symptoms, anxiety about health and symptoms, and significant time and energy dedicated to symptoms or health concerns
Psychological factors affecting a medical condition • an underlying medical condition exists but behavioral or psychological factors affect condition (i.e., someone with mild arthritis in C-spine experiences significant muscle tension in neck due to anxiety thus producing significant neck pain)
Factitious disorder (on self or other) • falsification of physical symptoms in self or another, with identified deception
Psychotic Disorder with somatic delusion or hallucination • most common somatic delusions are: foul order from body (i.e., halitosis), infestation in body, body part being misshapen, or body parts not functioning properly (e.g., circulatory system) [25] • the description or cause is likely to be bizarre (e.g., the pain is from an alien lifeform in my abdomen) • related behavioral observation present (e.g., damage to skin/tissue from self-treatment)
If patient in not particularly distressed from or limited by functional symptoms no diagnosis may be indicated

the physical symptoms or the perceived cause of the symptoms [25]. The DSM-5 transitioned away from the classification of somatoform disorders, which implied psychogenic origin, to somatic symptoms and related disorders.

The ICD system has similar diagnoses for distress from physical symptoms or anticipation of medical illness. The anticipated ICD-11 contains a proposed "bodily distress disorder" appearing in the mental health section, which is similar to the DSM-5 somatic symptom disorder [26]. A "bodily distress syndrome" is proposed to appear in the health care section as a replacement for medically unexplained somatic complaints [27].

Psychological Treatment of Functional Illness

There are a variety of psychological treatments that have been researched by category of physical symptom (i.e., pain and tinnitus), diagnosis (i.e., migraine, temporomandibular joint (TMJ), and fibromyalgia), and aligned psychological diagnosis (i.e., somatic symptom disorder). All therapies have in common a desire to intervene at the biopsychosocial level, by impacting the stress system and considering/targeting thoughts and interpretations, behavior, emotion, and physical sensations.

Below is a summary of different therapies that are designed to treat functional syndromes and functional limitations. Other treatments within each treatment orientation exist for comorbid diagnoses (i.e., generalized anxiety disorder) but are not reviewed here.

Cognitive-Behavioral Therapy

The cognitive-behavioral model is compatible (Fig. 19.2) with the biopsychosocial model in terms of the dynamic reciprocal relationship among physiological, psychological, social, and behavioral factors and how these variables function to predispose, precipitate, and perpetuate FSS [13, 14]. The model posits that there is a reciprocal and dynamic interplay of the thoughts, emotions, behavior, and physical sensations.

For example, an individual may be in a situation in which they notice physical sensations. Then these sensations may be catastrophically misinterpreted as being reflective of a serious disease, these responses will lead to emotional distress in the form of increased anxiety and/or depression, and the individual will make efforts to reduce the symptoms through avoiding daily activities or frequent symptom checking. These in turn can lead to increased preoccupation with symptoms, increased avoidance, physical deconditioning and disability, which in turn makes it more likely that anxiety and the physical symptoms will continue thus keeping this interplay continuing in a loop.

Furthermore, environmental/social variables such as how others respond to the individual and/or symptoms play an important role in whether maladaptive thoughts and behaviors are maintained. Cognitive behavioral treatment focuses on symptom reduction by helping the patient to identify, examine, and reshape thoughts and

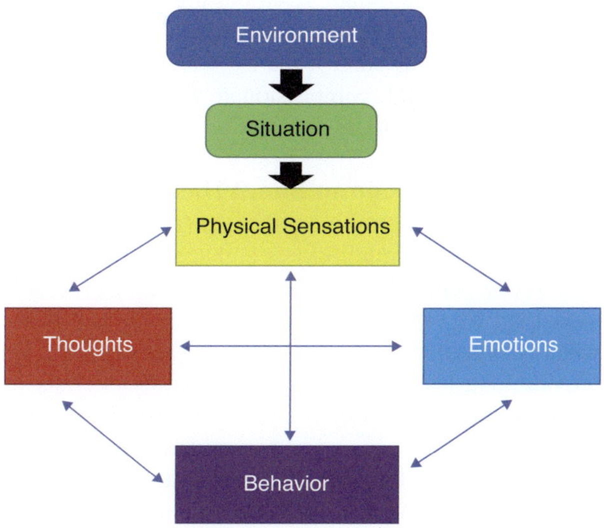

Fig. 19.2 Cognitive-behavioral model of treatment

beliefs about symptoms through education, guided discovery, setting up personal experiments, exposure to physical sensations, response prevention of bodily checking behavior, considering alternative explanations for the symptoms or perceived inability to cope with them, considering how the patient's behavior may be contributing to or maintaining symptoms, and increasing participation in functional activities of daily living. These strategies are often combined with relaxation training (or other emotion control strategies) aimed at reducing emotional distress. Treatment can range anywhere from 6 to 20 sessions depending on the severity and chronicity of bodily distress.

Cognitive behavioral treatment, in individual or group form, has been demonstrated to improve symptoms and functioning, with small to moderate effects sizes in meta-analytic reviews, for a variety of FSS presentations including generalized bodily distress [28–30], as well as singular syndromes such as fibromyalgia [31–33], chronic fatigue syndrome [34– 36], irritable bowel syndrome [37–40], burning mouth syndrome [41], noncardiac chest pain [42], dizziness [43], and tinnitus [44–46].

"Third-Wave" Cognitive-Behavioral Therapies

Mindfulness-based stress reduction (MBSR), mindfulness-based cognitive therapy (MBCT), and acceptance and commitment therapy (ACT) are psychological interventions that have at their core the practice of mindfulness, an acceptable way of relating to whatever is happening in the present moment without trying to change it, push the experience away, or cling to it. All three traditions agree that the purpose of meditative practice is not necessary to induce relaxation, but to facilitate the ability to notice (e.g., attention) and accept one's own experience and automatic reactions to that experience which may include thoughts, sensations, emotions, or behavior. These automatic reactions are thought to produce and/or amplify distress from an original experience. Through acceptance of one's experience (rather than trying to change or control the experience), including unpleasant aspects, one can cultivate intentional, compassionate responses to difficulties which then typically reduce distress and improve function.

Acceptance and Commitment Therapy

Acceptance and commitment therapy (ACT) (Fig. 19.3) is a newer approach within CBT consisting of mindfulness and acceptance intervention strategies. ACT is fundamentally guided by relational frame theory [47] and the psychological flexibility model (PFM; [48]). The PFM postulates that human suffering inevitably results when efforts to avoid distressing thoughts, feelings, and physical sensations fail to provide long-lasting relief. The PFM consists of six interrelated processes: acceptance, cognitive defusion, contact with the present moment, self as context, connecting with personal values, and committed action (see Fig. 19.3).

Acceptance is the willingness to embrace whatever internal experience shows up, be it a thought, feeling, or physical sensation without defense, regardless of whether it is positive or negative. Cognitive diffusion is the name given to the

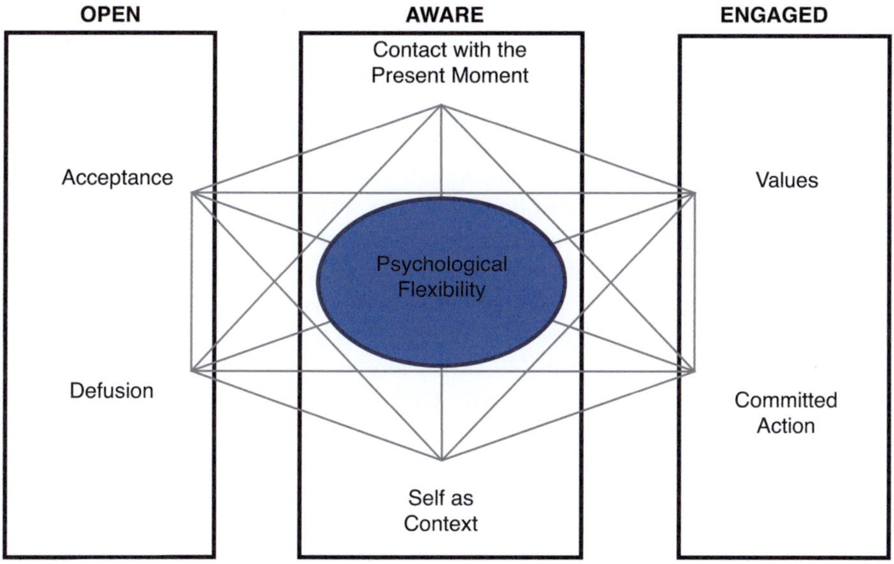

Fig. 19.3 ACT model of treatment

process of holding thoughts lightly and seeing them for what they are—mental representations of events rather than the events themselves. Gradually thoughts are seen from a distance and their literal importance is undermined in favor of doing what matters in life. Contact with the present moment reflects a willingness to stay with one's present moment experience regardless of distractions of the mind or urges to avoid unpleasant experiences. Self as context, or perspective taking, is the process of observing that there is a transcendent self that is separate from one's thoughts, feelings, physical sensations, roles, urges, or physical body. These aspects of experience change over time while the observing aspect of self does not. Values reflect the people and things that provide a deeply personal sense of meaning and purpose to the patient. They serve both an aspirational and motivational function for the patient. Committed action is the process of goal-directed action undertaken in the face of barriers that are guided and fueled by one's values.

ACT uses metaphors, experiential paradox, and experiential exercises to undermine the literal content of language and enhance contact with present moment experience in the service of living according to one's chosen values. It is considered a transdiagnostic, process-oriented approach to therapy that typically does not employ a session-by-session protocol. Rather it maintains a flexible approach that can be tailored to the individual needs of the patient.

In ACT for FSS, there are several therapeutic goals including helping the patient to identify previous attempts to control/avoid bodily symptoms and related emotional distress and come to their own conclusions regarding how successful these have been over time. In doing so, attachment to control strategies is undermined and willingness engendered, to abandon unworkable attempts to control/avoid distressing physical and emotional symptoms. Through this process, patients open up to alternative ways of responding to physical symptoms and related emotional distress in order to live more freely in accordance with their chosen values (i.e., psychological flexibility).

ACT is a relatively new approach to treatment in physical medicine compared to traditional cognitive behavioral therapy. However, in the past 15 years, in an effort to generally improve upon the relatively consistent but small effect sizes observed in studies of traditional cognitive behavioral treatments, there have been a considerable number of randomized controlled trials of ACT for FSS, particularly in the area of chronic pain. ACT for chronic pain, including fibromyalgia and headache, has been found to be more clinically effective than usual care or wait list control conditions on a range of outcome measures (i.e., pain, disability, quality of life, pain interference, anxiety, and depression) with small to large effect sizes at both post-treatment and follow up intervals [49, 50]. There have been an insufficient number of studies directly comparing ACT with CBT to determine whether one is more effective than the other at this point.

In a theoretical and empirical review of the cognitive behavioral model of treatment for medically unexplained symptoms, Deary et al. [13] suggested that because of its nature as a treatment for distress tolerance, ACT could be an effective treatment for FSS. Since that review, ACT has been investigated as a treatment for a variety of FSS in several randomized controlled trials including patients with health anxiety, generalized bodily distress, irritable bowel syndrome, and tinnitus. For health anxiety, ACT demonstrated large effect sizes regardless of it being compared to wait list [51] or an active control group [52], while for generalized bodily distress the effects were moderate [53, 54]. In three RCTs for IBS, ACT outperformed active control conditions with moderate to large effect sizes [55–57]. Finally, in the area of tinnitus, ACT conveyed a large effect over tinnitus retraining therapy (TRT) in one study [58], while in another [59], online ACT was as effective as online CBT, both with moderately large effect sizes.

There are several barriers to delivering effective behavioral treatments such as ACT for FSS, including the number of sessions, a dearth of trained clinicians and multidisciplinary treatment centers, the stigma associated with mental health care, poor treatment adherence, prohibitive costs, reduced mobility, prohibitive distance, and lack of transportation. One solution has been to offer ACT in a 1-day workshop format [60] that enables more flexible dissemination of treatment in clinical settings to enhance adherence. One-day ACT workshops have been implemented for a wide variety of conditions including diabetes [61], multiple sclerosis [62], migraine [63–65], vascular disease [66], post-surgical pain [67, 68], and inflammatory bowel disease [69], with encouraging results reflecting the improved quality of life, decreased emotional distress, and improved disease management.

Mindfulness-Based Stress Reduction (MBSR) and Mindfulness-Based Cognitive Therapy (MBCT)

MBSR was developed by Jon Kabat-Zinn primarily to provide stress reduction to individuals with medical conditions to see what they may be able to do for themselves (in addition to what medicine may be able to offer) after learning to notice and understand their bodies [70]. MBCT was developed as a way to prevent relapse in those with persistent depression who were triggered by difficult daily events [71].

MBSR and MBCT are typically led in 8-week group formats and include psychoeducation, and formal meditative practices, during which participants are encouraged to do practice between sessions. MBSR typically includes a yoga practice as a meditative component whereas MBCT integrates elements of more traditional cognitive-therapy such as identifying cognitive distortions. Both encourage body-oriented and experiential practices that encourage tolerating unpleasant physical sensations while encouraging movement and developing insight into one's patterns, behavior, symptoms, etc. [72].

The ongoing study of MBSR and MBCT into pain and other functional symptoms is driven by the effects of the treatment to reduce activation of sympathetic arousal including decreased blood pressure, reduction in immune-inflammatory markers through formal meditative practices and reduction in stress/anxiety generation through the acceptance techniques and psychological flexibility [73–76].

Systematic reviews and meta-analyses have concluded that the benefits of mindfulness-based interventions (MBIs) for patients with FSS, excluding tinnitus, have offered mixed results. For example, Veehoff et al. and Frostholm et al. have suggested the benefits are inconsistent at best and when there were benefits, they tended to be relatively small [50, 77]. However, others have reported moderate to large effect sizes for medically unexplained symptoms and FSS [78, 79]. Research has suggested that MBCT is superior to CBT in myalgic encephalomyelitis [80]. Several randomized controlled trials have demonstrated that MBCT is an effective treatment for tinnitus with small to moderately large effect sizes [81–83]. An RCT of MBCT for health anxiety reported a medium-sized positive outcome when compared to treatment as usual [84].

Compassion-focused therapy is another "third wave" treatment that incorporates aspects of mindfulness and cultivating compassion for oneself and adjusting to limitations associated with their pain [85]. Third-wave therapies may be recommended more often for individuals who have previous histories with CBT, and for whom efforts to control emotional and physical sensations (often seen through behavioral avoidance, high medication and/or substance use) are negatively impacting their life.

Hypnosis

Hypnosis is generally defined as "a therapeutic technique in which clinicians make suggestions to individuals who have undergone a procedure designed to relax them and focus their minds" [86]. During this state, an individual is more amenable to suggestions that can influence perception, thought processes and behavior, as modulated by the peripheral and central nervous systems regardless of organic cause [87]. As this relates to functional illness, suggestions can be provided to alter the perception of unpleasant stimuli and/or create a general sense of calm, thought processing that may amplify the sensations (i.e., interpretations of the nature of the symptoms, focus on limitations, and losses), or behavior that improves the comfort or quality of life of the sufferer. The effects of hypnosis can be objectively studied through PET scan imagery, changes in vascular activity, and inflammatory response [82]. Jensen (2011) suggests that truly psychogenic pain is best treated with psychotherapy with hypnosis as an adjunct [87]. Targets may be reducing symptom annoyance, improving symptom control, and reducing overall stress as examples. In a recent review of the use of hypnosis, Flynn (2018) suggested that hypnosis with or without additional relaxation strategies provided improvement reduction in headache activity, and improved quality of life with no adverse effects reports in a relatively short time (1–4 sessions) [88]. Maudouz, Bonnet, Lhonneux-Ledoux and Lefebvre (2007) used hypnosis to assist tinnitus patients in modulating sound intensity in 5–10 sessions and reported improvements for participants with mild through "catastrophic" impairment from tinnitus [89].

Several systematic reviews and meta-analyses have concluded that hypnotherapy/guided imagery training offers small to moderate benefits for irritable bowel syndrome [37, 38, 90–92] and strong evidence for efficacy for fibromyalgia [93, 94].

Biofeedback

Biofeedback is a treatment that focuses on building awareness of physiological processes associated with nervous system functioning (i.e., muscle tension, heart rate, and perspiration), through the use of externally located sensory equipment. Individuals can then learn to influence these processes, with the potential for symptom reduction and relief. Many have argued that its philosophy truly embodies the biopsychosocial model [95]. Treatment typically begins with a psychophysiological assessment which may include muscle tension (as measured by surface electromyography (sEMG)) in facial muscles, neck, and shoulders; heart rate; heart rate variability; breathing rate; finger temperature; and skin conductance in response to a series of stress-inducing tasks. Education is provided on the role of muscle use and emotional stress in producing muscle tension which can produce bothersome symptoms. The active phase of treatment involves breathing training, observing changes related to muscle-specific variables (i.e., posture, talking), along with using other relaxation skills, mindfulness, or noticing cognitions while attending to physiological readings (see [17, 96] for detailed protocols). Biofeedback-assisted training has been studied for tinnitus [97–100], temporomandibular joint [101], headaches [102], and fibromyalgia [103] among other anxiety, pain, functional conditions, and injury rehabilitation. A meta-analysis of self-management treatments concluded that biofeedback did not add additional benefit to other self-management interventions such as psychosocial and jaw relaxation and may not justify the added cost of the equipment [104]. These authors also consider whether the administration of biofeedback from a psychologist or medical provider may influence the receptivity of patients to the intervention.

Eye Movement Desensitization and Reprocessing (EMDR)

EMDR is a therapeutic approach that was originally developed for the treatment of PTSD and is based on the Adaptive Information Processing Model (AIP; [105]). In brief, the AIP posits that traumatic events are stored in a fragmented fashion in one's memory, and activation of the processing system through the EMDR procedures will lead to adaptive resolution of the event therefore reducing the PTSD symptoms. The goal of treatment is to reduce maladaptive learning and distress, and strengthen adaptive beliefs associated with traumatic events. The treatment itself follows standardized procedures. Initially affect regulation techniques are taught. Then the active component includes focusing simultaneously on images, thoughts, emotions, and/or bodily sensations associated with the traumatic event along with bilateral stimulation (BLS) such as lateral eye movements across the visual field. EMDR's use in treating functional symptoms would be targeting traumatic (if applicable) events that play a role in symptom onset such as previous injury or illness associated with symptom onset, unfortunate medical experiences, enhancing coping with symptoms by reducing distress related to thoughts of being helpless, worthless, etc., target the physical sensations themselves, reduce fears for the future, and/or challenge secondary gain. When distress and/or dysfunctional learning is removed from the above targets, then an adaptive belief (e.g., I can cope) is reinforced. Then the patient reports any residual physical sensations that are present while engaging in BLS. See Luber (2019) for EMDR protocols for treating somatic and medical-related conditions [106].

Several studies have suggested that EMDR is helpful in the treatment of chronic pain, reducing disability and associated anxious and depressive symptoms [107–109] EMDR has demonstrated success as an abortive treatment for migraine compared to standard care medications [110] and decreased migraine frequency and duration [111]. EMDR was compared to Duloxetine in women with SSD and found to provide greater symptom reduction relative to the duloxetine group at 6 weeks [112]. A recent review [113] suggested that EMDR has been effective at reducing tinnitus-related distress. Luyten et al. [114] reported that EMDR combined with tinnitus retraining therapy (TRT) was as effective as CBT with TRT. EMDR was found to be effective in treating functional neurological conditions in a recent description of case examples [115].

Generally, the literature base suggests that EMDR is a promising treatment for functional syndromes particularly if the pain is a symptom, but published evidence has been criticized for not having large-scale randomized clinical trials [104]. Individuals with functional symptoms that are clearly part of a trauma-related disorder should be offered psychological treatment specifically for PTSD in addition to treatment for functional distress.

Summary of Psychological Treatments

A variety of psychological treatments are continually being studied and developed for the treatment of FSS allowing the opportunity for choice to patients given their own conceptualization of functional symptoms, psychological comorbidities, as well as time and goals for treatment. Other models of psychological therapy, such as psychodynamic therapy, have been used in the management of functional syndromes, however, only treatments provided by the authors were presented here. Individuals with functional symptoms may still benefit from treatments targeting other comorbidities such as PTSD, conversion disorder, insomnia, major depression, personality disorders, and specific anxiety disorders.

Strategies for Health Care Providers (HCP)

Assessment

Functional somatic syndromes and non-specific bodily distress can account for up to 25% of primary care and 50% of specialist practice [9]. The interaction between the health care provider(s) and the patient can play a significant role in whether or not the patient will continue to seek further referral medical assessments or consider the role of psychosocial factors [116]. It is useful to physically examine the patient, even if medically unexplained symptoms are suspected. This will ensure that no clinical signs are missed and help to reassure the patient that the complaint has been taken seriously and adequate assessment has taken place. Once a patient has been carefully assessed, misdiagnosis is uncommon (estimated 0.5%) [117] but more likely to occur in patients with comorbid mental health presentations [118]. While investigations are important, a balance must be struck between the risk of misdiagnosis and the potential for increasing the patient's fear of disease (i.e., iatrogenic psychological harm). Initial impressions of functional symptoms can be offered. If additional tests are ordered, the reasons for the diagnostics should be explained with a sense of expected (negative) results [9].

The assessment should also explore the patient's beliefs and fears about the underlying disease, and acute anxiety towards the same. This information can inform the conceptualization of an additional psychological diagnosis and can provide guidance on areas to provide reassurance to the patient. The patient should also be asked about psychological symptoms, but this is best done only after taking a history of physical symptoms so that the patient will not feel that their concerns about the physical disease have been prematurely dismissed. This sequence allows for a logical inquiry into the understandable distress that has occurred following symptom onset. Self-report symptom measures may also provide helpful information and facilitate discussion between patients and health care providers.

Providing Diagnostic Feedback

When providing diagnostic feedback, above all else, it is crucial that patients know that the physician believes them. Communicate clearly to the patient that you believe the symptoms are real, as are the dysfunction and distress they are causing. Avoid psychogenic implications such as, "there is nothing wrong" that the patient could misinterpret. However, it is important to provide a clear message that no serious disease has been found. The dynamic interactions involving stress, mood state, and functional illness explained by the biopsychosocial model can also be useful in providing a plausible alternative explanation for the symptoms. The physician can also provide information about prognosis based on typical experiences with the symptom such as it usually goes away with time, it may come and go, or it may be persistent. However, in any case, ongoing care will be available through follow-up visits or referral for psychological treatment to learn self-management coping strategies. Sharpe (2020) has cautioned against making multiple medical specialist referrals for functional illnesses due to the potential for iatrogenic harms referenced earlier.

Treatment Plan

All patients should be given a treatment plan that includes a sense of ongoing support and follow-up be it with general practitioner, medical specialist, or psychologist. Many patients also respond well to advice on knowing when to be concerned about their symptoms (e.g., if symptoms get worse, additional symptoms present) and when not to be. Henningsen et al. [9] have suggested a stepped care plan based on the number of physical and psychological symptoms present and the severity of the symptoms. For example, patients with mild symptoms may respond to reassurance and are encouraged to maintain a healthy lifestyle.

Those with moderate symptoms may benefit from an additional discussion on coping resources (i.e., self-help organizations, and self-care), advice on complementary medicine and allied health providers, setting realistic goals, and consideration for anti-depressant medication, particularly for comorbid anxiety or depressive symptoms, or pain. They also may be amenable to suggestions to try relaxation training or mindfulness mediation from a reliable trainer.

For individuals with more severe symptoms, in addition to the above considerations for those with moderate symptoms, one should evaluate the current state of past traumas and any maintaining factors such as tumultuous living arrangements, current litigation issues, concerning medication use patterns, and consider more strongly the need for a referral to a psychologist or other mental health practitioner, or referral to multi-disciplinary service, if available. Patients should continue to receive physical assessments at regular intervals for persisting symptoms at follow-up visits. Some practitioners may prefer to schedule follow-up office visits at regular intervals (i.e., 4–6 weeks) rather than having patients schedule as needed. At follow-ups, physicians should reinforce education on the functional nature of symptoms, changes in symptoms that would be concerning, and additional professionals who may be able to provide treatment if needed (i.e., physiotherapy, occupational therapy, psychology, etc.).

Making Referrals

When considering referral for psychological treatment, it is important to know what services are available and what types of referrals will be accepted (e.g., a treatment service that offers brief CBT will not likely accept a patient who requires long-term therapy for a personality disorder) prior to making a referral. Another important consideration is making sure the patient understands why they are being referred. It should be clearly communicated that you are not making the referral because you believe the illness is a figment of the patient's imagination or "all in their head." Sharpe [119] has suggested using statements to encourage a referral such as "having physical symptoms can make anxiety and depression worse and turn into a vicious circle. I wonder if treating the anxiety/depression (or learning relaxation skills) may also be helpful. In my experience it has been". It is also prudent to indicate that the psychological treatment has empirical evidence to support its use and therefore has a reasonable chance of helping. When possible, explain what they may expect in therapy and that you are not "passing them off" to mental health, but will continue to follow them [119]. Attending to these considerations should maximize the likelihood that they will attend the initial appointment with the psychologist. Co-locating psychological services in primary care offices or specialty clinics can help normalize psychological treatment in FSS.

Summary

The development of FSS is a complex process of precipitating, perpetuating, and predisposing biopsychosocial factors. A psychological assessment aims at understanding these factors, past and present, in a patient's life. A number of evidence-based psychological treatments exist that can reduce symptoms, symptom distress, and associated loss of function. Health care providers are instrumental in explaining the complex role psychological factors may play in symptom development and encouraging participation in treatment.

References

1. Melzack R, Wall PD. Pain mechanisms: a new theory. Science. 1965;150:971–9. https://doi.org/10.1126/science.150.3699.971.
2. Melzack R, Casey KL. Sensory, motivational and central control determinants of pain: a new conceptual model. In: Kenshalo D, editor. The skin senses. Springfield, IL: Charles C Thomas; 1968. p. 423–43.
3. Melzack R. Pain and the neuromatrix in the brain. J Dent Educ. 2001;65:1378–82.
4. Engel GL. The need for a new medical model: a challenge for biomedical science. Science. 1977;196:129–36.
5. Kellner R. Functional somatic symptoms and hypochondriasis. Arch Gen Psychiatry. 1985;42:821–33.
6. Kellner R. Hypochondriasis and somatization. JAMA. 1987;258:2718–22.
7. Kellner R. Psychosomatic syndromes, somatization and somatoform disorders. Psychother Psychosom. 1994;61:4–24.
8. Barsky AJ, Borus JF. Functional somatic syndromes. Ann Intern Med. 1999;130:910–21.
9. Henningsen P, Zipfel S, Sattel H, Creed F. Management of functional somatic syndromes and bodily distress. Psychother Psychosom. 2018;87:12–31. https://doi.org/10.1159/0004844413.
10. Kleykamp BA, Ferguson MC, McNicol E, Bixho I, Arnold LM, Edwards RR, et al. The prevalence of psychiatric and chronic pain comorbidities in fibromyalgia: an ACTTION systematic review. Semin Arthritis Rheu. 2021;51:166–74. https://doi.org/10.1016/j.semarthrit.2020.10.006.

11. Carta MG, Moro MF, Pinna FL, Testa G, Cacace E, Ruggiero V, et al. The impact of fibromyalgia syndrome and the role of comorbidity with mood and post-traumatic stress disorder in worsening the quality of life. Int J Soc Psychiatry. 2018;64:647–55.
12. Janssens KAM, Zijlema WL, Joustra ML, Rosmalen JGM. Mood and anxiety disorders in chronic fatigue syndrome, fibromyalgia and irritable bowel syndrome: results from the LifeLines cohort study. Psychosom Med. 2015;77:449–57.
13. Deary V, Chalder T, Sharpe M. The cognitive behavioural model of medically unexplained symptoms: a theoretical and empirical review. Clin Psychol Rev. 2007;27:781–97. https://doi.org/10.1016/j.cpr.2007.07.002.
14. Sharpe M, Peveler R, Mayou R. The psychological treatment of patients with functional somatic symptoms: a practical guide. J Psychosom Res. 1992;36:515–29.
15. Van den Bergh O, Witthoft M, Petersen S, Brown R. Symptoms and the body: taking the inferential leap. Neurosci Biobehav Rev. 2017;74:185–203.
16. Kube T, Rozenkrantz L, Rief W, Barsky A. Understanding persistent physical symptoms: conceptual integration or psychological expectation models and predictive processing accounts. Clin Psychol Rev. 2020;76:101829.
17. Khazan IZ. The clinical handbook of biofeedback: a step-by-step guide for training and practice with mindfulness. Singapore: Wiley-Blackwell; 2013.
18. Woolfolk RL, Allen LA. Treating somatization: a cognitive-behavioral approach. New York: Guilford Press; 2007.
19. Pilowsky I. Dimensions of hypochondriasis. Br J Psychiatry. 1967;113:89–93.
20. Kellner R, Abbott P, Winslow WW, Pathak D. Fears, beliefs, and attitudes in dsm-iii hypochondriasis. J Nerv Ment Dis. 1987;175:20–5.
21. Salkovskis PM, Rimes KA, Warwick HM, Clark DM. The health anxiety inventory: development and validation of scales for the measurement of health anxiety and hypochondriasis. Psychol Med. 2002;32:843–53.
22. Hedman E, Lekander M, Ljótsson B, Lindefors N, Rück C, Andersson G, Andersson E. Optimal cut-off points on the health anxiety inventory, illness attitude scales and whiteley index to identify severe health anxiety. PLoS One. 2015;10(4):e0123412.
23. Reiss S, Peterson RA, Gursky DM, McNally RJ. Anxiety sensitivity, anxiety frequency and the prediction of fearfulness. Behav Res Ther. 1986;24(1):1–8. https://doi.org/10.1016/0005-7967(86)90143-9.
24. Sullivan MJL, Bishop S, Pivik J. The pain catastrophizing scale: development and validation. Psychol Assess. 1995;7:524–32.
25. American Psychiatric Association. Diagnostic and statistical manual of mental disorders. 5th ed. Washington, DC: Author; 2013.
26. Gureje O, Reed GM. Bodily distress disorder in ICD-11: problems and prospects. World Psychiatry. 2016;15:291–2.
27. Goldberg DP, Reed GM, Robles R, Bobes J, Iglesias C, Fortes S, et al. Multiple somatic symptoms in primary care: a field study for ICD-11 PHC, WHO's revised classification of mental disorders in primary care setting. J Psychosom Res. 2016;91:48–54.
28. Koelen JA, Houtveen JH, Abbass A, Luyten P, Eurelings-Bontekoe EH, Van Broeckhuysen-Kloth SA, Bühring ME, Geenen R. Effectiveness of psychotherapy for severe somatoform disorder: meta-analysis. Br J Psychiatry. 2014;204:12–9.
29. Menon V, Rajan TM, Kuppili PP, Sarkar S. Cognitive behavior therapy for medically unexplained symptoms: a systematic review and meta-analysis of published controlled trials. Indian J Psychol Med. 2017;39:399–406.
30. van Dessel N, den Boeft M, van der Wouden JC, Kleinstäuber M, Leone SS, Terluin B, Numans ME, van der Horst HE, van Marwijk H. Non-pharmacological interventions for somatoform disorders and medically unexplained physical symptoms (MUPS) in adults. Cochrane Database Syst Rev. 2014;11:CD011142.
31. Bernardy K, Füber N, Köllner V, Häuser W. Efficacy of cognitive-behavioral therapies in fibromyalgia syndrome—a systematic review and metaanalysis of randomized controlled trials. J Rheumatol. 2010;37:1991–2005.

32. Bernardy K, Klose P, Busch AJ, Choy EH, Häuser W. Cognitive behavioural therapies for fibromyalgia. Cochrane Database Syst Rev. 2013;9:CD009796.
33. Glombiewski JA, Sawyer AT, Gutermann J, Koenig K, Rief W, Hofmann SG. Psychological treatments for fibromyalgia: a metaanalysis. Pain. 2010;151:280–95.
34. Malouff JM, Thorsteinsson EB, Rooke SE, Bhullar N, Schutte NS. Efficacy of cognitive behavioral therapy for chronic fatigue syndrome: a meta-analysis. Clin Psychol Rev. 2008;28:736–45.
35. Marques MM, De Gucht V, Gouveia MJ, Leal I, Maes S. Differential effects of behavioral interventions with a graded physical activity component in patients suffering from chronic fatigue (syndrome): an updated systematic review and meta-analysis. Clin Psychol Rev. 2015;40:123–37.
36. Price JR, Mitchell E, Tidy E, Hunot V. Cognitive behaviour therapy for chronic fatigue syndrome in adults. Cochrane Database Syst Rev. 2008;3:CD001027.
37. Altayar O, Sharma V, Prokop LJ, Sood A, Murad MH. Psychological therapies in patients with irritable bowel syndrome: a systematic review and meta-analysis of randomized controlled trials. Gastroenterol Res Pract. 2015;2015:549308.
38. Laird KT, Tanner-Smith EE, Russell AC, Hollon SD, Walker LS. Comparative efficacy of psychological therapies for improving mental health and daily functioning in irritable. bowel syndrome: a systematic review and meta-analysis. Clin Psychol Rev. 2017;51:142–52.
39. Li L, Xiong L, Zhang S, Yu Q, Chen M. Cognitive-behavioral therapy for irritable bowel syndrome: a meta-analysis. J Psychosom Res. 2014;77:1–12.
40. Zijdenbos IL, de Wit NJ, van der Heijden GJ, Rubin G, Quartero AO. Psychological treatments for the management of irritable bowel syndrome. Cochrane Database Syst Rev. 2009;1:CD006442.
41. Kisely S, Forbes M, Sawyer E, Black E, Lalloo R. A systematic review of randomized trials for the treatment of burning mouth syndrome. J Psychosom Res. 2016;86:39–46.
42. Kisely SR, Campbell LA, Yelland MJ. Paydar A: psychological interventions for symptomatic management of non-specific chest pain in patients with normal coronary anatomy. Cochrane Database Syst Rev. 2015;6:CD004101.
43. Schmid G, Henningsen P, Dieterich M, Sattel H, Lahmann C. Psychotherapy in dizziness: a systematic review. J Neurol Neurosurg Psychiatry. 2011;82:601–6.
44. Cima RFF, Andersson G, Schmidt CJ, Henry JA. Cognitive-behavioral treatments for tinnitus: a review of the literature. J Am Acad Audiol. 2014;25:29–61.
45. Hesser H, Weise C, Westin VZ, Andersson G. A systematic review and meta-analysis of randomized controlled trials of cognitive behavioral therapy for tinnitus distress. Clin Psychol Rev. 2011;31:545–53.
46. Martinez-Devesa P, Perera R, Theodoulou M, Waddell A. Cognitive behavioural therapy for tinnitus. Cochrane Database Syst Rev. 2010;9:CD005233.
47. Hayes SC, Barnes-Holmes D, Roche B, editors. Relational frame theory: a post-Skinnerian account of human language and cognition. New York: Kluwer Academic/Plenum; 2001.
48. Hayes SC, Strosahl KD, Wilson KG. Acceptance and commitment therapy: an experiential approach to behavior change. 2nd ed. New York: Guilford Press; 2012.
49. Hughes LS, Clark J, Colclough JA, Dale E, McMillan D. Acceptance and commitment therapy (ACT) for chronic pain: a systematic review and meta-analyses. Clin J Pain. 2017;33:552–68.
50. Veehof MM, Trompetter HR, Bohlmeijer ET, Schreurs KMG. Acceptance- and mindfulness-based interventions for the treatment of chronic pain: a meta-analytic review. Cogn Behav Ther. 2016;45:5–31. https://doi.org/10.1080/16506073.2015.1098724.
51. Eilenberg T, Fink P, Jensen J, Rief W, Frostholm L. Acceptance and commitment group therapy (ACT-G) for health anxiety: a randomized controlled trial. Psychol Med. 2016;46:103–15.
52. Hoffmann D, Rask CU, Hedman-Lagerlöf E, Jensen JS, Frostholm L. Efficacy of internet-delivered acceptance and commitment therapy for severe health anxiety: results from a randomized, controlled trial. Psychol Med. 2020;51:1–11. https://doi.org/10.1017/S0033291720001312.

53. Maria Kleinstäuber M, Allwang C, Bailer J, Berking M, Brünahl C, Erkic M, et al. Cognitive behaviour therapy complemented with emotion regulation training for patients with persistent physical symptoms: a randomised clinical trial. Psychother Psychosom. 2019;88:287–99.
54. Pedersen HF, Agger JL, Frostholm L, Jensen JS, Ørnbøl E, Fink P, Schröder A. Acceptance and Commitment group Therapy for patients with multiple functional somatic syndromes: a three-armed trial comparing ACT in a brief and extended version with enhanced care. Psychol Med. 2019;2019(49):1005–14.
55. Ljótsson B, Falk L, Vesterlund AW, Hedman E, Lindfors P, Ruck C, et al. Internet-delivered exposure and mindfulness based therapy for irritable bowel syndrome—a randomized controlled trial. Behav Res Ther. 2010;48:531–9. https://doi.org/10.1016/j.brat.2010.03.003.
56. Ljótsson B, Hedman E, Andersson E, Hesser H, Lindfors P, Hursti T, et al. Internet-delivered exposure-based treatment vs. stress management for irritable bowel syndrome: a randomized trial. The Amer. J Gastroenterol. 2011;106:1481–91. https://doi.org/10.1038/ajg.2011.139.
57. Ljótsson B, Hesser H, Andersson E, Lackner JM, El Alaoui S, Falk L, et al. Provoking symptoms to relieve symptoms: a randomized controlled dismantling study of exposure therapy in irritable bowel syndrome. Behav Res Ther. 2014;55:27–39. https://doi.org/10.1016/j.brat.2014.01.007.
58. Westin V, Schulin M, Hesser H, Karlsson M, Noe R, Olofsson U, et al. Acceptance and Commitment Therapy versus Tinnitus Retraining Therapy in the treatment of tinnitus: a randomised controlled trial. Behav Res Ther. 2011;49:737–47.
59. Hesser H, Gustafsson T, Lunden C, Henrikson O, Fattahi K, Johnsson E, et al. A randomized controlled trial of internet-delivered cognitive behavior therapy and acceptance and commitment therapy in the treatment of tinnitus. J Consult Clin Psychol. 2012;80:649–61.
60. Dindo L, Van Liew JR, Arch JJ. Acceptance and commitment therapy: a transdiagnostic behavioral intervention for mental health and medical conditions. Neurotherapeutics. 2017;14:546–53.
61. Gregg JA, Callaghan GM, Hayes SC, Glenn-Lawson JL. Improving diabetes self-management through acceptance, mindfulness, and values: a randomized controlled trial. J Consult Clin Psychol. 2007;75:336–43.
62. Sheppard SC, Forsyth JP, Hickling EJ, Bianchi J. A novel application of Acceptance and Commitment Therapy for psychosocial problems associated with multiple sclerosis. Int J MS Care. 2010;12:200–6.
63. Dindo L, Recober A, Marchman JN, Turvey C, O'Hara M. One-day behavioral treatment for patients with comorbid depression and migraine: a pilot study. Behav Res Ther. 2012;50:537–43.
64. Dindo L, Recober A, Marchman JN, O'Hara M, Turvey C. One-day behavioral intervention for depressed migraine patients: effects on headache. Headache. 2014;54:528–38.
65. Huddleston C, Martin L, Woods K, Dindo L. One-day behavioral intervention for distressed veterans with migraine: results of a multimethod pilot study. Mil Med. 2018;183:e184–92.
66. Dindo L, Marchman J, Grindes H, Fiedorowicz JG. A brief behavioral intervention targeting mental health risk factors for vascular disease: a pilot study. Psychother Psychosom. 2015;84:183–5.
67. Dindo L, Zimmerman MB, Hadlandsmyth K, St. Marie B, Embree J, Marchman JN, Tripp-Reimer T, Rakel B. Acceptance and Commitment Therapy for the prevention of chronic postsurgical pain and opioid use in at-risk veterans: a pilot randomized controlled study. J Pain. 2018;19:1211–21.
68. Hadlandsmyth K, Dindo LN, Wajid R, Sugg SL, Zimmerman MB, Rakel BA. A single-session acceptance and commitment therapy intervention among women undergoing surgery for breast cancer: a randomized pilot trial to reduce persistent postsurgical pain. Psycho-Oncology. 2019;28:2210–7.
69. Hou JK, Vanga RR, Thakur E, Gonzalez I, Willis D, Dindo L. One-day behavioral intervention for patients with inflammatory bowel disease and co-occurring psychological distress. Clin Gastroenter Hepatol. 2017;15:1633–4.
70. Kabat-Zinn J. Mindfulness for beginners. Boulder: Sounds True; 2012.

71. Segal Z, Williams M, Teasdale J. Mindfulness-based cognitive therapy for depression. 2nd ed. New York: Guilford Press; 2013.
72. Van Ravesteijn H, Fjorback L. Mindfulness-based cognitive therapy: medically unexplained symptoms. In: Eisendrath SJ, editor. Mindfulness-based cognitive therapy: innovative applications. Cham: Springer; 2016. https://doi.org/10.1007/978-3-319-29866-5.
73. Conversano C, Orrù G, Pozza A, Miccoli M, Ciacchini R, Marchi L, Gemignani A. Is mindfulness-based stress reduction effective for people with hypertension? A systematic review and meta-analysis of 30 years of evidence. Int J Environ Res Public Health. 2021;18:2882. https://doi.org/10.3390/ijerph18062882.
74. Intarakamhang U, Macaskill A, Prasittichok P. Mindfulness interventions reduce blood pressure in patients with non-communicable diseases: a systematic review and meta-analysis. Heliyon. 2020;6:e03834. https://doi.org/10.1016/j.heliyon.2020.e03834.
75. Andrés-Rodríguez L, Borràs X, Feliu-Soler A, Pérez-Aranda A, Rozadilla-Sacanell A, Montero-Marin J, et al. Immune-inflammatory pathways and clinical changes in fibromyalgia patients treated with Mindfulness-Based Stress Reduction (MBSR): a randomized, controlled clinical trial. Brain Behav Immun. 2019;80:109–19. https://doi.org/10.1016/j.bbi.2019.02.030.
76. Pérez-Aranda A, Feliu-Soler A, Montero-Marín J, García-Campayo J, Andrés-Rodríguez L, Borràs X, et al. A randomized controlled efficacy trial of mindfulness-based stress reduction compared with an active control group and usual care for fibromyalgia: the EUDAIMON study. Pain. 2019;160:2508–23. https://doi.org/10.1097/j.pain.0000000000001655.
77. Frostholm L, Rask C. Third wave treatments for functional somatic syndromes and health anxiety across the age span: a narrative review. Clin Psychol Eur. 2019;1:e32217.
78. Billones R, Saligan L. What works in mindfulness interventions for medically unexplained symptoms? A systematic review. Asian Pac Isl Nurs J. 2020;5:1–11. https://doi.org/10.31372/20200501.1082.
79. Grossman P, Tiefenthaler-Gilmer U, Raysz A, Kesper U. Mindfulness training as an intervention for fibromyalgia: evidence of postintervention and 3-year follow-up benefits in well-being. Psychother Psychosom. 2007;76:226–33. https://doi.org/10.1159/000101501.
80. Rimes KA, Wingrove J. Mindfulness-based cognitive therapy for people with chronic fatigue syndrome still experiencing excessive fatigue after cognitive behaviour therapy: a pilot randomized study. Clin Psychol Psychother. 2013;20:107–17. https://doi.org/10.1002/cpp.793.
81. McKenna L, Marks EM, Hallsworth CA, Schaette R. Mindfulness-based cognitive therapy as a treatment for chronic tinnitus: a randomized controlled trial. Psychother Psychosom. 2017;86:351–61.
82. McKenna L, Marks EM, Vogt F. Mindfulness-based cognitive therapy for chronic tinnitus: evaluation of benefits in a large sample of patients attending a tinnitus clinic. Ear Hear. 2018;39:359–66.
83. Philippot P, Nef F, Clauw L, de Romrée M, Segal Z. A randomized controlled trial of mindfulness-based cognitive therapy for treating tinnitus. Clin Psychol Psychother. 2012;19:411–9.
84. McManus F, Surawy C, Muse K, Vazquez-Montes M, Williams JM. A randomized clinical trial of mindfulness-based cognitive therapy versus unrestricted services for health anxiety (hypochondriasis). J Consult Clin Psychol. 2012;80:817–28.
85. Gooding H, Stedmon J, Crix D. 'All these things don't take the pain away but they do help you to accept it': making the case for compassion-focused therapy in the management of persistent pain. Br J Pain. 2020;14:31–41. https://doi.org/10.1177/2049463719857099.
86. American Psychological Association. Hypnosis [Internet]. American Psychological Association; [cited 2021 Jun 24]. Available from https://www.apa.org/topics/hypnosis
87. Jensen MP. Hypnosis for chronic pain management: therapist guide. New York: Oxford University Press; 2011.
88. Flynn N. Systematic review of the effectiveness of hypnosis for the for the management of headache. Int J Clin Exp Hyp. 2018;66:343–52. https://doi.org/10.1080/00207144.2018.1494432.

89. Maudoux A, Bonnet S, Lhonneux-Ledoux F, Lefebvre P. Ericksonian hypnosis in tinnitus therapy. B-ENT. 2007;3(Suppl 7):75–7.
90. Lee HH, Choi YY, Choi MG. The efficacy of hypnotherapy in the treatment of irritable bowel syndrome: a systematic review and meta-analysis. J Neurogastroenterol Motil. 2014;20:152–62.
91. Schaefert R, Klose P, Moser G, Häuser W. Efficacy, tolerability, and safety of hypnosis in adult irritable bowel syndrome: systematic review and meta-analysis. Psychosom Med. 2014;76:389–98.
92. Webb AN, Kukuruzovic RH, Catto-Smith AG, Sawyer SM. Hypnotherapy for treatment of irritable bowel syndrome. Cochrane Database Syst Rev. 2007;4:CD005110.
93. Bernardy K, Füber N, Klose P, Häuser W. Efficacy of hypnosis/guided imagery in fibromyalgia syndrome—a systematic review and meta-analysis of controlled trials. BMC Musculoskelet Disord. 2011;12:133.
94. Zech N, Hansen E, Bernardy K, Häuser W. Efficacy, acceptability and safety of guided imagery/hypnosis in fibromyalgia—a systematic review and meta-analysis of randomized controlled trials. Eur J Pain. 2017;21:217–27.
95. Masters KS. Recurrent abdominal pain, medical intervention, and biofeedback: what happened to the biopsychosocial model? Appl Psychophysiol Biofeedback. 2006;31(2):155–65. https://doi.org/10.1007/s10484-006-9016-4.
96. Schwartz MS, Andrasik F, editors. Biofeedback. 4th ed. New York: Guilford Press; 2016.
97. Flor H, Schwartz MS. Tinnitus: nothing is as loud as a sound you are trying not to hear. In: Schwartz MS, Andrasik F, editors. Biofeedback. 3rd ed. New York: Guilford Press; 2003. p. 750–75.
98. Kutyana AM. Heart rate variability biofeedback for tinnitus: preliminary findings from multiple case studies. Biofeedback. 2015;43:142–8.
99. Rief W, Weise C, Kley N, Martin A. Psychophysiologic treatment of chronic tinnitus: a randomized clinical trial. Psychosom Med. 2005;67:833–8. https://doi.org/10.1097/01.psy.0000174174.38908.c6.
100. Weise C, Heinecke K, Rief W. Biofeedback-based behavioral treatment for chronic tinnitus: results of a randomized controlled trial. J Consult Clin Psych. 2008;76:1046–57. https://doi.org/10.1037/a0013811.
101. Glaros AG, Lausten L. Tempromandibular disorders. In: Schwartz MS, Andrasik F, editors. Biofeedback. 3rd ed. New York: Guilford Press; 2003. p. 349–68.
102. Schwartz MS, Andrasik F. Headache. In: Schwartz MS, Andrasik F, editors. Biofeedback. 3rd ed. New York, NY: Guilford Press; 2003. p. 275–348.
103. Schwartz MS, Thompson JM. Fibromyalgia syndrome. In: Schwartz MS, Andrasik F, editors. Biofeedback. 3rd ed. New York: Guilford Press; 2003. p. 776–94.
104. Aggarwal VR, Fu Y, Main CJ, Wu J. The effectiveness of self-management interventions in adults with chronic orofacial pain: a systematic review, meta-analysis and meta regression. Eur J Pain. 2019;23:849–65. https://doi.org/10.1002/ejp.1358.
105. Shapiro F. Eye movement desensitization and preprocessing: basic principles, protocols, and procedures. 2nd ed. New York: Guilford Press; 2001.
106. Luber M, editor. Eye movement desensitization and reprocessing (EMDR) therapy scripted protocols and summary sheets: treating trauma in somatic and medical-related conditions. New York: Springer; 2019.
107. Grant M, Threlfo C. EMDR in the treatment of chronic pain. J Clin Psychol. 2002 Dec;58(12):1505–20. https://doi.org/10.1002/jclp.10101.
108. Tefft AJ, Jordan IO. Eye movement desensitization reprocessing as treatment for chronic pain syndromes: a literature review. J Am Psychiatr Nurses Assoc. 2016;22:192–214. https://doi.org/10.1177/1078390316642519.
109. Tesarz J, Leisner S, Gerhardt A, Janke S, Seidler GH, Eich W, Hartmann M. Effects of eye movement desensitization and reprocessing (EMDR) treatment in chronic pain patients: a systematic review. Pain Med. 2014;15:247–63. https://doi.org/10.1111/pme.12303.

110. Marcus SV. Phase 1 of integrated EMDR: an abortive treatment for migraine headaches. J EMDR Pract Res. 2008;2:15–25.
111. Konuk E, Epozdemir H, Atceken SH, Aydin Y. EMDR treatment of migraine. J EMDR Pract Res. 2011;5:166–76.
112. Demirci OO, Sagaltici E, Yildirim A, Boysan M. Sleep Hypn. 2017;19:70–7. https://doi.org/10.5350/Sleep.Hypn.2017.19.0146.
113. Luyten T, van Rompaey V, van de Heyning P, van Looveran N, Jacquemin L, Cardon E, Declau F, et al. EMDR in the treatment of chronic subjective tinnitus: a systematic review. J EMDR Pract Res. 2020;14:135–49.
114. Luyten TR, Jacquemin L, Van Looveren N, Declau F, Fransen E, Cardon E, et al. Bimodal therapy for chronic subjective tinnitus: a randomized controlled trial of EMDR and TRT versus CBT and TRT. Front Psychol. 2020;10(11):2048. https://doi.org/10.3389/fpsyg.2020.02048.
115. Cope S. EMDR as an adjunctive psychological therapy for patients with functional neurological disorder: illustrative case examples. J EMDR Pract Res. 2020;14:76–89.
116. Page LA, Wessely S. Medically unexplained symptoms: exacerbating factors in the doctor-patient encounter. J R Soc Med. 2003;96:223–7. https://doi.org/10.1258/jrsm.96.5.223.
117. Stone J, Carson A, Duncan R, Coleman R, Roberts R, Warlow C, et al. Symptoms 'unexplained by organic disease' in 1144 new neurology outpatients: how often does the diagnosis change at follow-up? Brain. 2009;132:2878–88.
118. Sharpe M. Medically unexplained symptoms. In: Firth J, Conlon C, Cox T, editors. Oxford textbook of medicine. 6th ed. Oxford: Oxford University Press; 2020. p. 1–8. https://doi.org/10.1093/med/9780198746690.003.0623.
119. Sharpe M, Wessely S. Psychological treatments. In: Firth J, Conlon C, Cox T, editors. Oxford textbook of medicine. 6th ed. Oxford: Oxford University Press; 2020. p. 1–10. https://doi.org/10.1093/med/9780198746690.003.0626.

Pharmacologic Treatment Options in Functional Illness

20

Claire A. Abijay and Ashley D. Agan

Introduction

Few drugs are indicated for functional illness as the pathophysiology and etiology of the symptoms remain unknown. Pharmacological treatments mostly involve off-label use. To date, completed randomized controlled trials typically involve a small number of participants and report highly heterogenous outcomes; therefore, limited numbers of systematic reviews and meta-analysis are available. Drug administration has variable efficacy with moderate symptom improvement among patients who respond to treatment. Many of the drugs' mechanisms of action specific to functional illness remain under investigation. Thus, multidisciplinary treatment is strongly emphasized with pharmacotherapy primarily utilized as an adjunct to non-pharmacological interventions. The drug classes with published studies that are covered in this chapter are summarized in Table 20.1.

Many of the drugs discussed in this chapter are serotonergic and can precipitate the potentially fatal serotonin syndrome. Serotonin syndrome occurs when central and peripheral serotonin receptors (5HT-1A and 5HT-2A) are overactivated by a serotonergic drug used alone at therapeutic ranges or in excess or when used in combination with other serotonergic drugs [1]. Developing within 24 h after exposure to the serotonergic drug, the classic clinical triad includes cognitive changes (altered mental status, agitation, anxiety), autonomic dysfunction (tachycardia, mydriasis, hypertension, sweating), and neuromuscular abnormalities (hyperreflexia, tremor, myoclonus) [1]. It is a diagnosis of exclusion, and management entails withdrawal of all serotonergic drugs and supportive care [2]. For moderate to

C. A. Abijay
University of Texas Southwestern Medical Center, Dallas, TX, USA

A. D. Agan (✉)
Department of Otolaryngology-Head and Neck Surgery, University of Texas Southwestern Medical Center, Dallas, TX, USA
e-mail: ashley.agan@utsouthwestern.edu

© The Author(s), under exclusive license to Springer Nature Switzerland AG 2023

B. W. Blakley, J. E. Blakley (eds.), *Functional Illness of the Head and Neck*,
https://doi.org/10.1007/978-3-031-12998-8_20

Table 20.1 Chapter overview of the investigated drug classes for functional illness

Drug class	Drug examples	Investigated for	General adverse effects
Acetaminophen	Acetaminophen	Fibromyalgia (with tramadol)	Acute overdose liver failure
Antidepressants	Tricyclic Antidepressants (TCA) (amitriptyline, nortriptyline)	Chronic cough, chronic fatigue syndrome, fibromyalgia, functional dizziness, somatoform disorder, tinnitus	Drowsiness, anticholinergic effects (dry mouth, blurred vision, constipation, orthostatic hypotension). Serious AE: serotonin syndrome
	Selective Serotonin Reuptake Inhibitors (SSRI)(fluoxetine, paroxetine)	Functional dizziness, fibromyalgia, chronic fatigue syndrome, somatoform disorder, tinnitus	Headache, nausea/ vomiting, dry mouth, sleep disturbances, sexual disturbances, drowsiness. Serious AE: serotonin syndrome
	Serotonin and Norepinephrine Reuptake Inhibitors (SNRI) (duloxetine, milnacipran)	Fibromyalgia, functional dizziness (with migraine), chronic fatigue syndrome, somatoform disorder	
	Other (mirtazapine)	Chronic fatigue syndrome	Sedation, dry mouth, weight gain
Antiepileptic drugs (AED)	Gabapentin	Chronic cough, fibromyalgia, tinnitus	Sedation, dizziness, gait disturbance, headache
	Pregabalin	Chronic cough, fibromyalgia, fibromyalgia in children and adolescents	
	Other (lamotrigine, topiramate)	Fibromyalgia, vestibular migraine	
Antipsychotics (APs)	First-generation(haloperidol, chlorpromazine)	Fibromyalgia, somatoform pain disorder (flupentixol)	Sedation, sexual dysfunction, orthostatic hypotension, cardiac arrhythmias, QT interval prolongation. 1st generation: extrapyramidal effects. 2nd generation: weight gain, metabolic syndrome. Serious AE: neuroleptic malignant syndrome
	Second-generation (olanzapine, quetiapine)	Fibromyalgia (olanzapine, quetiapine, ziprasidone), tinnitus (sulpiride)	
Benzodiazepines	Clonazepam, alprazolam	Fibromyalgia, functional dizziness, tinnitus	Lethargy, drowsiness, fatigue, motor impairment, anterograde amnesia. Delirium and increased fall risk in elderly

Table 20.1 (continued)

Drug class	Drug examples	Investigated for	General adverse effects
Muscle relaxants	Cyclobenzaprine	Fibromyalgia, chronic orofacial pain, tinnitus	Drowsiness, fatigue, dizziness, dry mouth, reports of delirium. Serious AE: Serotonin syndrome
	Methocarbamol	Myofascial pain syndrome	Sedation, dizziness, headache
Nonsteroidal anti-inflammatory drugs (NSAIDs)	Naproxen, diclofenac	Fibromyalgia, myofascial pain syndrome (diclofenac injections/patches), temporomandibular disorders (naproxen)	Long-term oral use: peptic ulcer disease, acute renal failure, congestive heart failure exacerbation
Opioids	Tramadol	Fibromyalgia (monotherapy or with acetaminophen/ antidepressant), chronic cough	Nausea, vomiting, sedation, dry mouth, fatigue. Serious AE: serotonin syndrome, angioedema
Opioid antagonist	Low Dose Naltrexone (LDN)	Fibromyalgia, chronic fatigue syndrome, chronic pain syndromes	Vivid dreams, possible anxiety
Stimulants	Dextroamphetamine	Chronic fatigue syndrome	Anorexia, weight loss, insomnia, nausea, vomiting, increased heart rate/blood pressure
	Methylphenidate	Chronic fatigue syndrome	Similar to amphetamine, less associated with weight loss
	Modafinil	Chronic fatigue syndrome, fibromyalgia	Headache, nausea (less anorexia)

Abbreviations: *AE* adverse effects, *NMDA N*-methyl-D-aspartate

severe symptoms, a serotonin antagonist (cyproheptadine) may need to be given [1]. Examples of commonly prescribed drugs that can induce serotonin syndrome include tricyclic antidepressants, selective serotonin reuptake inhibitors, serotonin-norepinephrine reuptake inhibitors, tramadol, cyclobenzaprine, dopamine agonists, amphetamines, and monoamine oxidase inhibitors [2].

Acetaminophen

Acetaminophen, also known as paracetamol, is a non-salicylate analgesic with unclear mechanisms of action. Its central effects are thought to be mediated by inhibition of prostaglandin or nitric oxide synthesis [3]. It may act at the supraspinal and spinal level [4]. Acetaminophen formulations are available over the counter or in combination with prescription medications. It is commonly used as a fever reducer and for pain relief in mild to moderate headaches, myalgias, and back pain.

Acute acetaminophen overdose resulting in liver failure is one of the most concerning adverse effects. A potentially toxic dose for adults is a single ingestion of 7.5 g and for children 150 mg/kg [5]. Unintentional overdose can also occur when patients take combination compounds that contain acetaminophen.

The long-term effects of acetaminophen use are not well understood. McCrae et al. [6] reviewed the long-term adverse effects for chronic, regular acetaminophen use and determined that most evidence points to dose-dependent increased risks for gastrointestinal bleed and a small but possibly clinically significant increase in systolic blood pressure (approximately 4 mmHg) [6]. Due to the chronic nature of most functional illnesses, these risks should be considered.

Acetaminophen in Functional Illness

Acetaminophen monotherapy has few if, any roles, in long-term management for functional illnesses. A review for fibromyalgia pharmacotherapy by Kia et al. [7] noted potential utility for low-dose and short-term acetaminophen for patients with fibromyalgia and comorbid osteoarthritis. The review cited other possible mechanisms of action that may be useful for fibromyalgia, including acetaminophen's metabolites acting on the endogenous cannabinoid system [8] and acetaminophen's serotonin receptor antagonism [9]. However, there has been no evidence for use of acetaminophen monotherapy in fibromyalgia.

Acetaminophen is often combined in opioid formulations for pain relief. One randomized, double-blind, placebo-controlled trial with 313 patients with fibromyalgia reported that the combination of tramadol (37.5 mg) and acetaminophen (325 mg) improved quality of life measures after 3 months [10, 11]. The rationale for a 1:8 ratio of tramadol and acetaminophen was based on a synergy study utilizing animal models [12]. Though the study reported improved outcomes, 29 (19%) patients in the treatment group discontinued the medications due to adverse effects like nausea, dizziness, and somnolence, which were most likely side effects from tramadol.

Antidepressants

Antidepressants are used mostly off-label in chronic pain and somatic disorders including but not limited to fibromyalgia, chronic fatigue syndrome, neuropathic pain, functional dizziness, and chronic idiopathic cough. The investigated antidepressant medications covered in this section are summarized in Table 20.2. Known mechanisms of action depend on the category of antidepressant, which are primarily tricyclic antidepressants (TCA), selective serotonin reuptake inhibitors (SSRI), and serotonin and norepinephrine reuptake inhibitors (SNRI).

Table 20.2 Summary of investigated antidepressant medications for functional illness symptoms

Symptom	Drug class	Comments
Chronic cough	TCA	Amitriptyline considered initial pharmacologic option
Functional dizziness	SSRI	First-line pharmacologic treatment
	SNRI	Tried after failed SSRI trials
	TCA/SNRI	Can be tried for dizziness with migraine
Fibromyalgia	SNRI	Duloxetine, milnacipran are FDA-approved
	TCA	Amitriptyline may be useful for sleep disturbances
	SSRI	Consider for comorbid depression
Chronic fatigue syndrome	TCA	Nortriptyline/amitriptyline had positive effects in small RCT/ case reports
	SNRI	Venlafaxine/duloxetine had positive effects in case reports
	SSRI	Mixed results in RCTs
	Mirtazapine	Positive effects in one RCT
Somatoform disorders	SSRI/SNRI	Improved severity of symptoms over placebo
	TCA	Opipramol specifically indicated for somatoform disorder
Tinnitus	SSRI TCA	Likely aids in depression and anxiety and improves tinnitus tolerance

Abbreviations: *TCA* tricyclic antidepressant, *SSRI* selective serotonin reuptake inhibitor, *SNRI* serotonin and norepinephrine reuptake inhibitor, *FDA* Food and Drug Administration, *RCT* randomized controlled trial

TCAs are first-generation antidepressants that include amitriptyline, nortriptyline, desipramine, and imipramine. They are inhibitors of serotonin and norepinephrine reuptake at the presynaptic neuron terminals, resulting in increased levels and activity of the serotonin and norepinephrine neurotransmitters. The class is also known for its promiscuous receptor activity with antagonist effects on alpha1 and alpha2 cholinergic, muscarinic, and histaminergic receptors [13]. Due to these additional affinities, TCAs have several significant adverse effects. The anticholinergic effects include dry mouth, blurred vision, constipation, and orthostatic hypotension, and the anti-histaminergic effects can lead to drowsiness, increased appetite, and weight gain.

SSRIs are second-generation antidepressants that act at the presynaptic neurons and block serotonin transporters, thereby inhibiting serotonin reuptake and increasing serotonin activity. Commonly used SSRIs include fluoxetine, sertraline, paroxetine, citalopram, escitalopram, and fluvoxamine. This class includes the common first-line agents for many mental illnesses such as major depression and anxiety. Compared to the first-generation antidepressants, SSRIs have lower side effect profiles because these medications generally do not activate acetylcholine and histamine receptors [14]. SSRI half-lives vary by compound, and most last approximately 1 day. Fluoxetine has the longest half-life of 2–4 days, with an active metabolite half-life of 7–15 days [14]. Paroxetine has the shortest half-life at 21–24 h and has the highest rate of discontinuation symptoms [15].

SNRIs are also second-generation antidepressants that bind to serotonin and norepinephrine transporters with variable affinities based on the specific compound. The common drugs in this class are venlafaxine, duloxetine, and milnacipran. Typical indications for SNRI include severe depression that failed SSRI trials, anxiety, posttraumatic stress disorders, obsessive compulsive disorders, and chronic pain such as for diabetic neuropathy. Notably, duloxetine and milnacipran are FDA-approved medications for fibromyalgia [16]. SNRI's analgesic mechanism of action is currently unknown. Current evidence in animal models points towards the important effects of the noradrenergic system on pain [17], which appears to be reflected in human clinical trials that report SNRIs' greater effect on pain in comparison to SSRIs [18]. SNRIs are generally metabolized by the cytochrome P450 system. They have better tolerability compared to TCAs as they do not interact with histaminergic or alpha1-adrenergic receptors.

SSRI and SNRI compounds may also have anti-inflammatory and anti-oxidative effects [19]. Although the mechanisms of action are currently unknown, there are studies reporting improvements in immune system regulation and reductions in inflammatory markers after treatment [19].

Common adverse effects across all antidepressants include headache, nausea or vomiting, drowsiness, fatigue, anxiety, and gastrointestinal problems [20]. SSRI and SNRI side effects often include sleep disturbances, sexual dysfunction, and dry mouth. TCAs are particularly known for the anticholinergic and sedative effects. Nevertheless, antidepressants are generally more tolerable compared to the sedating and addictive benzodiazepines and barbiturates. However, many patients with functional disorders such as functional dizziness and fibromyalgia are sensitive to medication side effects. Adverse effects can amplify the patient's perception of symptoms and could lead to an early termination of a medication trial.

Nine antidepressants carry an FDA black box warning of an increased risk for suicidality in young people less than 24 years old. These medications include SSRIs (citalopram, paroxetine, fluoxetine, sertraline, fluvoxamine), SNRIs (venlafaxine), nefazodone, mirtazapine, and bupropion. However, observation of these black box warnings is controversial as it may have led to the unintentional decline in depression diagnoses and treatment [21].

As many antidepressants act by increasing serotonin activity, prescribers of antidepressants should be aware of serotonin syndrome, which was discussed in the introduction of this chapter, especially when considering combination of serotonergic drugs. Symptoms include altered mental status, tachycardia, sweating, myoclonus, and hyperreflexia.

Antidepressants in Functional Illness

Chronic Cough

Amitriptyline is often used as an initial pharmacotherapy option for idiopathic chronic cough. A 2016 review of neuromodulators for idiopathic cough by Giliberto et al. [22] identified one randomized controlled trial for amitriptyline [23]. Jeyakumar et al. [23] compared amitriptyline (10 mg/day for 10 days) to codeine/guaifenesin (opioid/expectorant) and reported that 13 out of 15 (87%) patients taking amitriptyline experienced at least a 50% reduction in their cough versus 1 out of 13 (8%) patients in the comparison group. A 2016 retrospective study by Ryan et al.

[24] concluded amitriptyline is effective for short and long-term management of idiopathic cough. In their cohort, 67% of patients reported at least a 50% improvement at the first follow-up (average 2.5 months), and 34% (13 of 38) of patients continued to take amitriptyline after 2–3 years. Among the 38 respondents at 2–3 years, 53% of patients reported at least a 50% improvement in cough symptoms. The authors emphasized that many patients required titrating dosages or even restarting the medication in order to balance cough symptoms and adverse effects. Side effect intolerance was a common reason for quitting amitriptyline, with most reporting sedation and dry mouth, followed by anxiety, difficulty sleeping, dizziness, and weight gain [24].

A 2018 paper on pharmacotherapy tachyphylaxis for chronic cough by Bowen et al. [25] reported that nearly 30% of their successfully treated patients developed drug dependence. For the patients who tried to stop or decrease the dosage, cough symptoms often returned, requiring patients to remain on the neuromodulator for several years. The authors advise that patients should be counseled on the possibility of long-term pharmacotherapy use. Additionally, improvements are expected to be seen shortly after medication initiation (1–3 months), although some patients can still respond even with later medication trials [25]. Chronic cough pharmacotherapy is also discussed under the antiepileptics section for gabapentin and pregabalin options.

Functional Dizziness

For functional dizziness such as chronic subjective dizziness (CSD) and persistent postural-perceptual dizziness (PPPD), SSRIs are the mainstay treatment based on several open label, prospective studies [26]. As summarized by Ruckenstein et al. [27], studies have reported approximately 70% of patients experiencing significant improvement in symptoms and about 50% of patients having full remission with SSRI treatment [28–30]. In the *Handbook of Clinical Neurology*'s chapter on chronic subjective dizziness, Dieterich et al. [31] recommended cognitive-behavioral therapy with or without pharmacologic treatment only if self-desensitization and explanation of functional disorder fail to reduce symptoms. If pharmacologic therapy is tried, one SSRI is attempted, followed by a second if the first was intolerable or ineffective. SNRIs are tried after failing the two trials of SSRI. Treatment should be initiated with low doses, generally a quarter to a half of doses used for major depression, and slowly titrated to a maximum that is in the lower half of the therapeutic range for major depression [26, 27]. The gradual dosing strategy is based on previous studies reporting 20% dropout rates due to medication intolerance. Ruckenstein et al. [27] emphasized that patients may experience an initial increase in anxiety, which can result in early termination of the medication trial. At least 8–12 weeks of treatment are required before patients experience a clinically significant response [27]. TCA use in functional dizziness has been mentioned as an option, although they do not appear to have been investigated systematically [26, 31, 32].

In patients with migraine and chronic subjective dizziness, utilizing either SNRIs (venlafaxine or duloxetine) or a TCA (amitriptyline) can target both symptoms [27].

Fibromyalgia

Duloxetine and milnacipran are two of three FDA-approved medications for fibromyalgia, with the antiepileptic pregabalin being the third. Duloxetine (60–120 mg/day) helps with pain reduction, sleep, and functional ability but not fatigue [16, 33]. Milnacipran (100–200 mg/day) also improved pain and fatigue [16, 33]. Both drugs appear to be effective in the long term. However, in the trials for both drugs, high placebo response rates (>30%) were noted [16]. A 2014 Cochrane review by Lunn et al. [34] on duloxetine reported 12.6% of participants dropping out due to adverse effects. Another systemic review and meta-analysis reported 60 mg/day of duloxetine had less withdrawal effects compared to 120 mg/day [35].

Amitriptyline has been widely investigated for fibromyalgia and improves pain (30% pain reduction) and sleep [33, 36]. The 2017 European League Against Rheumatism (EULAR) guidelines for fibromyalgia treatment weakly recommend amitriptyline, mostly for patients with sleep disturbances [37]. According to 2008 review by Nishishinya et al. [38], patients responded to 25 mg/day of amitriptyline in 6–8 weeks, while 50 mg/day did not appear useful. Nevertheless, only some patients (approximately 36%) are expected to benefit from TCAs [16].

SSRI efficacy in fibromyalgia has not been consistently demonstrated. The 2017 EULAR recommendations do not recommend the use of SSRIs [37]. A 2015 Cochrane review by Walitt et al. [39] did not find evidence that SSRIs were superior to placebo in improving fibromyalgia pain, fatigue, or sleep disturbances. However, due to the high prevalence of the comorbidity of depression in fibromyalgia patients, SSRIs still may be useful [16]. The difference in SSRI and SNRI efficacy further suggests norepinephrine's important role in pain modulation.

Chronic Fatigue Syndrome (CFS)

Investigations of TCAs for use with patients with Chronic Fatigue Syndrome (CFS) include a small, randomized control trial for nortriptyline (60 mg/day) and several case reports for amitriptyline and doxepin (25–50 mg at bedtime) [40]. While these studies report positive effects for fatigue, larger randomized control trials are needed.

The positive effects of SNRIs (venlafaxine and duloxetine) on CFS have been reported in human case reports and demonstrated in animal studies; however, there are no randomized control trials for CFS patients [40]. Among the case reports, venlafaxine (225 mg/day) for 6 weeks was utilized after failed SSRI trials [41], and use of duloxetine (120 mg/day) had improvements within 4 weeks [42]. The rationale for utilizing SNRIs is that CFS and fibromyalgia appear closely related in terms of symptoms and epidemiology, although whether these assumptions are applicable is unknown [40].

SSRI use in CFS has mixed results. In general, randomized controlled trials have not shown them to be superior to placebo, although open-label studies have reported significant improvement in symptoms. The 2009 review by Pae et al. [40] identified citalopram (20–40 mg/day for 1–2 months) [43] and escitalopram (10–20 mg/day for up to 12 weeks) [44] demonstrating some improvement in fatigue, although not always reaching statistical significance. Pae et al. [40] also covered fluoxetine (20 mg/day), which did not improve fatigue or other CFS-related symptoms in one randomized controlled trial [45], and sertraline (50 mg/day) which had a positive response in 65% of patients in one uncontrolled pilot study [46].

Mirtazapine is an alpha2-adrenergic receptor antagonist that increases serotonin and norepinephrine activity. One randomized controlled trial by Stubhaug et al. [47] (n = 72) found significant improvements for fatigue and symptom severity in the treatment arm of 12 weeks of cognitive behavioral therapy followed by 12 weeks of mirtazapine (standard dose 15–45 mg) in comparison to the other treatment combinations, which included mirtazapine followed by cognitive behavioral therapy. The study suggests that timing of pharmacological treatment may be an important factor to consider for CFS patients.

Somatoform Disorders

For somatoform disorders, SSRIs and SNRIs are the most studied pharmacotherapies. A 2014 Cochrane review by Kleinstauber et al. [48] reported that only low or very low-quality evidence existed for any drug class in regard to efficacy in somatoform disorders. Nevertheless, SSRI/SNRIs performed better than placebo in reducing severity of somatoform disorder symptoms. The review identified three studies in which SSRI/SNRIs were superior to placebo after 8–12 weeks of treatment and two studies in which SSRI/SNRI increased quality of life measures by improving depressive symptoms and functionality [48]. No study found an effect on anxiety. Generally, dropout rates were similar between the SSRI/SNRI treatment and placebo, and efficacy among the SSRI/SNRIs medications was also comparable. Another review by Somashekar et al. [18] noted SNRIs appearing to be more useful than SSRIs for somatoform pain disorder, which is a similar observation seen with fibromyalgia [16].

In the somatoform treatment review by Kleinstauber et al. [48], TCAs were not found to be superior to placebo in reducing symptoms (n = 239).

Tinnitus

Antidepressants can be tried for tinnitus, although their direct effect on tinnitus severity is unknown. A 2012 meta-analysis by Baldo et al. [49] found no evidence that antidepressants improved tinnitus. A 2016 tinnitus therapy review by Hesse [50] discussed how previous SSRIs and TCA studies that observed tinnitus improvements could not rule out the effect of improved depression and anxiety. The general recommendation is to initiate therapy for decompensated, chronic tinnitus, as improvement in depression and anxiety aids in the tolerance of tinnitus [50].

Antiepileptic Drugs (AED)

Antiepileptic drugs (AED) are used off-label as anxiolytics, mood stabilizers, and pain relievers in neuropathic pain syndromes and migraine. Common AEDs include gabapentin, pregabalin, lamotrigine, lacosamide, carbamazepine, valproate, topiramate, phenytoin, and clonazepam. In general, AEDs are thought to work by decreasing high frequency neuronal firing by modulating gamma-aminobutyric acid

(GABA) neurotransmission or stabilizing neuronal cell membrane potentials [51]. The exact mechanisms of action for how AEDs modulate pain are still under investigation. Analgesic effects of the gabapentinoids pregabalin and gabapentin are currently hypothesized to be related to the binding of the α2δ subunit of voltage-dependent calcium channels [52, 53]. Based on animal studies, the α2δ subunit is important in the nociceptive pathophysiology of neuropathic conditions [52, 53]. They are also known to modulate the noradrenergic pain pathways and may have indirect effects on proinflammatory cytokines [52]. Gabapentin has been used effectively for several peripheral neuropathies like postherpetic neuralgia and painful diabetic neuropathy [54]. The other AEDs also do not have clear mechanisms of action; known effects include interactions with voltage-gated sodium channels (lamotrigine, lacosamide, carbamazepine, topiramate), acetylcholine receptors (lamotrigine), and amino-3-hydroxy-5-methyl-4-isoxazolepropionic acid (AMPA) receptors (topiramate), and GABAergic pathways (valproate, clonazepam, topiramate) [55].

Common side effects include sedation, somnolence, dizziness, and gait disturbance, along with reports of headache and peripheral edema [54]. Typically, adverse effects are alleviated with dose tapering or drug discontinuation. Pregabalin is more potent than gabapentin, with greater bioavailability and should be administered at lower doses [48]. With the growing concern for the potential misuse and abuse of gabapentinoids, prescribers should carefully monitor for any signs of misuse, particularly in patients with a history of substance abuse [56, 57]. An article by Schifano et al. [57] included a qualitative review of online posts and observations describing a wide range of experiences in gabapentinoid abuse: a marijuana-like high, euphoria, sedation, and dissociative/psychedelic effects. Combinations with alcohol, benzodiazepines, lysergic acid diethylamide (LSD), heroin, and opiates have been reported [57]. These reports typically utilized gabapentinoids at significantly higher doses (3–20 times) than therapeutic use.

Antiepileptic Drugs in Functional Illness

Chronic Cough

Gabapentin is a reasonable initial choice for neurogenic cough, along with the TCAs nortriptyline and amitriptyline [22, 25]. A double-blind, randomized controlled trial ($n = 26$) using gabapentin (titrated to a maximum of 1800 mg/day for 10 weeks) demonstrated decreased cough frequency and severity and improved cough-specific quality of life measures [58]. However, these improvements did not persist after medication discontinuation.

Pregabalin (titrated to a maximum of 300 mg/day for 11 weeks) with speech therapy was compared with placebo and speech therapy in a randomized controlled trial ($n = 35$) [59]. Both the treatment and placebo arms improved cough severity, frequency, and quality of life measures, and the patients on pregabalin had greater improvements compared to speech therapy alone [59].

As discussed in the antidepressant section for chronic cough, patients should be counseled that medication response typically occurs early on with initial treatment, although successful outcomes are still possible with subsequent trials of other medications [25]. A retrospective review on unexplained chronic cough pharmacotherapy tachyphylaxis and dependence noted that patients who experienced few side effects on gabapentin and nortriptyline were more likely to have successful outcomes compared to amitriptyline [25]. However, patients experiencing more side effects on gabapentin and nortriptyline were more likely to quit the study compared to those on amitriptyline. Sedation was the most common experienced side effect [25]. The same study reported tachyphylaxis-induced failures typically occurring after an upper respiratory infection or allergy exacerbation, which may be an area for further investigation to determine interventions for drug failure prevention.

Fibromyalgia/Chronic Pain

Pregabalin was the first FDA-approved medication for fibromyalgia in 2007. Based on several randomized clinical trials, pregabalin improves overall quality of life through decreased pain and improved sleep [16]. However, it does not appear to affect depression, mood, anxiety, or fatigue [60]. One randomized controlled trial by Arnold et al. [52] ($n = 750$) reported improvements with pregabalin monotherapy (300 mg/day, 450 mg/day, or 600 mg/day for up to 14 weeks). Optimal dosing is unclear, but the recommended ranges are between 300 mg/day and 600 mg/day [61]. The 2017 EULAR recommendations [37] support pregabalin's use, citing a 2013 Cochrane meta-analysis of randomized controlled trials ($n = 3579$) that concluded a small benefit of pregabalin over placebo for sleep and pain (50% pain reduction, risk ratio = 1.59, confidence interval CI 95% = 1.33–1.90, number needed to benefit = 12; CI 95% = 9–21) [62]. However, this Cochrane review was withdrawn in 2017 due to conflicts of interest.

One cross-over, randomized controlled trial by Gilron et al. [63] ($n = 41$) investigated a combination of pregabalin-duloxetine (maximum 450 mg/day of pregabalin, maximum 120 mg/day of duloxetine) for 6 weeks. The study demonstrated superior improvements in combination therapy for pain intensity over pregabalin monotherapy, although the improvements did not reach statistical significance for duloxetine monotherapy. Nevertheless, combination therapy improvements were superior to either monotherapy for quality-of-life measures, functional improvements, and global pain relief. Combination therapy also had a higher frequency of drowsiness compared to duloxetine alone.

Gabapentin is considered an alternative for patients who cannot tolerate pregabalin. Only one randomized controlled trial by Arnold et al. [64] ($n = 150$) has been published using gabapentin for fibromyalgia. Patients were treated with 1200–2400 mg/day of gabapentin; 51% of patients treated with gabapentin reported at least a 30% reduction in pain versus 31% of patients on placebo ($P = 0.014$) [64]. Twelve of 75 patients (16%) discontinued gabapentin due to side effects. The EULAR 2017 guidelines recommend gabapentin for research purposes only [37].

A 2013 Cochrane review by Wiffen et al. [55] for AED use in fibromyalgia and neuropathic pain conditions determined only gabapentin and pregabalin had evidence of efficacy with little to no evidence for lacosamide, clonazepam, phenytoin, carbamazepine, lamotrigine, oxcarbazepine, and topiramate. The authors emphasized only a minority of patients will respond to AEDs and knowing which patients will respond to certain drugs is unknown. Nevertheless, patients who do respond and can achieve a 50% reduction in pain are known to improve significantly in terms of quality of life.

Vestibular Migraine

AEDs are commonly used in migraine prophylaxis, and some studies have shown efficacy in improving the vestibular symptoms of vestibular migraine. A 2014 review of vestibular migraine treatment by Obermann et al. [65] identified a retrospective observational study (n = 19) of lamotrigine (100 mg/day for 3–4 months after 4-week titration) in which average vertigo frequency was reduced from 18.1 to 5.4 episodes per month [66]. Average headache frequency also decreased from 8.7 to 4.4 episodes per month, but did not reach statistical significance [66]. A retrospective review by Mikulec et al. [67] evaluated caffeine cessation and pharmacotherapy options for patients with vestibular migraine or "complex dizziness of undetermined etiology". A small number of patients (6/44 or 14%) found caffeine cessation alone effective for reduction in symptoms. Otherwise, nortriptyline (TCA) was effective (at least a 50% improvement) in 11 of 26 patients (46%), and topiramate reduced symptoms in 4 of 16 patients (25%) [67].

Antipsychotics (APs)

Antipsychotics (APs), formerly known as neuroleptics, are primarily indicated for management of psychosis in schizophrenia and have various off-label uses for anxiety, insomnia, bipolar depression, and treatment-refractory depression. The class is divided into the "typical" first-generation (e.g., haloperidol, chlorpromazine) and "atypical" second-generation drugs (e.g., clozapine, risperidone, olanzapine, quetiapine). First-generation APs are primarily dopamine D2 antagonists that also inhibit noradrenergic, cholinergic, and histaminergic receptors. Second-generation APs are generally also D2 antagonists with additional serotonin receptor antagonist activity. The analgesic mechanism of APs is unknown. Animal models have suggested that multiple pathways are involved including the intrinsic opioid system and alpha2-adrenergic receptor action [68].

In terms of pain management, the advantage of APs over opioids is that they are not addictive and are less strictly controlled [68]. However, the class' use is generally limited in chronic, functional illnesses due to the high rates of dose-dependent side effects. Common adverse effects for both first- and second-generation APs include sedation, sexual dysfunction, orthostatic hypotension, and cardiac arrhythmias [69]. APs can cause QT interval prolongation, which can lead to Torsades de Pointes and cardiac death, although this side effect is more concerning for patients with severe psychotic disorders on maximum dosages. With use of first-generation, high potency APs (e.g., haloperidol), patients must be monitored for extrapyramidal side effects and irreversible tardive dyskinesia. In second-generation APs (clozapine, olanzapine), prescribers must monitor for weight gain and metabolic syndrome.

Considerations of these side effects are important in determining whether to initiate or continue utilization of APs. Although rare, neuroleptic malignant syndrome (NMS) is a potentially fatal adverse effect of all APs that occurs due to D2 receptor antagonism. NMS requires rapid recognition and can present with altered mental status, "lead pipe" muscle rigidity, tremor, myoclonus, hyperthermia, and autonomic dysfunction [70]. Withdrawal of the offending antipsychotic medication is the critical step in NMS management followed by aggressive supportive care (volume replacement, careful monitoring for electrolyte imbalances, renal failure, cardiorespiratory failure, and aspiration pneumonia) [70].

APs in Functional Illness

Fibromyalgia

Early studies for fibromyalgia have reported variable efficacy of APs depending on the compound used. First-generation APs have not been found to be a clinically useful analgesic for pain management in general [71, 72]. In contrast, a 2018 review by Jimenez et al. [68] concluded that second-generation APs may be helpful options or additions for chronic pain conditions like fibromyalgia and headache. The review identified studies for olanzapine, quetiapine, and ziprasidone in fibromyalgia.

Olanzapine appears to have efficacy for fibromyalgia based on 2 case series and a retrospective review [68]. In a retrospective review ($n = 51$) by Freedenfeld et al. [73], most patients experienced some pain relief and improved daily life function at doses less than 5 mg/day, with some requiring doses 10 mg/day, and a small minority at 20 mg/day. However, half (53%) of patients discontinued olanzapine within 2 months, with the most cited reasons being weight gain, sedation, or no perceived benefit.

A 2016 Cochrane review by Walitt et al. [74] on APs for fibromyalgia reported very low-quality evidence for quetiapine's superiority over placebo and did not find evidence for its superiority to amitriptyline. The meta-analysis concluded that short-term quetiapine trials (50–300 mg at bedtime for 4–12 weeks) could be useful for patients with comorbid fibromyalgia, depression, and sleep disturbances [74]. One double-blind, randomized controlled trial by McIntyre et al. [75] determined an extended-release quetiapine formulation (max titration to 150–300 mg/day) to be efficacious for patients with both fibromyalgia and major depressive disorder. Nevertheless, the risk and benefits must be thoroughly considered due to the high rates of weight gain and metabolic syndrome [74]. For patients with fibromyalgia and depression who failed duloxetine trials, Walitt et al. [74] recommended a limited trial of quetiapine (4–12 weeks) with a definitive stopping point to reduce adverse effects. Ziprasidone (20 mg/day for 12 weeks) was not found to be effective for fibromyalgia symptoms or sleep in one case series ($n = 32$) [76].

AP side effect rates are high, with 1 in 4 patients dropping out of studies due to intolerance of side effects [68, 77] It should be emphasized that most patients with fibromyalgia are particularly sensitive to adverse effects. If APs are tried, low doses and slow titration are recommended.

Tinnitus

Sulpiride is an atypical antipsychotic with dose-dependent D2 antagonism that has been investigated for tinnitus. A single-blinded, randomized, prospective, placebo-controlled trial ($n = 120$) by Lopez-Gonzalez et al. [78] reported that low dose sulpiride (50 mg/8 h) combined with the anti-histamine hydroxyzine (25 mg/12 h) decreased the perception of tinnitus. Based on a subjective grading of tinnitus perception, a decrease in tinnitus perception was reported by 35 of 43 (81%) patients with the combination sulpiride/hydroxyzine, 23 of 41 patients (56%) on sulpiride alone, and 8 of 38 (21%) patients on placebo. The authors noted that sulpiride is for short-term management (1 month) of intolerable tinnitus, and once the perception of tinnitus is more controlled, other management options like cognitive-behavioral therapy and sound treatment are emphasized. Sulpiride's effects may occur through modulation of the D2-mediated audito-limbic system [78]. The rationale for hydroxyzine's use was based on its utility for generalized anxiety [79].

Benzodiazepines (BZD)

Benzodiazepines (BZD) are the first-line drugs for status epilepticus, alcohol withdrawal, and anxiety crisis without psychosis. BZDs are also utilized as an amnestic and anxiolytic intraoperatively. Common drugs in this class include alprazolam, lorazepam, clonazepam, and diazepam. This drug class acts throughout the central nervous system by enhancing the inhibitory effect of the neurotransmitter gamma amino butyric acid's (GABA). BZDs bind to the GABA-A receptor, a chloride channel, which results in hyperpolarization of the cell [80]. Reviewed by Griffin et al. [80], different BZD receptors on the GABA-A complex are responsible for a variety of effects—sedative, amnestic, anticonvulsant, anxiolytic, and myorelaxant.

Benzodiazepines can be short-acting (half-life of 1–12 h; midazolam), intermediate-acting (half-life of 12–40 h; alprazolam, lorazepam), or long-acting (half-life of 40–250 h; clonazepam), with some long-acting drugs producing active metabolites. Most BZDs are metabolized by the cytochrome P450 system and excreted via the urine; therefore, renal and hepatic diseases along with drug-drug interactions can greatly affect elimination half-life [80]. Although approximately 40% of patients on chronic opioid therapy for pain are also prescribed BZDs, concurrent use of opioids and BZDs may lead to overdose and result in death from respiratory depression [81]. Gudin et al. [81] suggest managing this risk by adjusting pharmacotherapy plans to replace BZDs with antidepressants, atypical antipsychotics, or buspirone (anxiolytic, partial serotonin agonist).

Common side effects include lethargy, drowsiness, fatigue, motor impairment, and anterograde amnesia. Delirium and an increase risk of falls are especially common for the elderly, due to the slowed metabolism of the drugs [80].

BZDs in Functional Illness

Benzodiazepine use generally is discouraged for many functional illnesses due to their serious adverse effects with long-term use. Tolerance and physical dependence can occur within 4 weeks of treatment, with approximately 20–100% of patients developing dependence after 1 month of taking BZDs [82]. This class should only be considered as an alternative option for clear indications, mainly the comorbidities of severe anxiety or insomnia. If BZDs are initiated, prescribers should prioritize educating and establishing a definitive plan with the patient. Best practices include limiting the duration to 2–4 weeks and anticipating slow tapers of 12–18 months or longer [82].

A narrative review by Wright [82] concluded that among chronic pain syndromes, only patients with burning mouth syndrome and stiff person syndrome have been shown to respond to the analgesic benefits of BZDs. Otherwise, insufficient evidence exists for BZD efficacy in relieving neck pain, fibromyalgia, and temporomandibular dysfunction [82].

Fibromyalgia

The American Pain Society, European League Against Rheumatism, and Association of the Scientific Medical Societies in Germany do not recommend BZD use in fibromyalgia [83]. A 2018 Cochrane review by Thorpe et al. [84] identified three studies combining NSAIDs and various BZDs and reported conflicting results on the alleviation of fibromyalgia symptoms. In the study by Russell et al. [85], the combination of alprazolam and ibuprofen performed better than the placebo, but not better than the monotherapy arms. In a different study by Quijada-Carrera et al. [86], combination therapy of tenoxicam and bromazepam performed better than the monotherapy, but not better than the placebo. Finally, Kravitz et al. [87] concluded that the monotherapies of alprazolam and ibuprofen performed better than in combination. Another systematic review by Corrigan et al. [88] did not find enough evidence to support use of clonazepam for fibromyalgia or chronic neuropathic pain, noting that the adverse effects could overshadow any benefits that do exist. In addition, the "Z-drugs" zolpidem and zopiclone (nonbenzodiazepine sedative-hypnotics) did not improve fibromyalgia symptoms, but had some subjective improvements in sleep [16, 89].

Functional Dizziness

For functional dizziness, Dieterich et al. [31] recommend that only a small number of patients attempt a short duration (no more than a few weeks) of an anxiolytic like lorazepam as an adjunct to antidepressants (SSRI or TCA). While BZDs are not effective primary treatments for functional dizziness, they are options for patients with severe comorbid anxiety to help alleviate anxiety symptoms [26].

Tinnitus

A review for tinnitus therapy by Hesse [50] identified two studies in which patients with chronic tinnitus were treated with BZDs in combination with other drugs:

clonazepam (1 mg/day) with melitracen (TCA) [90] and clonazepam (0.5 mg/day) with ginkgo [91]. Although tinnitus severity and disturbances appeared to be reduced in both studies, Hesse [50] criticized these studies for failing to warn against the adverse effects of BZDs, particularly cognitive impairment and risk of falls. In addition, the reduction of symptoms could likely be attributed to the sedative properties of these drugs.

Muscle Relaxants

Muscle relaxants are given to reduce skeletal muscle tone for muscle spasms and pain. The common muscle relaxants with potential use in functional illnesses are cyclobenzaprine and methocarbamol. These drugs are considered to be "centrally" acting agents, although their mechanisms are unclear. Cyclobenzaprine is structurally similar to amitriptyline (TCA) and was initially investigated for use in depression [92]. Based on animal models, it is a serotonin 5-HT2 and alpha-2 adrenergic blocker with central anticholinergic effects, and its actions ultimately result in decreased activity of spinal cord interneurons [92]. Methocarbamol is thought to work as central nervous system depressant, although its mechanism of action is also currently unknown [93].

Cyclobenzaprine shares some of its side effects with amitriptyline. These side effects are covered in depth in the 2009 review by Cimolai [92]. Drowsiness and fatigue are commonly reported, which are the reasons for its bedtime dosing. Other adverse effects include dizziness, lightheadedness, and some anticholinergic effects like xerostomia. Caution is advised for patients with urinary retention or glaucoma due to these possible anticholinergic side effects. Contraindications include patients with hyperthyroidism, congestive heart failure, cardiac arrythmia, and patients recovering from myocardial infarction. Serotonin syndrome has been observed with cyclobenzaprine when combined with duloxetine, SSRIs, and monoamine oxidase inhibitors. There have been case reports of delirium, psychosis, and mania, all of which resolved after discontinuation [92].

Methocarbamol's side effects are primarily drowsiness, headache, and dizziness [93]. Urine color changing to black, brown, or green may occur as well.

Muscle Relaxants in Functional Illness

Fibromyalgia

Cyclobenzaprine is used for fibromyalgia, although there is weak evidence for its efficacy. A 2004 meta-analysis by Tofferi et al. [94] identified five randomized controlled trials with 312 patients utilizing doses between 10–40 mg/day for 2–24 weeks. The review concluded that patients could expect modest pain improvement early in the treatment course and moderate sleep benefits. However, they noted a high dropout rate of 29% of patients, with 85% of them reporting adverse effects. A 2011 randomized, double-blind, placebo-controlled study by Moldofsky et al. [95] ($n = 36$) reported that a low dose of cyclobenzaprine (2–4 mg) at bedtime improved pain, mood, and sleep for patients with fibromyalgia. Overall, the 2017 EULAR guidelines for fibromyalgia recommend cyclobenzaprine in patients with fibromyalgia and sleep disturbances [37]. As of 2020, a sublingual low-dose cyclobenzaprine formulation (TNX-102 SL, 2 × 2.8 mg/day) completed its phase three clinical trial (NCT04172831) for fibromyalgia pain, although results are not yet available [96].

Chronic Orofacial Pain

As reviewed by Hersh et al. [97], muscle relaxants are also tried for chronic orofacial pain due to their efficacy for treating muscle spasms in the cervical and lumbar region [98]. A randomized controlled trial by Herman et al. [99] for temporomandibular pain reported cyclobenzaprine (10 mg at bedtime) when added to self-care and management education to be superior to either placebo or 0.5 mg clonazepam. A more recent pharmacologic review for temporomandibular disorders by Ouanounou et al. [100] suggests cyclobenzaprine doses starting at 10 mg with a 30-day trial and 2-week washout period before assessing its efficacy.

Myofascial Pain Syndrome

For myofascial pain syndrome, Nicol et al.'s [61] review of opioid alternatives for chronic pain identified one older study by Valtonen [101] from 1975 involving methocarbamol. The study ($n = 118$) had patients on 1500 mg four times a day for 1-week and deemed methocarbamol superior to placebo for pain relief [101]. Note that typical dosing for methocarbamol in painful muscle spasms is 6 g daily (1.5 g four times daily) for the first 2–3 days and lowering afterwards to 4–4.5 g daily in 3–6 divided doses [102].

Tinnitus

Cyclobenzaprine has been tried in a multicenter, open-label pilot study by Coelho et al. [103] with 14 patients with chronic tinnitus. The high dose of 30 mg had significant improvements in the Tinnitus Handicap Inventory after 12-weeks. Reported side effects included xerostomia, drowsiness, and constipation. Coelho et al. [103] emphasized a need for placebo-controlled trials. However, a tinnitus pharmacology review by Hesse [50] criticized the study for a lack of adequate justification for the drug's use.

Nonsteroidal Anti-inflammatory Drugs (NSAIDs)

NSAIDs are known to reduce prostaglandin and thromboxane synthesis by inhibiting the cyclooxygenase enzymes, which results in their peripheral anti-inflammatory effects. Commonly used NSAIDs include ibuprofen, naproxen, celecoxib, and diclofenac. Based on animal models, NSAIDs' central effects may play a role in the modulation of pain pathways via spinal prostaglandins like PGE_2 [104]. Topical

NSAIDs have also been used effectively for pain management in acute and chronic musculoskeletal pain [105, 106].

The adverse effects of long-term NSAID use are well documented and limit their utility for chronic functional illnesses. Major affected organ systems include gastrointestinal (peptic ulcer disease), renal (decreased glomerular perfusion and acute renal failure), cardiovascular (myocardial infarction, hypertension exacerbation, congestive heart failure exacerbation), and cerebrovascular (stroke) [107]. Particularly for older adults with chronic conditions, alternative options such as acetaminophen are often recommended for patients with mild-moderate pain, such as in osteoarthritis.

NSAIDS in Functional Illness

Myofascial Pain Syndrome

In myofascial pain, the review by Nicol et al. [61] identified two studies for injected or topical NSAID use. One older study in 1986 by Frost et al. [108] reported diclofenac trigger point injections to be superior over lidocaine for pain improvement. A double-blind, randomized, placebo-controlled study in 2010 by Hsieh et al. [109] determined diclofenac sodium patches (60 mg, 10 cm × 14 cm) effective in reducing pain and improving functional outcomes for myofascial pain in the upper trapezius.

Opioids

Opioids typically are indicated for short-term moderate-to-severe pain. In the context of cancer pain relief, the World Health Organization categorizes weak opioids (e.g., codeine, tramadol, dihydrocodeine) for mild to moderate pain and strong opioids (e.g., morphine, methadone, fentanyl, oxycodone, hydromorphone) for moderate to severe pain [110]. With the chronic nature of most functional illnesses, the use of strong opioids is discouraged. Rather, the main opioid of interest is tramadol, which has dual actions as a weak μ-receptor agonist and a norepinephrine and serotonin reuptake inhibitor [2]. Tramadol is reviewed in-depth by Beakley et al. [2]. Compared to other opiates, tramadol has less potential for abuse and respiratory depression, although there is still a risk. Tramadol goes through an extensive first-pass metabolism in the liver and is mostly eliminated renally. Its half-life is 5–6 h, and the M1 metabolite with analgesic properties has a half-life of 8 h [2]. Common side effects for tramadol include nausea and vomiting, sedation, dry mouth, and fatigue. Severe adverse effects include increased anticoagulant effects, angioedema, and serotonin syndrome, particularly in combination with other serotonergic medications [2]. Despite tramadol's lower risk for addiction, dependence has been observed with doses as low as 50 mg/day with history of drug abuse being an important risk factor [111].

Opioids in Functional Illness

Fibromyalgia

Chronic use of strong opioids is not recommended for fibromyalgia due to the lack of data for its long-term efficacy, its high potential for abuse, and risk of death via respiratory depression [16, 37].

The 2017 EULAR guidelines for fibromyalgia weakly recommend tramadol's use [39]. A systematic review by da Rocha et al. [112] identified four randomized controlled trials involving tramadol alone or in combination with acetaminophen or an antidepressant. Overall, the review concluded that not enough high-quality evidence was available to support or refute the routine use of tramadol for patients with fibromyalgia. A randomized, double-blind, placebo-controlled trial with 313 patients with fibromyalgia reported that the combination of tramadol and acetaminophen improved quality of life after 3 months [13, 14]. With each tablet containing 37.5 mg of tramadol and 325 mg of acetaminophen, the mean use was 4.0 tablets per day with a maximum use of 8 tablets per day (300 mg tramadol/2600 mg acetaminophen). However, 29 patients (19%) discontinued the combination treatment due to adverse effects like nausea, dizziness, and somnolence [13].

A cross-sectional study by Scott et al. [113] suggested that caffeine may act as an opioid adjuvant for fibromyalgia-like chronic pain. Users of any type of opioid consuming low to moderate amounts of caffeine were found to have less pain severity and improved physical function compared to opioid users who were not consuming caffeine. No effects were seen for non-opioid users. How caffeine may potentiate the analgesic properties of opioids is unknown. The authors discussed caffeine's involvement with the adrenergic and noradrenergic system and increased release of endogenous opioid as possible explanations. Caffeine may also be countering the negative effects of opioids by reducing fatigue and improving mood and attention [113].

Chronic Cough

A 2017 pilot study by Dion et al. [114] treated 16 patients with 50 mg of tramadol every 8 h as needed. The study reported improvements in quality of life and cough severity and emphasized the need for a controlled trial. Four patients reported somnolence. A retrospective review by Bowen et al. [28] reported 4 out of 13 patients (31%) successfully responded to tramadol with median doses of 50 mg/day. Two patients stopped tramadol due to tachyphylaxis, three patients from side effects, and four from no perceived benefits. The median time taken to develop tachyphylaxis was 11 months [28].

Opioid Antagonist

Naltrexone and its active metabolite 6-β-naltrexol are long-acting μ-opioid and κ-opioid receptor antagonists, with higher affinities for the μ-opioid receptor [115].

The drug is FDA-approved for treatment of opioid dependence and alcohol dependence, with standard doses typically between 50 and 150 mg. Due to significant first-pass metabolism, its oral bioavailability ranges from 5 to 40% [115]. Naltrexone and its metabolites are renally eliminated.

Low dose naltrexone (LDN) is considered a promising new therapy for chronic pain due to its limited adverse effects and relatively low cost. As reviewed by Trofimovitch et al. [116], LDN has multiple mechanisms of action that may be relevant for pain syndromes. At low doses of 1–5 mg, naltrexone has anti-inflammatory and analgesic properties through its inhibition of the central nervous system (CNS) microglial cells [117]. Activated microglial cells respond to CNS injury and produce proinflammatory cytokines. LDN is an antagonist of Toll-like receptor 4 (TLR4) that interrupts signaling cascades and ultimately decreases the production of these proinflammatory cytokines. LDN also increases endogenous opioid signaling, with the increased levels of endorphins producing positive effects [116].

A 2014 review article by Younger et al. [117] reported a low side effect profile for LDN, with vivid dreams being the most commonly reported. The authors had not observed cases of severe adverse effects, although they emphasized the need for larger trials. Anecdotally, anxiety was another side effect, although its incidence is unknown.

Opioid Antagonists in Functional Illness

Fibromyalgia

A double-blind, randomized, placebo-controlled study ($n = 31$) by Younger et al. [118] for LDN (3.0–4.5 mg/day) reported 57% of participants experiencing at least a 30% reduction in pain, with improvements in mood and general satisfaction in life. The most common side effects were vivid dreams and headaches. Side effects were reduced when switching to the 3.0 mg/day dose. Other reported adverse effects include nausea, nightmares, and agitation. A single-blind, 10-week crossover study by Parkitny et al. [119] with 8 women found reductions in plasma proinflammatory cytokines and a 15% reduction in fibromyalgia pain.

Chronic Fatigue Syndrome

Bolton et al. [120] reviewed a series of three case reports of LDN utilization in patients with chronic fatigue syndrome and myalgic encephalomyelitis. A range of responses were observed. One patient returned to a normal quality of life with improved mood, while another patient experienced minimal changes in functionality. Nevertheless, even the patient with the lowest response reported improvements in sleep and pain levels. Dosing was initiated at very low doses (0.25–1.5 mg/day) and increased as tolerated. The highest maintenance dose of 6 mg twice a day was taken by the patient with the greatest improvements. Bolton et al. [120] emphasized the need for randomized controlled trials to assess LDN's efficacy and hoped that the case report series would help motivate such clinical studies.

Chronic Pain Syndromes

Reviewed by Trofimovitch et al. [116], case reports have described LDN being successfully utilized for patients with refractory chronic pain syndromes like chronic low back pain and diabetic neuropathy. LDN was initiated with 2 mg/day for 2 weeks, followed by 4 mg/day [121, 122]. However, there have yet to be large randomized, clinical trials assessing efficacy and safety.

Stimulants

Stimulant drugs generally increase alertness and include methylphenidate, dextroamphetamine, and modafinil.

Methylphenidate and amphetamine are used in the treatment for attention deficit hyperactive disorder (ADHD). Methylphenidate is the first-line medication used for ADHD and second-line for narcolepsy. It is a norepinephrine and dopamine reuptake inhibitor that increases norepinephrine and dopamine in the synaptic cleft; methylphenidate also has a weak affinity for the 5-HT1A receptor [123].

Dextroamphetamine, also known as dexamphetamine, is the more potent of the two amphetamine enantiomers [124]. It increases wakefulness and is known to improve alertness and fatigue in healthy subjects [125]. Dextroamphetamine is a highly regulated medication due to its high potential for drug dependence and abuse [124]. Common adverse effects for amphetamines include anorexia, weight loss, and insomnia; other reported effects include nausea, vomiting, increased blood pressure and heart rate, and possible motor tic exacerbation [124]. Methylphenidate has similar side effects, although it is less associated with weight loss [123]. For both drugs, the side effect of increased heart rate and blood pressure should be considered out of concern for adverse cardiovascular events such as stroke and myocardial infarction. However, recent studies have not found an increased risk between ADHD medication users versus non-users [126, 127].

Modafinil is a non-amphetamine first-line waking drug for narcolepsy, although its waking mechanism is not well understood [125]. Armodafinil, the R-enantiomer of modafinil, is known to have a longer waking effect compared to the S-enantiomer (10–14 h v. 3–4 h) [125]. Modafinil has a lower potential for abuse, and the most common reported side effects are headaches and, on higher doses, nausea [128].

Stimulants in Functional Illness

Chronic Fatigue Syndrome

Stimulants have been tried in chronic fatigue syndrome (CFS) due to the common symptom of concentration disturbances similar in ADHD, although the pathophysiology for the mechanism of action in CFS remains unknown. A randomized, placebo-controlled study (n = 60) by Blockmans et al. [129] gave methylphenidate 10 mg twice a day for 4 weeks and reported improvements in fatigue and concentration with a number needed to treat (NNT) of 6. The same authors used a questionnaire to study long-term methylphenidate use in their CFS patients [130]. Fifty out of 144 (35%) patients who voluntarily continued to take the medication reported improvements in fatigue (48% of patients), concentration (62%), and functionality in the home and at work. No rebound fatigue was experienced, and tachyphylaxis and addiction were not major issues [130]. Patients who discontinued the medication more frequently reported side effects such as agitation, palpitations, increased fatigue, dry mouth, headache, and upset stomach. The study noted that a trial to determine if the treatment will be effective for an individual requires only 2 days. Suggested dosing is 10 mg twice a day for the first day, followed on the second day by either lowering to 5 mg twice a day if there are side effects, increasing to 20 mg twice a day if there is no effect, or maintaining the dose if there is a positive effect [130].

Dexamphetamine (5 or 10 mg/day for 4 weeks) was tried in one randomized controlled pilot study ($n = 20$) [131]. The pilot concluded that dexamphetamine is effective in reducing fatigue symptoms and led to clinically improved quality-of-life scores. Anorexia was the most common adverse event with five out of ten patients reporting decreased food consumption and three reporting weight loss.

In a CFS pharmacology review by Pae et al. [42], the authors noted benefits from modafinil use based on clinical experience when used alone or as an adjunct to antidepressants. However, they note that current evidence does not support its use. A small placebo-controlled, randomized, crossover study ($n = 14$) using modafinil (200 mg or 400 mg/day for 20 days) reported no effects on fatigue, quality-of-life, or mood [128].

Fibromyalgia

Fatigue is a common symptom reported by fibromyalgia patients. Modafinil was studied in a retrospective review of 98 fibromyalgia patients [132]. Patients were excluded if they were initiated on other off-label use drugs for fibromyalgia such as duloxetine, amitriptyline, and tramadol. Patients reported reduced fatigue with modafinil use. The same authors conducted a randomized placebo-controlled study of armodafinil (flexible dosing 50–250 mg/day for 8 weeks) for fibromyalgia patients ($n = 60$) [133]. However, no differences were seen between armodafinil and placebo, and high placebo effects were observed. Common side effects in the armodafinil group were headache, dry mouth, concentration disturbance, and fatigue. Limitations of the study included possibly high population heterogeneity with patients being on multiple medications and having multiple medical conditions.

Conclusion

A wide range of pharmacological treatments have been studied for functional illness symptoms. Except for a select few regimens, such as SSRI use in chronic subjective dizziness, the efficacy of most medication trials is highly variable depending on the individual, with the few available randomized controlled trials reporting weak evidence of positive effects over placebo. Discussing with the patient a treatment's potential benefits and the known adverse effects is especially important in establishing expectations. In general, antidepressants appear to have the broadest scope for clinical utility, particularly for patients with comorbid depression and anxiety. Investigators are continually exploring alternative options such as low-dose naltrexone, especially for the treatment of pain-dominant disorders. The management of functional illnesses can be challenging for practitioners, and multimodal therapy with non-pharmacologic options is strongly emphasized. Nevertheless, patients may seek and request counsel on the vast array of pharmacological treatments, and thus clinicians will need to maintain an awareness of the available options in order to provide proper guidance.

References

1. Volpi-Abadie J, Kaye AM, Kaye AD. Serotonin syndrome. Ochsner J. 2013;13(4):533–40.
2. Beakley BD, Kaye AM, Kaye AD. Tramadol, pharmacology, side effects, and serotonin syndrome: a review. Pain Physician. 2015;18(4):395–400.
3. Toussaint K, Yang XC, Zielinski MA, Reigle KL, Sacavage SD, Nagar S, et al. What do we (not) know about how paracetamol (acetaminophen) works? J Clin Pharm Ther. 2010;35(6):617–38.
4. Raffa RB, Stone DJ Jr, Tallarida RJ. Discovery of "self-synergistic" spinal/supraspinal antinociception produced by acetaminophen (paracetamol). J Pharmacol Exp Ther. 2000;295(1):291–4.
5. Hodgman MJ, Garrard AR. A review of acetaminophen poisoning. Crit Care Clin. 2012;28(4):499–516.
6. McCrae JC, Morrison EE, MacIntyre IM, Dear JW, Webb DJ. Long-term adverse effects of paracetamol—a review. Br J Clin Pharmacol. 2018;84(10):2218–30.
7. Kia S, Choy E. Update on treatment guideline in fibromyalgia syndrome with focus on pharmacology. Biomedicines. 2017;5(2):20.
8. Högestätt ED, Jönsson BA, Ermund A, Andersson DA, Björk H, Alexander JP, et al. Conversion of acetaminophen to the bioactive N-acylphenolamine AM404 via fatty acid amide hydrolase-dependent arachidonic acid conjugation in the nervous system. J Biol Chem. 2005;280(36):31405–12.
9. Gould GG, Seillier A, Weiss G, Giuffrida A, Burke TF, Hensler JG, et al. Acetaminophen differentially enhances social behavior and cortical cannabinoid levels in inbred mice. Prog Neuro-Psychopharmacol Biol Psychiatry. 2012;38(2):260–9.
10. Bennett RM, Kamin M, Karim R, Rosenthal N. Tramadol and acetaminophen combination tablets in the treatment of fibromyalgia pain: a double-blind, randomized, placebo-controlled study. Am J Med. 2003;114(7):537–45.
11. Bennett RM, Schein J, Kosinski MR, Hewitt DJ, Jordan DM, Rosenthal NR. Impact of fibromyalgia pain on health-related quality of life before and after treatment with tramadol/acetaminophen. Arthritis Rheum. 2005;53(4):519–27.
12. Tallarida RJ, Raffa RB. Testing for synergism over a range of fixed ratio drug combinations: replacing the isobologram. Life Sci. 1996;58(2):Pl 23-8.
13. Hillhouse TM, Porter JH. A brief history of the development of antidepressant drugs: from monoamines to glutamate. Exp Clin Psychopharmacol. 2015;23(1):1–21.
14. Preskorn SH. Clinically relevant pharmacology of selective serotonin reuptake inhibitors. An overview with emphasis on pharmacokinetics and effects on oxidative drug metabolism. Clin Pharmacokinet. 1997;32(Suppl 1):1–21.
15. Rosenbaum JF, Fava M, Hoog SL, Ascroft RC, Krebs WB. Selective serotonin reuptake inhibitor discontinuation syndrome: a randomized clinical trial. Biol Psychiatry. 1998;44(2):77–87.
16. Okifuji A, Gao J, Bokat C, Hare BD. Management of fibromyalgia syndrome in 2016. Pain Manag. 2016;6(4):383–400.

17. Obata H. Analgesic mechanisms of antidepressants for neuropathic pain. Int J Mol Sci. 2017;18(11):2483.
18. Somashekar B, Jainer A, Wuntakal B. Psychopharmacotherapy of somatic symptoms disorders. Int Rev Psychiatry. 2013;25(1):107–15.
19. Gałecki P, Mossakowska-Wójcik J, Talarowska M. The anti-inflammatory mechanism of antidepressants—SSRIs, SNRIs. Prog Neuro-Psychopharmacol Biol Psychiatry. 2018;80:291–4.
20. Anderson HD, Pace WD, Libby AM, West DR, Valuck RJ. Rates of 5 common antidepressant side effects among new adult and adolescent cases of depression: a retrospective US claims study. Clin Ther. 2012;34(1):113–23.
21. Friedman RA. Antidepressants' black-box warning—10 years later. N Engl J Med. 2014;371(18):1666–8.
22. Giliberto JP, Cohen SM, Misono S. Are neuromodulating medications effective for the treatment of chronic neurogenic cough? Laryngoscope. 2017;127(5):1007–8.
23. Jeyakumar A, Brickman TM, Haben M. Effectiveness of amitriptyline versus cough suppressants in the treatment of chronic cough resulting from postviral vagal neuropathy. Laryngoscope. 2006;116(12):2108–12.
24. Ryan MA, Cohen SM. Long-term follow-up of amitriptyline treatment for idiopathic cough. Laryngoscope. 2016;126(12):2758–63.
25. Bowen AJ, Huang TL, Nowacki AS, Trask D, Kaltenbach J, Taliercio R, et al. Tachyphylaxis and dependence in pharmacotherapy for unexplained chronic cough. Otolaryngol Head Neck Surg. 2018;159(4):705–11.
26. Staab JP. Chronic subjective dizziness. Continuum (Minneap Minn). 2012;18(5 Neuro-otology):1118–41.
27. Ruckenstein MJ, Staab JP. Chronic subjective dizziness. Otolaryngol Clin N Am. 2009;42(1):71–7, ix.
28. Staab JP, Ruckenstein MJ, Amsterdam JD. A prospective trial of sertraline for chronic subjective dizziness. Laryngoscope. 2004;114(9):1637–41.
29. Staab JP, Ruckenstein MJ. Chronic dizziness and anxiety: effect of course of illness on treatment outcome. Arch Otolaryngol Head Neck Surg. 2005;131(8):675–9.
30. Staab JP, Ruckenstein MJ, Solomon D, Shepard NT. Serotonin reuptake inhibitors for dizziness with psychiatric symptoms. Arch Otolaryngol Head Neck Surg. 2002;128(5):554–60.
31. Dieterich M, Staab JP, Brandt T. Chapter 37—Functional (psychogenic) dizziness. In: Hallett M, Stone J, Carson A, editors. Handbook of clinical neurology, vol. 139. Amsterdam: Elsevier; 2016. p. 447–68.
32. Lapira A. Vestibular migraine treatment and prevention. HNO. 2019;67(6):425–8.
33. Tzadok R, Ablin JN. Current and emerging pharmacotherapy for fibromyalgia. Pain Res Manag. 2020;2020:6541798.
34. Lunn MP, Hughes RA, Wiffen PJ. Duloxetine for treating painful neuropathy, chronic pain or fibromyalgia. Cochrane Database Syst Rev. 2014;(1):Cd007115.
35. Lian YN, Wang Y, Zhang Y, Yang CX. Duloxetine for pain in fibromyalgia in adults: a systematic review and a meta-analysis. Int J Neurosci. 2020;130(1):71–82.
36. Häuser W, Petzke F, Üçeyler N, Sommer C. Comparative efficacy and acceptability of amitriptyline, duloxetine and milnacipran in fibromyalgia syndrome: a systematic review with meta-analysis. Rheumatology. 2010;50(3):532–43.
37. Macfarlane GJ, Kronisch C, Dean LE, Atzeni F, Häuser W, Fluß E, et al. EULAR revised recommendations for the management of fibromyalgia. Ann Rheum Dis. 2017;76(2):318–28.
38. Nishishinya B, Urrútia G, Walitt B, Rodriguez A, Bonfill X, Alegre C, et al. Amitriptyline in the treatment of fibromyalgia: a systematic review of its efficacy. Rheumatology (Oxford). 2008;47(12):1741–6.
39. Walitt B, Urrútia G, Nishishinya MB, Cantrell SE, Häuser W. Selective serotonin reuptake inhibitors for fibromyalgia syndrome. Cochrane Database Syst Rev. 2015;2015(6):Cd011735.
40. Pae CU, Marks DM, Patkar AA, Masand PS, Luyten P, Serretti A. Pharmacological treatment of chronic fatigue syndrome: focusing on the role of antidepressants. Expert Opin Pharmacother. 2009;10(10):1561–70.

41. Goodnick PJ. Treatment of chronic fatigue syndrome with venlafaxine. Am J Psychiatry. 1996;153(2):294.
42. Rosenhagen MC, Schmidt U, Ebinger M, Nickel T, Uhr M. Successful treatment of chronic fatigue syndrome with duloxetine and trijodthyronine—a case study. J Clin Psychopharmacol. 2008;28(1):105–7.
43. Hartz AJ, Bentler SE, Brake KA, Kelly MW. The effectiveness of citalopram for idiopathic chronic fatigue. J Clin Psychiatry. 2003;64(8):927–35.
44. Amsterdam JD, Shults J, Rutherford N. Open-label study of s-citalopram therapy of chronic fatigue syndrome and co-morbid major depressive disorder. Prog Neuropsychopharmacol Biol Psychiatry. 2008;32(1):100–6.
45. Vercoulen JH, Swanink CM, Zitman FG, Vreden SG, Hoofs MP, Fennis JF, et al. Randomised, double-blind, placebo-controlled study of fluoxetine in chronic fatigue syndrome. Lancet. 1996;347(9005):858–61.
46. Behan PO, Haniffah BAG, Doogan DP, Loudon M. A pilot study of sertraline for the treatment of chronic fatigue syndrome. Clin Infect Dis. 1994;18(Supplement_1):S111.
47. Stubhaug B, Lie SA, Ursin H, Eriksen HR. Cognitive-behavioural therapy v. mirtazapine for chronic fatigue and neurasthenia: randomised placebo-controlled trial. Br J Psychiatry. 2008;192(3):217–23.
48. Kleinstäuber M, Witthöft M, Steffanowski A, van Marwijk H, Hiller W, Lambert MJ. Pharmacological interventions for somatoform disorders in adults. Cochrane Database Syst Rev. 2014;11:CD010628.
49. Baldo P, Doree C, Molin P, McFerran D, Cecco S. Antidepressants for patients with tinnitus. Cochrane Database Syst Rev. 2012;2012(9):Cd003853.
50. Hesse G. Evidence and evidence gaps in tinnitus therapy. GMS Curr Top Otorhinolaryngol Head Neck Surg. 2016;15:Doc04.
51. Dickenson AH, Ghandehari J. Anti-convulsants and anti-depressants. In: Stein C, editor. Analgesia. Berlin: Springer; 2007. p. 145–77.
52. Arnold LM, Russell IJ, Diri EW, Duan WR, Young JP, Sharma U, et al. A 14-week, randomized, double-blinded, placebo-controlled monotherapy trial of pregabalin in patients with fibromyalgia. J Pain. 2008;9(9):792–805.
53. Patel R, Dickenson AH. Mechanisms of the gabapentinoids and α 2 δ-1 calcium channel subunit in neuropathic pain. Pharmacol Res Perspect. 2016;4(2):e00205.
54. Moore RA, Wiffen PJ, Derry S, Toelle T, Rice AS. Gabapentin for chronic neuropathic pain and fibromyalgia in adults. Cochrane Database Syst Rev. 2014;2014(4):Cd007938.
55. Wiffen PJ, Derry S, Moore RA, Aldington D, Cole P, Rice AS, et al. Antiepileptic drugs for neuropathic pain and fibromyalgia—an overview of Cochrane reviews. Cochrane Database Syst Rev. 2013;2013(11):Cd010567.
56. Chiappini S, Schifano F. A decade of gabapentinoid misuse: an analysis of the european medicines agency's 'suspected adverse drug reactions' database. CNS Drugs. 2016;30(7):647–54.
57. Schifano F. Misuse and abuse of pregabalin and gabapentin: cause for concern? CNS Drugs. 2014;28(6):491–6.
58. Ryan NM, Birring SS, Gibson PG. Gabapentin for refractory chronic cough: a randomised, double-blind, placebo-controlled trial. Lancet. 2012;380(9853):1583–9.
59. Vertigan AE, Kapela SL, Ryan NM, Birring SS, McElduff P, Gibson PG. Pregabalin and speech pathology combination therapy for refractory chronic cough: a randomized controlled trial. Chest. 2016;149(3):639–48.
60. Häuser W, Bernardy K, Uçeyler N, Sommer C. Treatment of fibromyalgia syndrome with gabapentin and pregabalin—a meta-analysis of randomized controlled trials. Pain. 2009;145(1–2):69–81.
61. Nicol AL, Hurley RW, Benzon HT. Alternatives to opioids in the pharmacologic management of chronic pain syndromes: a narrative review of randomized, controlled, and blinded clinical trials. Anesth Analg. 2017;125(5):1682–703.
62. Üçeyler N, Sommer C, Walitt B, Häuser W. WITHDRAWN: anticonvulsants for fibromyalgia. Cochrane Database Syst Rev. 2017;10(10):CD010782-CD.

63. Gilron I, Chaparro LE, Tu D, Holden RR, Milev R, Towheed T, et al. Combination of pregabalin with duloxetine for fibromyalgia: a randomized controlled trial. Pain. 2016;157(7):1532–40.
64. Arnold LM, Goldenberg DL, Stanford SB, Lalonde JK, Sandhu HS, Keck PE Jr, et al. Gabapentin in the treatment of fibromyalgia: a randomized, double-blind, placebo-controlled, multicenter trial. Arthritis Rheum. 2007;56(4):1336–44.
65. Obermann M, Strupp M. Current treatment options in vestibular migraine. Front Neurol. 2014;5:257.
66. Bisdorff AR. Treatment of migraine related vertigo with lamotrigine an observational study. Bull Soc Sci Med Grand Duche Luxemb. 2004;2:103–8.
67. Mikulec AA, Faraji F, Kinsella LJ. Evaluation of the efficacy of caffeine cessation, nortriptyline, and topiramate therapy in vestibular migraine and complex dizziness of unknown etiology. Am J Otolaryngol. 2012;33(1):121–7.
68. Jimenez XF, Sundararajan T, Covington EC. A systematic review of atypical antipsychotics in chronic pain management: olanzapine demonstrates potential in central sensitization, fibromyalgia, and headache/migraine. Clin J Pain. 2018;34(6):585–91.
69. Muench J, Hamer AM. Adverse effects of antipsychotic medications. Am Fam Physician. 2010;81(5):617–22.
70. Ware MR, Feller DB, Hall KL. Neuroleptic malignant syndrome: diagnosis and management. Prim Care Companion CNS Disord. 2018;20(1):17r02185.
71. Patt RB, Proper G, Reddy S. The neuroleptics as adjuvant analgesics. J Pain Symptom Manag. 1994;9(7):446–53.
72. Hanks GW, Thomas PJ, Trueman T, Weeks E. The myth of haloperidol potentiation. Lancet. 1983;2(8348):523–4.
73. Freedenfeld RN, Murray M, Fuchs PN, Kiser RS. Decreased pain and improved quality of life in fibromyalgia patients treated with olanzapine, an atypical neuroleptic. Pain Pract. 2006;6(2):112–8.
74. Walitt B, Klose P, Üçeyler N, Phillips T, Häuser W. Antipsychotics for fibromyalgia in adults. Cochrane Database Syst Rev. 2016;2016(6):CD011804.
75. McIntyre A, Paisley D, Kouassi E, Gendron A. Quetiapine fumarate extended-release for the treatment of major depression with comorbid fibromyalgia syndrome: a double-blind, randomized, placebo-controlled study. Arthritis Rheumatol. 2014;66(2):451–61.
76. Calandre EP, Hidalgo J, Rico-Villademoros F. Use of ziprasidone in patients with fibromyalgia: a case series. Rheumatol Int. 2007;27(5):473–6.
77. Calandre EP, Rico-Villademoros F. The role of antipsychotics in the management of fibromyalgia. CNS Drugs. 2012;26(2):135–53.
78. Lopez-Gonzalez MA, Moliner-Peiro F, Alfaro-Garcia J, Esteban-Ortega F. Sulpiride plus hydroxyzine decrease tinnitus perception. Auris Nasus Larynx. 2007;34(1):23–7.
79. Ferreri M, Hantouche E-G. Recent clinical trials of hydroxyzine in generalized anxiety disorder. Acta Psychiatr Scand. 1998;98(s393):102–8.
80. Griffin CE 3rd, Kaye AM, Bueno FR, Kaye AD. Benzodiazepine pharmacology and central nervous system-mediated effects. Ochsner J. 2013;13(2):214–23.
81. Gudin JA, Mogali S, Jones JD, Comer SD. Risks, management, and monitoring of combination opioid, benzodiazepines, and/or alcohol use. Postgrad Med. 2013;125(4):115–30.
82. Wright SL. Limited utility for benzodiazepines in chronic pain management: a narrative review. Adv Ther. 2020;37(6):2604–19.
83. Häuser W, Thieme K, Turk DC. Guidelines on the management of fibromyalgia syndrome—a systematic review. Eur J Pain. 2010;14(1):5–10.
84. Thorpe J, Shum B, Moore RA, Wiffen PJ, Gilron I. Combination pharmacotherapy for the treatment of fibromyalgia in adults. Cochrane Database Syst Rev. 2018;2(2):CD010585.
85. Russell IJ, Fletcher EM, Michalek JE, McBroom PC, Hester GG. Treatment of primary fibrositis/fibromyalgia syndrome with ibuprofen and alprazolam. A double-blind, placebo-controlled study. Arthritis Rheum. 1991;34(5):552–60.

86. Quijada-Carrera J, Valenzuela-Castaño A, Povedano-Gómez J, Fernández-Rodriguez A, Hernánz-Mediano W, Gutierrez-Rubio A, et al. Comparison of tenoxicam and bromazepan in the treatment of fibromyalgia: a randomized, double-blind, placebo-controlled trial. Pain. 1996;65(2-3):221–5.
87. Kravitz HM, Katz RS, Helmke N, Jeffriess H, Bukovsky J, Fawcett J. Alprazolam and ibuprofen in the treatment of fibromyalgia-report of a double-blind placebo-controlled study. J Musculoskelet Pain. 1994;2(1):3–27.
88. Corrigan R, Derry S, Wiffen PJ, Moore RA. Clonazepam for neuropathic pain and fibromyalgia in adults. Cochrane Database Syst Rev. 2012;2012(5):CD009486-CD.
89. Moldofsky H. The significance of dysfunctions of the sleeping/waking brain to the pathogenesis and treatment of fibromyalgia syndrome. Rheum Dis Clin N Am. 2009;35(2):275–83.
90. Meeus O, De Ridder D, Van de Heyning P. Administration of the combination clonazepam-Deanxit as treatment for tinnitus. Otol Neurotol. 2011;32(4):701–9.
91. Han SS, Nam EC, Won JY, Lee KU, Chun W, Choi HK, et al. Clonazepam quiets tinnitus: a randomised crossover study with Ginkgo biloba. J Neurol Neurosurg Psychiatry. 2012;83(8):821–7.
92. Cimolai N. Cyclobenzaprine: a new look at an old pharmacological agent. Expert Rev Clin Pharmacol. 2009;2(3):255–63.
93. Witenko C, Moorman-Li R, Motycka C, Duane K, Hincapie-Castillo J, Leonard P, et al. Considerations for the appropriate use of skeletal muscle relaxants for the management of acute low back pain. P T. 2014;39(6):427–35.
94. Tofferi JK, Jackson JL, O'Malley PG. Treatment of fibromyalgia with cyclobenzaprine: a meta-analysis. Arthritis Rheum. 2004;51(1):9–13.
95. Moldofsky H, Harris HW, Archambault WT, Kwong T, Lederman S. Effects of bedtime very low dose cyclobenzaprine on symptoms and sleep physiology in patients with fibromyalgia syndrome: a double-blind randomized placebo-controlled study. J Rheumatol. 2011;38(12):2653–63.
96. ClinicalTrials.gov [Internet]. Bethesda, MD: National Library of Medicine (US). 2000 Feb 29. Identifier NCT04172831, A Study To Evaluate The Efficacy And Safety Of TNX-102 SL In Patients With Fibromyalgia (RELIEF); 2019 Nov 21 [cited 2021 Feb 20]. Available from https://ClinicalTrials.gov/show/NCT04172831
97. Hersh EV, Balasubramaniam R, Pinto A. Pharmacologic management of temporomandibular disorders. Oral Maxillofac Surg Clin North Am. 2008;20(2):197–210, vi.
98. Borenstein DG, Korn S. Efficacy of a low-dose regimen of cyclobenzaprine hydrochloride in acute skeletal muscle spasm: results of two placebo-controlled trials. Clin Ther. 2003;25(4):1056–73.
99. Herman CR, Schiffman EL, Look JO, Rindal DB. The effectiveness of adding pharmacologic treatment with clonazepam or cyclobenzaprine to patient education and self-care for the treatment of jaw pain upon awakening: a randomized clinical trial. J Orofac Pain. 2002;16(1):64–70.
100. Ouanounou A, Goldberg M, Haas DA. Pharmacotherapy in temporomandibular disorders: a review. J Can Dent Assoc. 2017;83:h7.
101. Valtonen EJ. A double-blind trial of methocarbamol versus placebo in painful muscle spasm. Curr Med Res Opin. 1975;3(6):382–5.
102. Methocarbamol Tablets, USP (methocarbamol) [package insert on the Internet]. Charlotte, NC: Prinston Laboratories; 2020. [revised 2020 Jul 31; cited 2021 Mar 15]. Available from https://dailymed.nlm.nih.gov/dailymed/lookup.cfm?setid=32863f21-30ff-4a8b-a2e6-8ab14a37af0d
103. Coelho C, Figueiredo R, Frank E, Burger J, Schecklmann M, Landgrebe M, et al. Reduction of tinnitus severity by the centrally acting muscle relaxant cyclobenzaprine: an open-label pilot study. Audiol Neurootol. 2012;17(3):179–88.
104. Vuilleumier PH, Schliessbach J, Curatolo M. Current evidence for central analgesic effects of NSAIDs: an overview of the literature. Minerva Anestesiol. 2018;84(7):865–70.

105. Mason L, Moore RA, Edwards JE, Derry S, McQuay HJ. Topical NSAIDs for acute pain: a meta-analysis. BMC Fam Pract. 2004;5:10.
106. Mason L, Moore RA, Edwards JE, Derry S, McQuay HJ. Topical NSAIDs for chronic musculoskeletal pain: systematic review and meta-analysis. BMC Musculoskelet Disord. 2004;5:28.
107. Marcum ZA, Hanlon JT. Recognizing the risks of chronic nonsteroidal anti-inflammatory drug use in older adults. Ann Longterm Care. 2010;18(9):24–7.
108. Frost A. Diclofenac versus lidocaine as injection therapy in myofascial pain. Scand J Rheumatol. 1986;15(2):153–6.
109. Hsieh LF, Hong CZ, Chern SH, Chen CC. Efficacy and side effects of diclofenac patch in treatment of patients with myofascial pain syndrome of the upper trapezius. J Pain Symptom Manag. 2010;39(1):116–25.
110. World Health Organization. Cancer pain relief: with a guide to opioid availability. 2nd ed. Geneva: World Health Organization; 1996.
111. Tjäderborn M, Jönsson AK, Ahlner J, Hägg S. Tramadol dependence: a survey of spontaneously reported cases in Sweden. Pharmacoepidemiol Drug Saf. 2009;18(12):1192–8.
112. da Rocha AP, Mizzaci CC, Nunes Pinto ACP, da Silva Vieira AG, Civile V, Trevisani VFM. Tramadol for management of fibromyalgia pain and symptoms: systematic review. Int J Clin Pract. 2020;74(3):e13455.
113. Scott JR, Hassett AL, Brummett CM, Harris RE, Clauw DJ, Harte SE. Caffeine as an opioid analgesic adjuvant in fibromyalgia. J Pain Res. 2017;10:1801–9.
114. Dion GR, Teng SE, Achlatis E, Fang Y, Amin MR. Treatment of neurogenic cough with tramadol: a pilot study. Otolaryngol Head Neck Surg. 2017;157(1):77–9.
115. Toljan K, Vrooman B. Low-dose naltrexone (LDN)—review of therapeutic utilization. Med Sci. 2018;6(4):82.
116. Trofimovitch D, Baumrucker SJ. Pharmacology update: low-dose naltrexone as a possible nonopioid modality for some chronic, nonmalignant pain syndromes. Am J Hosp Palliat Care. 2019;36(10):907–12.
117. Younger J, Parkitny L, McLain D. The use of low-dose naltrexone (LDN) as a novel anti-inflammatory treatment for chronic pain. Clin Rheumatol. 2014;33(4):451–9.
118. Younger J, Noor N, McCue R, Mackey S. Low-dose naltrexone for the treatment of fibromyalgia: findings of a small, randomized, double-blind, placebo-controlled, counterbalanced, crossover trial assessing daily pain levels. Arthritis Rheum. 2013;65(2):529–38.
119. Parkitny L, Younger J. Reduced pro-inflammatory cytokines after eight weeks of low-dose naltrexone for fibromyalgia. Biomedicines. 2017;5(2):16.
120. Bolton MJ, Chapman BP, Van Marwijk H. Low-dose naltrexone as a treatment for chronic fatigue syndrome. BMJ Case Rep. 2020;13(1):e232502.
121. Ghai B, Bansal D, Hota D, Shah CS. Off-label, low-dose naltrexone for refractory chronic low back pain. Pain Med. 2014;15(5):883–4.
122. Hota D, Srinivasan A, Dutta P, Bhansali A, Chakrabarti A. Off-label, low-dose naltrexone for refractory painful diabetic neuropathy. Pain Med. 2016;17(4):790–1.
123. Faraone SV. The pharmacology of amphetamine and methylphenidate: relevance to the neurobiology of attention-deficit/hyperactivity disorder and other psychiatric comorbidities. Neurosci Biobehav Rev. 2018;87:255–70.
124. Heal DJ, Smith SL, Gosden J, Nutt DJ. Amphetamine, past and present—a pharmacological and clinical perspective. J Psychopharmacol. 2013;27(6):479–96.
125. Ballas C, Dinges DF. Stimulant and wake-promoting substances. In: Squire LR, editor. Encyclopedia of neuroscience. Oxford: Academic Press; 2009. p. 419–24.
126. Cooper WO, Habel LA, Sox CM, Chan KA, Arbogast PG, Cheetham TC, et al. ADHD drugs and serious cardiovascular events in children and young adults. N Engl J Med. 2011;365(20):1896–904.
127. Habel LA, Cooper WO, Sox CM, Chan KA, Fireman BH, Arbogast PG, et al. ADHD medications and risk of serious cardiovascular events in young and middle-aged adults. JAMA. 2011;306(24):2673–83.

128. Randall DC, Cafferty FH, Shneerson JM, Smith IE, Llewelyn MB, File SE. Chronic treatment with modafinil may not be beneficial in patients with chronic fatigue syndrome. J Psychopharmacol. 2005;19(6):647–60.
129. Blockmans D, Persoons P, Van Houdenhove B, Bobbaers H. Does methylphenidate reduce the symptoms of chronic fatigue syndrome? Am J Med. 2006;119(2):167.e23–30.
130. Blockmans D, Persoons P. Long-term methylphenidate intake in chronic fatigue syndrome. Acta Clin Belg. 2016;71(6):407–14.
131. Olson LG, Ambrogetti A, Sutherland DC. A pilot randomized controlled trial of dexamphetamine in patients with chronic fatigue syndrome. Psychosomatics. 2003;44(1):38–43.
132. Schwartz TL, Rayancha S, Rashid A, Chlebowksi S, Chilton M, Morell M. Modafinil treatment for fatigue associated with fibromyalgia. J Clin Rheumatol. 2007;13(1):52.
133. Schwartz TL, Siddiqui UA, Raza S, Morell M. Armodafinil for fibromyalgia fatigue. Ann Pharmacother. 2010;44(7-8):1347–8.

Pharmacology of Cannabis 21

Luxman Srikantha and Nathan J. Gonik

Introduction

Herbal cannabis or marijuana is a substance utilized medicinally and recreationally by large portions of the population, from all walks of life. Our knowledge of its potency and effects is burgeoning as new research uncovers its chemical and pharmacokinetic properties. Currently, the Food and Drug Administration (FDA) has approved its use only for the conditions of chronic pain, spasticity in multiple sclerosis, refractory seizures in the pediatric population, and chemotherapy-induced nausea and vomiting [1]. However, there are multiple ways in which strains of this plant are being utilized in other disease processes. Cannabis is now often seen as a tool for all practitioners. For those practicing Functional Medicine, marijuana may help extend the barriers of treatment to identify and treat antecedents and triggers of disease states [2].

It should be mentioned early in this discussion that as clinicians begin to incorporate cannabis in patient care, they must become familiar with all facets of this herbal remedy and consider it similar to other prescribed medications and supplements. A thorough medical and psychiatric history should precede any prescription, in order to identify patients at higher risk of adverse effects. Additionally, one should obtain a history of substance abuse and avoid fostering dependence or addiction. Recommendations also must account for regional legal, logistical, and social

L. Srikantha (✉)
College of Osteopathic Medicine, Michigan State University, Detroit, MI, USA

Department of Otolaryngology, Miami Valley Hospital, Dayton, OH, USA

N. J. Gonik
Department of Otolaryngology-Head and Neck Surgery, Wayne State University School of Medicine, Detroit, MI, USA

Children's Hospital of Michigan, Detroit, MI, USA

© The Author(s), under exclusive license to Springer Nature Switzerland AG 2023

B. W. Blakley, J. E. Blakley (eds.), *Functional Illness of the Head and Neck*,
https://doi.org/10.1007/978-3-031-12998-8_21

ramifications for those obtaining cannabis. Lastly, patients need to be educated on where to obtain and how to use the desired product.

History of Cannabis Use

Cannabis sativa is indigenous to Central Asia and the Indian subcontinent. Its use is well-documented throughout history [3–8]. Aged cannabis achenes found in Japan have been dated back to 8000 BC [4]. It was used in hallucinogenic drinks around 1500 BC in India. Altars in Tel Arad contained cannabis residue from 800 BC [5, 6]. Herodotus (480 BC) mentioned widespread use in Scythia for rituals and pleasure [7]. Later, an English botanist and physician, Nicholas Culpepper, summarized analgesic and anti-inflammatory benefits of "hemp" in his most famous work, *The English Physician* [8].

Discovering Its Chemical Effects

While cannabis has been used for millennia, our understanding of its effects on the human body is much more recent. Over 60 chemical compounds have been derived from the Cannabis plant. The main psychoactive compound delta-9 tetrahdyrocannabinol (THC) was isolated in 1964 [9]. In 1986, Agurell et al. described the pharmacokinetics of THC in human physiology and endogenous receptors were discovered in 1988 [10, 11]. To best understand the effects of exogenous cannabis administration, it is critical to realize that all vertebrate species possess an endogenous cannabinoid system [12].

CB1 receptors have been found in the brain, spinal cord, and peripheral nervous system. They are distributed, differentially, within the cerebral cortex, limbic areas, basal ganglia, cerebellum, thalamus, and brainstem [13]. CB2 receptors are found in macrophages in the spleen and throughout the immune system [14]. The first endogenous ligand for CB1 was discovered in 1992, which was noted to be slightly different from the plant cannabinoid [15]. This substance was derived from fatty acid arachidonic acid related to prostaglandins and was named anandamide after the Sanskrit word, *ananda*, meaning bliss. It has a high affinity for CB1 and mimics most of the actions of 9-THC.

Pharmacology

When cannabis is burned and THC inhaled, it is easily absorbed in the lungs [16]. On average, the effects can be felt within 9 min following usage. Bioavailability after oral ingestion is much less, and blood concentrations reach 25–30% of a similar inhaled dose [10]. This can be attributed to first-pass metabolism of the liver. Cannabinoids are lipophilic molecules and reach peak concentration in fatty tissue within 4–5 days [10]. Tissue elimination half-life of THC is about 7 days, and complete elimination of a single dose may take up to 30 days [17]. THC undergoes hepatic metabolism, resulting in more than 20 by-products. Twenty-five percent of these metabolites are excreted in the urine and the remaining 75% are excreted in the intestine where they can be resorbed, further prolonging their effects [16].

THC is a partial agonist of both CB1 and CB2 receptors [18, 19]. There are many downstream effects of CB activation, including modulation of serotonin, acetylcholine, dopamine, glutamate, and GABA, as well as NMDA and opioid receptor systems [13].

Through these systems, THC has been shown to have analgesic, anxiolytic, sedative, psychedelic, and anti-inflammatory properties [20, 21]. Nocioeffects or analgesia is generally attributed to the neurotropic CB1 receptor, whereas anti-inflammatory effects are tied to the CB2 receptors based on their disparate distributions [14]. They may also work in concert in cases of acute and chronic neuropathic pain of inflammatory origin [12]. Both in vitro and in vivo, cannabidiol (CBD) agonists have shown modulation of TNF-alpha, IL-12, IL-1, IL-6, and IL-10 [22]. Cannabinoid ligands also impact hormonal pathways. For instance, CBD analogs act similar to capsaicin as agonists at the TRPV1 receptor [23]. There are also agonist properties at 5HT1A that may explain anxiolytic properties of cannabis. Cannabinoid agonists may also release endogenous opioids, and interaction between the CBD and opioid systems has been shown in numerous studies.

Clinical Implication

With regard to cannabis use in the Otolaryngology patient, there are two sides to the story. There is mounting evidence of efficacy in treating a growing number of conditions. There is also evidence that overuse and abuse can have impacts on physical health and emotional or social well-being. We will discuss both the potential positive and negative impacts of its use.

THC- and CBD-infused products do exist with great variability in dosage, makeup, and efficacy. Currently, the FDA does not approve the ingestion of any THC or CBD-derived food products. At the authoring of this chapter, four cannabis-derived medications have been approved by the FDA [1]. Both Marinol® and Syndros® contain the active ingredient dronabinol, which is synthetic THC. Both of these have been approved for anorexia in AIDS patients and chemotherapy-induced nausea and vomiting. Cesamet® includes nabilone, which is a close derivative of THC and is indicated for the same symptoms. The newest FDA-approved medication is Epidiolex®, a purified concentrated form of CBD. This has been shown to be highly efficacious in intractable seizures in certain pediatric epileptic syndromes including Dravet syndrome, Lennox-Gastaut syndrome, and Tuberous Sclerosis Complex. Sativex®, with the active ingredient nabiximol, a 1:1 mixture of THC and CBD, has undergone clinical trials for the treatment of multiple sclerosis-related spasticity, but is not currently approved.

Multiple Sclerosis (MS)

There have been a myriad of studies looking into the potential uses of cannabis prior to and after FDA approvals. In 2018, a meta-analysis of 17 randomized controlled trials for the use of cannabis for spasticity due to multiple sclerosis looked at over 3000 patients and noted improvement in pain, spasticity, and bladder dysfunction [24]. In 2014, the American Academy of Neurology published specialty guidelines on nabiximols and noted the highest level of evidence for treating pain and spasticity in MS [25]. Currently, the medication is available for treatment for neuropathic pain in the European Union, but not in the United States.

Pain

In humans, the analgesic activity of THC is unclear. Endocannabinoids, as previously discussed, modulate pain threshold directly and indirectly. Varying studies have shown beneficial effects of THC in pain associated with MS, cancer, neuropathies, and HIV. A meta-analysis of orally administered synthetic cannabinoids, in which patients were separated into postoperative, posttraumatic, cancer-related pain, and spastic pain, showed that it was not more effective than codeine in controlling pain [26]. Another meta-analysis examining 79 randomized controlled trials including 6462 patients noted difficulty in making clear recommendations for the medical use of THC or CBD, due to small sample sizes, inadequate randomization, and poor blinding in the included studies [27]. They found moderate quality of evidence for CBD use in neuropathic and cancer pain as well as spasticity in MS, and low quality of evidence for other conditions including chemotherapy-associated nausea and vomiting, sleep disorders, and several mental health conditions.

Recent trials with Sativex® showed mixed results [28]. Although known for treating neuropathic pain, reduction in pain severity scores after brachial plexus avulsion injuries was limited. Oral THC did not improve postoperative or neuropathic pain [29]. Other studies did show some improvement of traumatic neuropathic injury with THC or Sativex®.

Ultimately, the research is still mixed. A 2017 meta-analysis of 27 studies examining the effectiveness in treating chronic pain found only weak evidence that it alleviates neuropathic pain and no evidence that cannabis was useful in other types of pain [30]. In one study, the number needed to treat (NNT) for non-cancer-related chronic pain was 24, whereas the number needed to harm (NNH) for any adverse effect was 6 [31]. Stated another way, with careful patient selection, where risks are reduced, there may be a role in utilizing cannabis to treat pain.

Glaucoma

The American Academy of Ophthalmology (AAO) released a position statement in 2010, stating that the risks associated with chronic use of cannabis outweighed the benefits and thus they didn't recommend the use of cannabis for glaucoma [32].

The reduction of intraocular pressure (IOP) only lasted 3–4 h. At higher doses, it had significant cardiovascular and neurological effects that ultimately could reduce ocular blood flow [33].

Cannabis in Otolaryngology

Within Otolaryngology, there is a paucity of literature discussing positive or negative clinical implications of cannabis use [34]. There are ongoing trials and accumulating anecdotal evidence elucidating its role in head and neck pathology.

Head and Neck Cancer

Most literature in Otolaryngology has been focused on cannabis use as a risk factor for head and neck cancer (HNC). The overall effect of cannabis on the incidence of head and neck cancer is unclear. Zhang et al. showed that marijuana use had an odds ratio of 2.6 compared to non-users and risk may be higher based on a dose-response relationship [35]. It has been proposed that marijuana is a significant risk factor for oral HPV in patients without HIV; however, there is conflicting data [36–38]. Looking more broadly at all aerodigestive cancers, one study demonstrated no increased risk of malignancy after 60 or more joint-years [39]. An International Head and Neck Cancer Epidemiology Consortium study noted that infrequent marijuana smoking did not confer a risk of HNC, especially in those who did not smoke tobacco or use alcohol [40]. A large meta-analysis in 2015 also revealed no association between lifetime marijuana use and the development of HNC [41]. The majority of studies show little evidence of malignant potential from the isolated consumption of marijuana products.

Otology

Due to the presence of cannabinoid receptors in the dorsal and ventral cochlear nuclei, studies have attempted to determine the effects of THC on the auditory pathway. Ghosh et al. suggested the endocannabinoid system may be protective against cisplatin-induced hearing loss [42]. Randomized studies have shown no lasting negative effects from short-term use on hearing or vestibular function [43, 44]. Chronic use, however, may be associated with more audiologic and vestibular symptoms [45]. Dizziness was noted as the most common adverse effect when analyzing the efficacy of CBD in treating non-cancer pain [46]. National Surveys on Drug Use and Health showed a positive association between duration of marijuana use and tinnitus [47].

Sleep Medicine

Dronabinol has been tested as a medical treatment option for obstructive sleep apnea (OSA). Prasad et al. showed a mean reduction of apnea-hypopnea index

(AHI) of −14 after 3 weeks of daily administration; no degradation of sleep architecture or serious adverse events was noted [48]. Other authors have shown that dronabinol suppresses serotonin-induced apnea and increased activation of genioglossus muscle. A double blind RCT conducted by the Pharmacotherapy of Apnea by Cannabimimetic Enhancement (PACE) group followed 73 adults with moderate or severe OSA [49]. Various dosages of dronabinol were given 1 h before sleep and an average AHI reduction between 10.7 and 12.9 was observed; Epworth Sleepiness Scores also decreased. However, the American Academy of Sleep Medicine has formally stated that synthetic cannabis should not be used for OSA, as there is still insufficient evidence of tolerability and safety [50].

Regulation

Studying cannabis is often a challenge due to federal regulations [51]. California became the first state to legalize the use of cannabis with the approval of a physician and the term “medical marijuana” was coined [52]. As of January 2021, 36 states and DC have legalized the use of cannabis for medical purposes [53]. It is listed as a schedule I narcotic by the Drug Enforcement Agency and is the most widely used recreational drug in the United States [54]. The listing of a schedule I narcotic implies that there is no acknowledged medical use, although the FDA has approved multiple formulations of THC and CBD-derived products. This anachronism highlights the contentious political nature surrounding its use and regulation. The American Medical Association, Institute of Medicine, American College of Physicians, and the American Academy of Pediatrics have formally supported the declassification of cannabis as schedule I [55].

Dosing is very complicated as there are varying proportions of THC and CBD within each strain of cannabis. The percentage of THC in cannabis sativa has been increasing every year due to advanced breeding processes; the average percentage was noted to be 4% in 1995 and rose to 12% in 2014 [56]. Percentages of THC and CBD content advertised in dispensaries are not regulated and are highly variable. This means that two patients using medical cannabis may be utilizing very different drugs depending on their marijuana strains and preparations. Also, there is a very limited understanding of the therapeutic ranges for each indication. Since 2001, Canada has authorized sale of cannabis for medical purposes and allowed registered individuals or their designates to grow their own marijuana for medical purposes. In 2018, recreational use of cannabis became legal.

Abuse

As with every drug, medicinal and recreational, there are often unwanted side effects. Cannabis has increasingly been seen as harmless, and this has contributed to its widespread use. However, the use of cannabis can cause adverse effects that must be acknowledged as a prescribing provider.

Cannabis Use Disorder (CUD) is a recognized condition in the Diagnostic and Statistical Manual of Mental Disorders V (DSM V) [57]. Ten percent of cannabis users meet criteria for CUD [58, 59]. A cannabis withdrawal syndrome also exists within DSM, which manifests with irritability, sleeping difficulty, dysphoria, craving, and anxiety [60]. These disorders are more pronounced in adolescents. Due to continued brain development into adulthood, adolescents are more vulnerable to adverse long-term outcomes from marijuana [61, 62]. Prenatal and childhood exposure to THC can result in impaired neural connectivity. The endocannabinoid and mesolimbic reward systems are still in development until 21 years old; these developmental changes make adolescents 2-4 times more likely to have symptoms of cannabis dependence within the first 2 years of use compared to adults [63, 64]. It is of the utmost importance that youthful minds be protected against disruptions in neural development.

Short-term side effects related to cannabis consumption include tachycardia, hypotension, xerostomia, xerophthalmia, and euphoria, as well as impaired attention, coordination, and judgment [21]. THC has not been found to induce any respiratory depression, and it is postulated that the lack of CB1 receptors in the midbrain may protect against these effects. Lower doses tend to have fewer side effects, but chronic adverse effects may be more pronounced; these adverse effects are broken into neuropsychiatric and systemic side effects [65]. These conditions include depression, anxiety, and may even manifest as a brief psychotic episode, which can develop into schizophrenia [66–68]. However, this link with psychosis and schizophrenia may also be related to preexisting psychiatric conditions and genetic vulnerability [69].

Marijuana is the most often reported drug associated with impaired driving accidents and fatal accidents [70, 71]. As the spread of recreational marijuana continues, it is important to note this risk and discuss this with patients. In controlled driving simulation studies, elevated THC blood content was associated with poorer performance [72]. A blood concentration of 2–5 ng/mL, typically associated with the sensation of euphoria, was shown to impair cognitive and psychomotor performance similar to alcohol and benzodiazepine consumption [73].

Long-term negative effects of low-level exposure do not appear to be common [74]. However, associations with inflammation of large airways, increased airway resistance, lung hyperinflation, and chronic bronchitis have been proposed [75]. Immunologic competence of the respiratory system may also be compromised and predispose to a higher rate of respiratory infections and pneumonia [76]. Additionally, vascular conditions such as myocardial infarction, stroke, and transient ischemic attacks during intoxication are well-documented, but causality has not been demonstrated [77].

Conclusion

The summary presented above should foster a more informed conversation between physicians and patients regarding marijuana use recreationally and medicinally. When possible, patients should consider more traditional approaches before attempting treatment with cannabis-derived products. However, the knowledge and willingness to explore these options may be meaningful in helping patients through difficult physical and emotional conditions. Additionally, due to the implications of adverse effects, obtaining a thorough medical and psychiatric history cannot be stressed enough. Patients at high risk of abuse or complications should be counseled effectively.

Within the field of Otolaryngology, there is little evidence to suggest efficacy in the prescription of cannabis or its analogs as therapeutic treatment. However, in cases of severe nausea and chronic pain, it may be a reasonable option and its use is better supported. As discussed above, obtaining consistent dosages and determining appropriate therapeutic levels are still the evolving commercial and research frontiers. Unlike most off-label use scenarios, patients must be aware of safe and reliable methods of obtaining the desired product and legal ramifications of its use.

As patients continue to inquire about more natural and holistic approaches to medicine, providers need to be aware of these options and signs of abuse, to bolster their armamentarium of alternative treatment modalities.

References

1. Office of the Commissioner. FDA regulation of cannabis and cannabis-derived products: Q&A. U.S. Food and Drug Administration, FDA. www.fda.gov/news-events/public-health-focus/fda-regulation-cannabis-and-cannabis-derived-products-including-cannabidiol
2. The Institute for Functional Medicine. Functional medicine: IFM. 17 Dec 2019. www.ifm.org/functional-medicine/
3. Datwyler SL, Weiblen GD. Genetic variation in hemp and marijuana (*Cannabis sativa L.*) according to amplified fragment length polymorphisms. J Forensic Sci. 2006;51(2):371–5.
4. Long T, et al. Cannabis in Eurasia: origin of human use and Bronze Age trans-continental connections. Veg Hist Archaeobotany. 2017;26(2):245–58.
5. Russo E. Cannabis in India: ancient lore and modern medicine. In: Cannabinoids as therapeutics. Basel: Birkhäuser; 2005. p. 1–22.
6. Arie E, Rosen B, Namdar D. Cannabis and frankincense at the Judahite Shrine of Arad. Tel Aviv. 2020;47(1):5–28.
7. Butrica JL. The medical use of cannabis among the Greeks and Romans. J Cannabis Ther. 2002;2(2):51–70.
8. Culpeper N. The English physician enlarged with three hundred and sixty-nine medicines, made of English herbs... By Nicholas Culpepper, John Binns. 1799.
9. Gaoni Y, Mechoulam R. Isolation, structure, and partial synthesis of an active constituent of hashish. J Am Chem Soc. 1964;86(8):1646–7.
10. Agurell S, et al. Pharmacokinetics and metabolism of delta 1-tetrahydrocannabinol and other cannabinoids with emphasis on man. Pharmacol Rev. 1986;38(1):21–43.
11. Devane WA, et al. Determination and characterization of a cannabinoid receptor in rat brain. Mol Pharmacol. 1988;34(5):605–13.
12. Pacher P, Bátkai S, Kunos G. The endocannabinoid system as an emerging target of pharmacotherapy. Pharmacol Rev. 2006;58(3):389–462.
13. Pertwee RG. Pharmacological actions of cannabinoids. In: Cannabinoids. Berlin: Springer; 2005. p. 1–51.
14. Munro S, Thomas KL, Abu-Shaar M. Molecular characterization of a peripheral receptor for cannabinoids. Nature. 1993;365(6441):61–5.

15. Devane WA, et al. Isolation and structure of a brain constituent that binds to the cannabinoid receptor. Science. 1992;258(5090):1946–9.
16. Ashton CH. Pharmacology and effects of cannabis: a brief review. Br J Psychiatry. 2001;178(2):101–6.
17. Maykut MO. Health consequences of acute and chronic marihuana use. Prog Neuro-Psychopharmacol Biol Psychiatry. 1985;9(3):209–38.
18. Paton WDM, Pertwee RG. The actions of cannabis in man. In: Marijuana: chemistry, pharmacology, metabolism and clinical effects. New York: Academic Press; 1973. p. 287–333.
19. Herkenham M. Localization of cannabinoid receptors in brain and periphery. Cannabinoid receptors. 1995.
20. Morales P, Jagerovic N. Novel approaches and current challenges with targeting the endocannabinoid system. Expert Opin Drug Discovery. 2020;15(8):917–30.
21. Ebbert JO, Scharf EL, Hurt RT. Medical cannabis. Mayo Clin Proc. 2018;93(12):1842.
22. Carrier EJ, Auchampach JA, Hillard CJ. Inhibition of an equilibrative nucleoside transporter by cannabidiol: a mechanism of cannabinoid immunosuppression. Proc Natl Acad Sci. 2006;103(20):7895–900.
23. Pisanti S, et al. Cannabidiol: state of the art and new challenges for therapeutic applications. Pharmacol Ther. 2017;175:133–50.
24. Torres-Moreno MC, et al. Assessment of efficacy and tolerability of medicinal cannabinoids in patients with multiple sclerosis: a systematic review and meta-analysis. JAMA Netw Open. 2018;1(6):–e183485.
25. Yadav V, et al. Summary of evidence-based guideline: complementary and alternative medicine in multiple sclerosis: report of the guideline development subcommittee of the American Academy of Neurology. Neurology. 2014;82(12):1083–92.
26. Campbell FA, et al. Are cannabinoids an effective and safe treatment option in the management of pain? A qualitative systematic review. BMJ. 2001;323(7303):13.
27. Whiting PF, et al. Cannabinoids for medical use: a systematic review and meta-analysis. JAMA. 2015;313(24):2456–73.
28. Berman JS, Symonds C, Birch R. Efficacy of two cannabis based medicinal extracts for relief of central neuropathic pain from brachial plexus avulsion: results of a randomised controlled trial. Pain. 2004;112(3):299–306.
29. Buggy DJ, et al. Lack of analgesic efficacy of oral δ-9-tetrahydrocannabinol in postoperative pain. Pain. 2003;106(1-2):169–72.
30. Nugent SM, et al. The effects of cannabis among adults with chronic pain and an overview of general harms: a systematic review. Ann Intern Med. 2017;167(5):319–31.
31. Stockings E, et al. Cannabis and cannabinoids for the treatment of people with chronic non-cancer pain conditions: a systematic review and meta-analysis of controlled and observational studies. Pain. 2018;159(10):1932–54.
32. Jampel H. American glaucoma society position statement: marijuana and the treatment of glaucoma. J Glaucoma. 2010;19(2):75–6.
33. Novack GD. Cannabinoids for treatment of glaucoma. Curr Opin Ophthalmol. 2016;27(2):146–50.
34. Valentino WL, McKinnon BJ. What is the evidence for cannabis use in otolaryngology? A narrative review. Am J Otolaryngol. 2019;40(5):770–5.
35. Zhang Z-F, et al. Marijuana use and increased risk of squamous cell carcinoma of the head and neck. Cancer Epidemiol Biomarkers Prev. 1999;8(12):1071–8.
36. Muller K, et al. Oral human papillomavirus infection and oral lesions in HIV-positive and HIV-negative dental patients. J Infect Dis. 2015;212(5):760–8.
37. Llewellyn CD, et al. An analysis of risk factors for oral cancer in young people: a case-control study. Oral Oncol. 2004;40(3):304–13.
38. Rosenblatt KA, et al. Marijuana use and risk of oral squamous cell carcinoma. Cancer Res. 2004;64(11):4049–54.

39. Hashibe M, et al. Marijuana use and the risk of lung and upper aerodigestive tract cancers: results of a population-based case-control study. Cancer Epidemiology and Prevention. Cancer Epidemiol Biomarkers Prev. 2006;15(10):1829–34.
40. Berthiller J, et al. Marijuana smoking and the risk of head and neck cancer: pooled analysis in the INHANCE consortium. Cancer Epidemiol Biomarkers Prev. 2009;18(5):1544–51.
41. De Carvalho MFF, et al. Head and neck cancer among marijuana users: a meta-analysis of matched case–control studies. Arch Oral Biol. 2015;60(12):1750–5.
42. Ghosh S, et al. The endocannabinoid/cannabinoid receptor 2 system protects against cisplatin-induced hearing loss. Front Cell Neurosci. 2018;12:271.
43. Spector M. Acute vestibular effects of marijuana. J Clin Pharmacol. 1973;13(5–6):214–7.
44. Liedgren SR, et al. Effect of marihuana on hearing. J Otolaryngol. 1976;5(3):233–7.
45. Spector M. Chronic vestibular and auditory effects of marijuana. Laryngoscope. 1974;84(5):816–20.
46. Johal H, et al. Cannabinoids in chronic non-cancer pain: a systematic review and meta-analysis. Clin Med Insights Arthritis Musculoskeletal Disord. 2020;13:1179544120906461.
47. Han B, Gfroerer JC, Colliver JD. Associations between duration of illicit drug use and health conditions: results from the 2005–2007 national surveys on drug use and health. Ann Epidemiol. 2010;20(4):289–97.
48. Prasad B, Radulovacki MG, Carley DW. Proof of concept trial of dronabinol in obstructive sleep apnea. Front Psychiatry. 2013;4:1.
49. Carley DW, et al. Pharmacotherapy of apnea by cannabimimetic enhancement, the PACE clinical trial: effects of dronabinol in obstructive sleep apnea. Sleep. 2018;41:1.
50. Ramar K, et al. Medical cannabis and the treatment of obstructive sleep apnea: an American Academy of Sleep Medicine position statement. J Clin Sleep Med. 2018;14(4):679–81.
51. Bryant LM, et al. Therapeutic cannabis and endocannabinoid signaling system modulator use in otolaryngology patients. Laryngoscope Investig Otolaryngol. 2018;3(3):169–77.
52. Chadi N, Weitzman ER, Levy S. Understanding the impact of national and state medical marijuana policies on adolescents. Curr Addict Rep. 2018;5(2):93–101.
53. Legal Medical Marijuana States and DC—Medical Marijuana—ProCon.org. Medical Marijuana. 1 Jan 2021. medicalmarijuana.procon.org/legal-medical-marijuana-states-and-dc/
54. Lopez MJ, Tadi P. Drug enforcement administration drug scheduling. StatPearls [Internet]. 2020.
55. Bostwick JM. Blurred boundaries: the therapeutics and politics of medical marijuana. Mayo Clin Proc. 2012;87(2):172.
56. ElSohly MA, et al. Changes in cannabis potency over the last 2 decades (1995–2014): analysis of current data in the United States. Biol Psychiatry. 2016;79(7):613–9.
57. American Psychiatric Association. DSM-IV: diagnostic and statistical manual of mental disorders. 1980.
58. World Health Organization. WHO Expert Committee on Drug Dependence: forty-second report. 2020.
59. Lopez-Quintero C, et al. Probability and predictors of transition from first use to dependence on nicotine, alcohol, cannabis, and cocaine: results of the National Epidemiologic Survey on Alcohol and Related Conditions (NESARC). Drug Alcohol Depend. 2011;115(1-2):120–30.
60. Gorelick DA, et al. Diagnostic criteria for cannabis withdrawal syndrome. Drug Alcohol Depend. 2012;123(1–3):141–7.
61. Mechoulam R, Parker LA. The endocannabinoid system and the brain. Annu Rev Psychol. 2013;64:21–47.
62. Zalesky A, et al. Effect of long-term cannabis use on axonal fibre connectivity. Brain. 2012;135(7):2245–55.
63. Hall W, Degenhardt L. Prevalence and correlates of cannabis use in developed and developing countries. Curr Opin Psychiatry. 2007;20(4):393–7.
64. Gogtay N, et al. Dynamic mapping of human cortical development during childhood through early adulthood. Proc Natl Acad Sci. 2004;101(21):8174–9.

65. Levinsohn EA, Hill KP. Clinical uses of cannabis and cannabinoids in the United States. J Neurol Sci. 2020;411:116717.
66. Haney M, Eden Evins A. Does cannabis cause, exacerbate or ameliorate psychiatric disorders? An oversimplified debate discussed. Neuropsychopharmacology. 2016;41(2):393–401.
67. Patton GC, et al. Cannabis use and mental health in young people: cohort study. BMJ. 2002;325(7374):1195–8.
68. Di Forti M, et al. Daily use, especially of high-potency cannabis, drives the earlier onset of psychosis in cannabis users. Schizophr Bull. 2014;40(6):1509–17.
69. Caspi A, et al. Moderation of the effect of adolescent-onset cannabis use on adult psychosis by a functional polymorphism in the catechol-O-methyltransferase gene: longitudinal evidence of a gene X environment interaction. Biol Psychiatry. 2005;57(10):1117–27.
70. Brady JE, Li G. Trends in alcohol and other drugs detected in fatally injured drivers in the United States, 1999–2010. Am J Epidemiol. 2014;179(6):692–9.
71. Lenné MG, et al. The effects of cannabis and alcohol on simulated arterial driving: influences of driving experience and task demand. Accid Anal Prev. 2010;42(3):859–66.
72. Hartman RL, Huestis MA. Cannabis effects on driving skills. Clin Chem. 2013;59(3):478–92.
73. Asbridge M, Hayden JA, Cartwright JL. Acute cannabis consumption and motor vehicle collision risk: systematic review of observational studies and meta-analysis. BMJ. 2012;344:e536.
74. Pletcher MJ, et al. Association between marijuana exposure and pulmonary function over 20 years. JAMA. 2012;307(2):173–81.
75. Tashkin DP. Effects of marijuana smoking on the lung. Ann Am Thorac Soc. 2013;10(3):239–47.
76. Owen KP, Sutter ME, Albertson TE. Marijuana: respiratory tract effects. Clin Rev Allergy Immunol. 2014;46(1):65–81.
77. Thomas G, Kloner RA, Rezkalla S. Adverse cardiovascular, cerebrovascular, and peripheral vascular effects of marijuana inhalation: what cardiologists need to know. Am J Cardiol. 2014;113(1):187–90.

22 Complementary and Alternative Therapies

Joan E. Blakley

Definitions

Health care that is described as mainstream in North America may also be called Western, evidence-based, conventional, biomedical, or allopathic medicine. Mainstream medicine bases treatment on physiological and pathological phenomena that are scientifically proven and reproducible. Opponents argue that mainstream medicine is reductionist and diminishes an individual to their smallest components without consideration of the whole person, excluding factors that influence an individual's overall state of well-being. Mainstream medicine is typically government-regulated. Services provided by physicians, nurses, hospitals, pharmacists, physiotherapists, rehabilitation therapists, and medical social service providers are usually paid for by insurers. In many jurisdictions, chiropractic and massage are also regulated as mainstream therapies and may be paid for as insured services.

There are numerous therapeutic approaches to healthcare that are not considered mainstream. The names used for these therapies include natural, complementary, traditional, holistic, naturopathic, homeopathic, and alternative. Complementary and alternative medicine (CAM) is designed to be individualized and purports to support optimal health through balance of the body, mind, and spirit. Complementary therapies may be indigenous to a geographic area and practiced within a specific cultural setting or adopted from other cultures and other geographic regions. Therapies included as complementary vary depending on how definitions are applied and by whom. Acceptance of CAM by mainstream medicine and the general public is also perceived variably depending on one's viewpoint. Proponents declare that because it is individualized to a person's specific needs, CAM therapy is more beneficial and less injurious than mainstream medicine. CAM providers acknowledge that there are health conditions outside their scope. Opponents to

J. E. Blakley (✉)
Winnipeg, Manitoba, Canada

© The Author(s), under exclusive license to Springer Nature Switzerland AG 2023
B. W. Blakley, J. E. Blakley (eds.), *Functional Illness of the Head and Neck*,
https://doi.org/10.1007/978-3-031-12998-8_22

complementary therapies raise concerns that patients may be subjected to unproven or disproven quackery or may injuriously delay mainstream therapies.

Where CAM therapies are used in conjunction with mainstream therapies in treatment of patients, this is described as integrative medicine. This frequently occurs when mainstream therapies are insufficient to manage or eliminate illness, especially chronic illnesses.

Historical Development of CAM

In early ages, there were specialized healers who likely used animals, plants, and minerals to provide therapies. Therapies were often combined with spiritual practices in recognition of the presence of powers that seemed to have influence beyond what could be overtly seen in the human body. Medical therapies grew from these early practices.

CAM proponents point to Rene Descartes, in the early 1600s, as having a strong influence on divergence of mainstream from complementary medicine. Descartes supported the concept of mind and body as separate entities. Adherence to his way of thinking led to the current mainstream model of medicine with distinct organ or system-specific medical specialities.

Over time, technologic and scientific advances led to improved understanding of physiology and pathology. Many therapeutic practices were provable and adopted as mainstream therapies. Many traditional therapies remained unproven and did not become part of mainstream medicine. Practitioners and patients continued to embrace these still unproven traditional therapies which came to be known as alternative or complementary or traditional.

In addition to lack of scientific proof for CAM therapies, regulation of health professions in the twentieth century is said to have had a significant negative effect on current perceptions of CAM. Complementary therapy proponents assert that regulatory efforts to standardize health care resulted in suppression of CAM therapies because they did not conform to the new requirements. Health professional regulation cemented the role of mainstream practitioners and marginalized complementary health care providers. Limited published evidence to validate efficacy of many CAM therapies resulted in insurers and policymakers being hesitant to embrace them in spite of their popularity with patients [1]. All of this contributed to dissonance between CAM supporters and those who advocated mainstream practices.

Popularity of Complementary and Alternative Medicine (CAM) Today

One might think that as the body of information and scientific evidence [2] for mainstream medicine is accumulated, complementary and alternative medical therapies would die out. However, they appear to be growing and flourishing. There are several things to consider when looking at reports of CAM utilization and prevalence. First, data reported for complementary therapies must be viewed cautiously as definitions of CAM vary widely between users and between researchers. What is reported may reflect different inclusion/exclusion criteria. Second, people may not reliably report their use of CAM therapies—either because they do not consider them as "therapies" but rather healthy life choices or because they think that mainstream health care providers will be prejudiced against CAM use by their patients.

One way that prevalence of CAM use can be validated is by the amount of money that people pay for CAM. In 2007, a U.S. National Institutes of Health report stated that adult Americans spent $33.9 billion on CAM therapist visits and products in a single year [3]. CAM expenditures included the cost of visits to CAM practitioners and purchase of products, classes, and materials. Almost all of these costs were out-of-pocket and unreimbursed by health care plans. In 2016, the National Center for Complementary and Integrative Health reported that "Americans spent $30.2 billion out-of-pocket on complementary health approaches" [4], showing that spending remains strong.

Another measure is in reported use of CAM. In 2016, The Fraser Institute reported that 79% of Canadians used at least one complementary or alternative therapy at some time in their lives and that this number has steadily increased over the last 20 years [5]. A systematic review of use of complementary medicine in the UK documented use by approximately 41% of people in any given year, but 52% of those surveyed indicated having used complementary medicine at some point in their life [6]. A 2017 National Health Interview Survey conducted by the US Centers for Disease Control and Prevention reported that use of yoga, meditation, and chiropractic increased among US adults [7]. A 2013 US military report noted that approximately 45% of respondents used a complementary medicine therapy in the past year as compared to civilian surveys that found between 36 and 38% usage [8]. According to the World Health Organization, approximately 65% to 85% of the world's population currently relies on traditional medicine (CAM) as their *primary form* of health care [9].

An increase has been seen in research [10] published about use of integrative medicine therapies to manage many chronic illnesses. By 2011, approximately 42% of U.S. hospitals offered complementary and alternative medicine therapies; research funds for CAM therapies exceeded $225 million per year; and more than 43% of medical schools across the US offered CAM in their curriculum [11].

Why CAM Thrives

There are many possible reasons for the continuing and increasing popularity and general acceptance of complementary therapies including:

little or no access to mainstream healthcare and/or unaffordability in many parts of the world.

persistence or rediscovery of practice of traditional medicine by ancient cultures.

patients have a sense of personal control through use of CAM.
ready access to information globally through the Internet.
perception of CAM therapies as holistic, addressing the whole person, promoting prevention and wellness over medicalization, being safer and more natural.
many chronic conditions with no cure and/or little symptom relief despite advances in mainstream medicine.
integration and perceived acceptance of some CAM therapies by mainstream care providers, especially for conditions with no mainstream medicine solution.

Organizations with a Dedicated Focus on Complementary Medicine

Since CAM therapies are not going away and continue to be sought to manage health issues, world health leaders established agencies to support CAM research and build an evidence base to inform choices by health care consumers and providers. These agencies support development of policies and regulation for increased safety and consistent quality of CAM therapies.

The World Health Organization (WHO) has promoted health and safety since 1948 with a particular goal to serving the vulnerable. WHO published their first Traditional Medicine Strategy in 2002. This recognized the growing use of Traditional Medicine as an accessible and affordable option for many people and urged governments to develop policy that would support safe, high-quality, and efficacious traditional and complementary medical care. The WHO Strategy update in 2014 confirmed widespread use of traditional medicine. The updated strategy paid tribute to countries where policy development and standards have improved safety and reliability of traditional medicine practices. The WHO differentiates between "traditional" and "complementary" medicine, saying that traditional medicine is specific to a culture and can be traced back historically, often through oral teachings over many generations, whereas complementary medicine practices did not originate in the country where they are employed and may be comparatively recent in emerging. Neither traditional nor complementary medicine are considered by the WHO as part of conventional or mainstream medicine.

The National Center for Complementary and Integrative Health (NCCIH) was created in 1992 by the National Institutes of Health as part of their mandate to support scientific study and improve health care. They separate therapies into complementary" (used alongside conventional medicine), "alternative" (used instead of conventional medicine), and "integrative" (using both conventional and complementary therapies). Current NCCIH objectives are to:

Advance fundamental science and methods development.
Improve care for hard-to-manage symptoms.
Foster health promotion and disease prevention.
Enhance the complementary and integrative health research workforce.
Disseminate objective evidence-based information on complementary and integrative health interventions [12].

The Cochrane Collaboration established a complementary medicine division [13] in 1996 to focus on systematic reviews of complementary, alternative, and integrative therapies. As with other Cochrane focus groups, their goal is to gather and evaluate scientific research in order to inform patient care—in this setting to inform complementary patient care.

Complementary Medicine Practices Prevalent Worldwide

Every region of the world has health care practices dating back thousands of years that can be described as traditional or indigenous to that area. The WHO assessed prevalence of traditional and complementary medicine practices in its 2019 survey of member states [9]. Acupuncture, herbal medicine, and indigenous traditional medicine were the three most common forms of traditional practice reported. Next in frequency were homeopathy and traditional Chinese medicine, followed by naturopathy, chiropractic, osteopathy and ayurvedic medicine, and Unani medicine. Other practices reported by WHO member states included prayer, spiritualism, traditional midwives, therapeutic massage, hypnotherapy, reiki, reflexology, hands-on healing, hydrotherapy, Feldenkrais, biofeedback, Rolfing, Bach flower remedies, anthroposophic medicine, neural therapy, gSoba Rig-pa (traditional Bhutanese medicine), Siddha medicine, Iranian TM, cupping, and ozone therapy.

On the following pages, some of the more common complementary and alternative therapies are listed with brief descriptions of use, claimed benefits, and risks or cautions. Although there are numerous published reports, findings are often contradictory or deemed of inadequate quality to be reliable. Use of any of these CAM therapies by mainstream health care providers should be associated with careful research and patient monitoring.

Acupuncture

Acupuncture involves inserting thin needles through the skin at specific points along lines called meridians which are believed to control the flow of energy through the body. The belief is that disease is caused by disruption or imbalance in the flow of energy, called qi (chee) [14]. Needles stimulate the point of insertion to unblock energy pathways or redirect sensation. Acupuncture is possibly most often associated with traditional Chinese medicine, but it is also used prominently in naturopathy and gSo-BA Rig-PA. Many mainstream medical practices include acupuncture in their approaches to treatment.

Many sources report success using acupuncture to treat pain [15], especially chronic pain such as low back pain or neck pain, but do not identify clear indications for acupuncture in preference to other therapies. Acupuncture has been reported for management of nausea and vomiting, as a smoking cessation aid, to reduce stress, insomnia, tension, osteoarthritis, migraines [16], and fibromyalgia [17]. Some providers recommend acupuncture to manage labor pain but, in general, acupuncture is not recommended for use in pregnancy or for children.

When performed by a skilled practitioner, acupuncture is deemed to be of low risk. However, there is always the possibility of infection, punctured organs, or nerve injury if acupuncture is done incorrectly.

Acupressure

The principles of acupressure are similar to acupuncture but use hands, elbows, or feet—not needles—to put pressure on specific points along the body's meridians or energy channels to clear blockage or restore balance.

Acupressure has been reported to reduce anxiety related to being transported by ambulance to hospital [18], to relieve lower back pain [19], to relieve neck pain when used with aromatic lavender oil [20], for improving movement in stroke patients [21], and for motion sickness [22].

Cupping

Cupping is used in traditional medicine, especially in China and the Middle East. Negative pressure is created on the skin using a cup either by applying a flame to the cup to remove oxygen before placing it on the skin or by attaching a suction device to the cup after it is placed on the skin. In "wet cupping," the skin is pierced, and blood flows into the cup. "Dry cupping" doesn't involve piercing the skin. One meta-analysis states that cupping reduces neck pain and improves function [23], although this is reported cautiously due to low quality of evidence. Overall, there is not enough high-quality research to allow conclusions to be reached about whether cupping is helpful for other conditions.

Cupping leaves temporary marks on the skin and may cause persistent skin discoloration, scars, burns, and infections and may worsen eczema or psoriasis. Rare risks of cupping include anemia from repeated wet cupping, bleeding in the skull after scalp cupping, and infections such as hepatitis from poorly cleaned equipment.

Herbal Medicine

Herbal medicine is one of the earliest forms of health care practiced. It can be a stand-alone practice, but administration of herbal preparations is also a major component of many traditional and complementary medicine practices. By definition, a herbal medicine is simply something that is made from a plant and this definition encompasses a very broad range of products. Herbal medications are very widely available and can be purchased in prepared forms in grocery stores, pharmacies, health food stores, and online. They are available as special preparations compounded by CAM providers; compounds are typically made specially when products are not readily available in the form or strength required by a consumer. Plant-based medicines are estimated to be used by 80% of the people in developing countries and in the US, $52 billion was spent in 2019 on dietary supplements [24].

Generally, there is little published peer-reviewed, high-quality research to support the many and varied benefits claimed by herbal medicine manufacturers. Unsubstantiated internet information abounds, but there are websites that provide reliable information about uses, proven benefits, and safety risks associated with herbal medicines. Better sites to check include:

The National Center for Complementary and Integrative Medicine.
https://www.nccih.nih.gov/health/how-safe-is-this-product-or-practice
The Mayo Clinic.
https://www.mayoclinic.org/healthy-lifestyle/consumer-health/in-depth/herbal-supplements/art-20046488?p=1
University of Rochester Medical Center.
https://www.urmc.rochester.edu/encyclopedia/content.aspx?contenttypeid=1&contentid=1169
Cochrane Complementary Medicine.
https://cam.cochrane.org/cochrane-reviews-related-complementary-medicine

Regulation of herbal medications is being strengthened as concern about safety and efficacy is addressed by governments. In Canada, under the Natural Health Products Regulation of The Food and Drugs Act [25], The Natural and Nonprescription Health Products Directorate manages regulation of natural products including herbal medicines. Their policy aims "to provide reasonable assurance that natural health products (NHPs) offered for sale in Canada are safe and effective when used under their recommended conditions of use" [26]. Distinctions are made in the Regulation based on claims being put forward with products. Application requirements for NHP licensing under the Natural Health Products Regulation distinguish products that: (1) make modern claims based on current published research, or (2) are traditional medicines with claims of long time use within one specific form of traditional medicine. NHP licensing requirements do not apply to products compounded by health care providers as those are covered under a separate policy. That policy, although not regulating the health care provider, states that the provider is responsible for products that they compound.

In the US, herbal medicines are regulated as dietary supplements by the US Food and Drug Administration (FDA) under the Federal Food, Drug and Cosmetic Act [27]. Dietary supplements include vitamins, minerals, herbs or other botanicals, amino acids, dietary substances to supplement the diet by increasing total dietary intake, or a concentrate, metabolite, constituent, extract, or combination of the preceding substances. They do not need assessment or evaluation before they are marketed. However, supplement manufacturers cannot claim that their products cure, treat, prevent, or diagnose disease. If the FDA finds that products are contaminated or falsely labeled (making unjustified health claims), they can remove products from the market.

There may be benefit from some herbal therapies, but there are also possible risks. Some herbal preparations interfere with prescribed medications and cause significant problems. Although derived from natural sources, herbal preparations may contain harmful contaminants. Also, it is possible to overdose on herbal preparations and cause harm. One review study reported that the media tends to downplay risks of herbal therapies and report inaccurately on clinical trial quality which may then skew a consumer's decision-making in favor of a CAM alternative [28]. Barrett observed that herbal medicines are easier than most CAM therapies to scientifically evaluate [29]. Posadzki reported on systematic reviews of adverse effects of herbal medicines and identified four herbal medicines with serious adverse effects—*Herbae pulvis standardisatus, Larrea tridentate, Piper methysticum,* and *Cassia senna*—with results including "liver or kidney damage, colon perforation, carcinoma, coma and death" [6]. The bottom line is that use of any herbal product requires careful benefit/risk analysis. Before initiating use, consumers (and their prescribers) are encouraged to review the pharmacology literature to be aware of any potential risks, interactions or interference with other therapies, and contraindications for use.

Here is a small sampling of well-known herbs, traditional uses, and a few potential safety risks …

Common Name	Source	Standard Use	Safety/Risk
Chamomile	Chamomile flowers	Antioxidant (few animal studies—Limited human evidence) [30], ↓cholesterol, ↓anxiety	Problem if allergic to daisies.
Echinacia	Purple cone-flower (root and flower)	Weak evidence of benefit for treating or preventing colds [24, 31, 32] ↑immunity [29], ↑wound healing	Mild symptoms such as rash, GI upset; avoid if immune-deficient or taking immunosuppressants; no effect on warfarin pharmacodynamics or clotting in healthy people
Garlic	Allium sativum—Bulb	↓blood pressure [29, 33] (findings mixed—Maybe better for uncontrolled hypertension); ↓hyperlipidemia [29] maybe	May interfere with drug absorption and metabolism [34]; may cause nausea, hypotension, or rarely bleeding [24]
Ginger	Root of ginger plant	↑digestive function (weak evidence), ↓nausea [29] and vomiting (weak), ↑anti-inflammatory response	May cause heartburn, diarrhea, unknown effect on pregnancy so be cautious
Ginkgo biloba	Ginkgo tree leaves	↑blood circulation, improve memory, ↓dementia [29], ↓anxiety, ↓dizziness; no use for tinnitus [35]	May cause dizziness, stomach upset, headache; roasted seeds may cause seizures; eating fresh seeds may cause death; exacerbates bleeding disorders [24], possibly carcinogenic [36]
Ginseng	Root of ginseng—Asian or American	↑immune system (weak evidence [32]), improve focus, ↑energy, ↓blood pressure [33] (mixed evidence)	Few adverse events [33]

Common Name	Source	Standard Use	Safety/Risk
Green tea		In combination with exercise and diet→↓blood glucose [37], anti-inflammatory and anti-oxidation	Unknown but potential drug-herb interactions [37]
St. John's wort		↓mild-moderate depression [29, 38]	May interact with immunosuppressants, anticancer agents, cardiovascular drugs, oral contraceptives, lipid-lowering agents—Severe outcomes possible [29, 39]

Indigenous Traditional Medicine

Every geographic area has indigenous traditional medicine practices that go back to earliest civilizations. Prehistoric people recognized links between consumption or application of specific herbs, animal, or mineral products and maintenance of health, prevention of illness, or recovery from illness. Healing systems developed from these observations were collected over generations and have been handed down as the oral teachings of respected healers and elders. Every culture has knowledge keepers and healers who are recognized and respected for these skills. Healing practices may be physical or have religious components where a healer has specialized spiritual skills; healing practices may include a shaman with specific training.

Much of health or illness is not apparent to the naked eye and may be attributed to unknown forces within the individual or the environment. Balance and harmony are key principles of indigenous traditional medicine which frequently include healing practices to heighten or restore harmony. A circle or wheel is often used symbolically to represent oneness and unity and, in some cultures, to represent realms of being (often physical, emotional, mental, and spiritual). Traditional healing is focused on treating the entire person and often involves the whole community in resolving illness.

In the Western Hemisphere, Canadian First Nations, Metis, Inuit, American Indians, Alaska Natives, and Aztecs have traditional practices based on an underlying belief of kinship with the earth and the creatures that inhabit it. Balance is maintained through respectful interaction of all creatures within the environment. Illness is perceived as a disruption of balance and the whole community might be involved in restoring a healing balance. Healing practices may include ceremonial burning of herbs such as sage, tobacco, and sweetgrass, cleansing ceremonies such as sweats and smudges, healing circles and sings, preparation of medicinal herbs for topical use or internal consumption, and counselling.

Traditional medicine practices especially prevalent in the southern US and Central America include use, for their psychotropic effects, of mescaline (extracted from peyote cactus), psilocybin mushrooms, and ayahuasca (brewed from the leaves of Psychotria viridis shrubs) [40]. Mescaline is legal in the US only when used by Native Americans for religious ceremonies. Psilocybin has been legalized in several US cities, but is generally not permitted; ayahuasca is also illegal in the US. Although pilot studies [41, 42] have indicated that psychedelic drugs may be effective in treating psychiatric disorders, early work shows altered molecular mechanisms and changes in cognition and brain connectivity. Renewed interest in testing these drugs may bring more information about their safety and efficacy.

Curanderismo is a Latin American indigenous healing system which blends beliefs from the Aztecs and Incas with practices brought from Europe (including Spanish, Arabic, and Christian beliefs) [43]. It is practiced in Mexico and is also said to be widespread among Latino communities in the US. It is a holistic system broadly based on the connection between a person's body and the health of the earth. Achieving a healthy state requires balance and harmony between natural illnesses (due to germs, genetics, psychological conditions) and supernaturally induced illnesses (due to evil spirits, antisocial magic). Healing practices include special diets, herbal remedies, prayer, healing rituals, spiritualism, massage, and psychic healing. As a person who practices Curanderismo holds very specific beliefs about health and healing, a mainstream care provider may find it difficult to interact without first learning about some of the Curanderismo patient's expectations.

South Africa has deeply entrenched traditional healing practices involving knowledge passed down orally for many generations [44]. The traditional healer intercedes on behalf of a patient in helping them find health through regaining balance which has been disrupted due to psychological conflict or disturbed social relationships (with someone alive or dead). Healing practices include cleanses, herbal remedies, appeasing of spirits, warding off evil spirits, and eliminating curses. Some traditional healers use drumming and dancing rituals as well as "throwing the bones" to diagnose and treat a patient's condition.

Polynesian traditional health beliefs (within an area bounded by Hawaii [native Hawaiians], Easter Island [Rapa Nui], and New Zealand [Maori]) emphasize extended family cooperation, helping, and responsibility [45]. Illness is said to arise from imbalance in relationships or life roles and affects the entire family, so all must be involved in decision-making and treatment plans. Health depends on balance or harmony of three points—body, mind, and spirit—represented as a triangle [46]. Healing practices involve the body, the physical environment (land or water), relationships with others, particularly family members, ancestors, and gods, and mental and emotional states. Practices are holistic and emphasize setting right any problems within the mental or spiritual realm. Treatment involves prayers, herbs, and repairing relationships. Although guided by traditional healers and teachers, success depends on the willingness of the individual to make amends in their life. Easter Island healers use strong massage, steam baths, sea baths, and cleanses [47].

Australian Aboriginals and Torres Strait Islanders hold traditional healing beliefs handed down through oral teaching that may go back 50,000 years. One fundamental belief is animism; everything—objects, places, creatures—possesses a distinct spiritual essence which must be respected. Spiritual and physical are very strongly interconnected. Illness may be attributed to a supernatural intervention or sorcery in response to an offense by an individual or someone associated with them [48]. Traditional healers' practices are very symbolic and ritualistic [49]. Bush medicine practiced by traditional healers can involve herbal preparations and traditional actions to remove evil that is believed to cause the illness. There are strong social strictures that define roles and guide interactions between men and women. This may be problematic when health care is to be provided to Australian Aboriginals by the opposite gender. Also, mainstream medicine beliefs may not align with traditional beliefs and may bring conflict to a relationship between care provider and patient.

There has been limited study of the impact of patients accessing indigenous traditional healers while in the care of mainstream health care providers, but there is concern that some traditional herbs may interfere with mainstream prescriptions and/or cause toxicity from active ingredients or additives [50]. As noted above, there may be tension and mistrust between expectations and practices of mainstream health care providers and indigenous traditional beliefs that will negatively impact health outcomes. Initiatives are underway currently to identify ways that indigenous healing practices can be integrated into mainstream care in recognition of their value in improving the health and well-being of their followers [51].

Homeopathy

Homeopathy was founded by a German physician, Samuel Christian Hahnemann, based on the "principle of similars". Hahnemann claimed that if a patient had an illness, it could be cured by giving a medicine which would produce similar symptoms to that illness if given to a healthy person [52]. Smaller exposure would allow a patient to react to the stimulus of the medicine and resist the illness. A care provider could prepare and administer the smallest amount of the appropriate "drug" to produce the slightest symptoms of the disease being treated. Medications were repeatedly diluted to end up with a product said to contain 1 part of medication per 100,000,000.

Homeopathic products are extracted from plants (such as red onion, poison ivy, belladonna from deadly nightshade, stinging nettle), minerals (such as white arsenic), or animals (such as crushed whole bees) and can be formulated as sugar pellets to place under the tongue, tablets to take orally, or ointments, gels, drops, and creams for topical application. Treatment is tailored to the individual, so people with the same condition could receive different treatments. There does not appear to be empirical support for use of homeopathy. Cochrane found homeopathic therapy had no benefit for chronic asthma [53] or in children with acute respiratory tract infections [54]. In fact, the NCCIH says, "there is no reliable evidence that homeopathy is effective for any health condition" [55].

Though homeopathic remedies appear to be ineffective in treating illness, there may be a risk of substance overdose from treatments that contain heavy metals or significant amounts of active ingredients such as belladonna (which may even be found in pediatric preparations) and alcohol.

Traditional Chinese Medicine

Traditional Chinese medicine emerged in the Shang dynasty (between 3000 and 1000 BC). It emphasizes the proper balance of qi (pronounced chee) or vital energy that flows through the body in health; imbalance or blockage of the energy flow results in disease. Qi consists of complementary forces called yin and yang which must be in balance for health. Traditional Chinese medicine consists of a group of techniques and methods that seek to regain balance to restore health. There must be balance between internal (body organs) and external (earth, fire, water, wood, and metal) elements. Techniques to regain balance include acupuncture, cupping, moxibustion, herbal medicine, massage, and movement exercises such as Tai Chi. China, Korea, Japan, India, and Vietnam have all developed their own unique versions of traditional medicine.

As with any herbal treatment, there is a risk of overdose and/or interference with the function of prescription drugs. Of note, in 2004, the FDA banned the sale of dietary supplements containing ephedra (a Chinese herb used in dietary supplements for weight loss and performance enhancement) and plants containing ephedra group alkaloids due to complications, such as heart attack and stroke. The ban does not apply to certain herbal products prepared under Traditional Chinese medicine guidelines intended only for short-term use rather than long-term dosing. It also does not apply to over-the-counter and prescription drugs or to herbal teas.

Naturopathy

Naturopathic medicine began in Germany and was popularized in the last century in the US by Dr. John Scheel [15]. Scheel is said to have given naturopathy its name. It is now widely practiced in North America, Britain, Australia, and New Zealand. Naturopathy is said to have grown out of traditional practices such as Ayurveda, traditional Chinese medicine, Native American, and the Greek medical teachings of Hippocrates. Naturopathic practices are intended to support the body to heal itself naturally through diet, herbal therapies, massage, joint manipulation, homeopathy, acupuncture, ultrasound, light therapy, counselling, pharmacology, and lifestyle management.

Naturopathy involves the belief that the body has an intrinsic ability to heal itself and disease is a sign of inability of the body to heal itself. The role of naturopathic medicine is to figure out what is impeding the body's natural ability to be healthy. Illness prevention and healthy living are stressed and, as with many other healing systems, holism is a central theme with balance and complex interactions between many elements playing significant roles.

A subset of naturopathy is hydrotherapy that uses hot and cold water to cure disease and to maintain health. Other offshoots of naturopathy focus on natural living, vegetarianism, and hygienic lifestyle that stresses moderation and light and air for healing.

A Cochrane review of naturopathic anesthetic ear drops and herbal installations used for acute otitis media [56] suggests that there may be benefit from using anesthetic ear drops, but that herbal drops did not help. Another systematic review looked at naturopathic therapies for surgery patients [57] and noted that there was benefit for using acupressure or acupuncture to relieve postoperative nausea, vomiting, or pain; aromatherapy and music therapy seemed to reduce pain, stress, and anxiety.

Chiropractic

Chiropractic is a manual therapy based on realigning the body to allow self-healing. It was defined by its founder, D. D. Palmer, as "a science of healing without drugs." [58] Chiropractors look at how the spine structure is able to work—and how that impacts health. Chiropractic focuses on the musculoskeletal and nervous systems, treating issues in the back, neck, joints, arms, legs, and head. It is believed that injury causes tissues around the joints to restrict movement, and this causes illness. The chiropractor uses spinal manipulation to "adjust" the joints using controlled force to mobilize and loosen them and, thereby, restore health.

In many jurisdictions, chiropractic is a well-accepted, regulated health profession and, as such, may be considered mainstream. Cochrane reviews found no or only weak benefit from chiropractic for lower back pain or carpal tunnel. However, other systematic reviews suggest that chiropractic is at least as effective as other therapies in treating migraine or neck pain that leads to headache [59] or low back pain [60]. One systematic review concluded that maintenance care—in this instance, preventive therapy for patients with previous pain—had good outcomes for patients with previous episodes of low back pain if they had good results from initial treatment [61].

Risks of Chiropractic include disk herniation, nerve compression in the lower spine, or vertebral artery dissection after neck manipulation.

Osteopathy

Osteopathic medicine is a manipulative therapy founded by Dr. Andrew Taylor Still in the late 1800s. It is holistic and premised on the concept of interconnectedness of all body systems. Doctors of Osteopathy use manipulation to assess health issues and then use manipulation to treat diseases, improve circulation, and support the individual's return to health. Touch is a significant component of therapy. Osteopathy is distinguished from chiropractic in that an osteopath looks at the effect on the entire body when they evaluate bones, muscle, and soft tissues, whereas a chiropractor looks at the effects of bones, muscle, and soft tissues on nerve function and healing [62].

PubMed did not have osteopathic research publications. A Cochrane systematic review did not find evidence of there being benefit to osteopathic manipulation for infantile colic, asthma, or other illnesses [63].

Ayurvedic Medicine

Ayurveda, which means "The Science of Life", originated in India from an ancient culture handed down through oral tradition for thousands of years. About 2000 years ago, practitioners documented the first known Ayurvedic teachings [64], The Charaka Samhita. It is not known whether this represents a compilation or one person's work but it appears to explain the theoretical foundation of Aurveda, especially Internal Medicine and is still widely used today. Another writing possibly from the same time period, the *Sushruta Samhita,* focuses on the field of Ayurvedic surgery and likely was developed in relation to war and how to cope with injuries from wars. Several later books of Ayurveda include emphasis on physiology and therapeutics.

Followers of Ayurveda believe that there are five states of matter each of which has its own characteristics. Depending on how these states of matter predominate or combine, they believe one can understand cause and effect [64]. Knowing the composition of a substance, you can predict its effect or counter an effect with something that has the opposite qualities. Ayurveda is based on prevention of illness through balance of mind, body, and consciousness or spirit. Patient assessment involves examining the tongue (considered to be a map of internal organs functioning), eyes, pulse, physical form, and vocal tone. Diet, lifestyle, exercise, and herbal therapies are tailored to an individual to support health. Massage, yoga, meditation, and controlled breathing are Ayurvedic practices. Practitioners treat illness with cleansing to remove toxins.

Cochrane systematic reviews cautiously suggest that Ayurvedic herbal therapies provide some benefit for type 2 diabetes [65] and irritable bowel disease [66]. NCCIH reports also suggest that there may be benefit to Ayurvedic herbal therapies when used for rheumatoid arthritis and type 2 diabetes. Turmeric, an Ayurvedic herb, may benefit people with ulcerative colitis [67].

Ayurvedic herbal products can be dangerous: researchers found toxic minerals or metals, such as lead or mercury, in some of the products [15]. Also, as many Ayurvedic preparations are very complex and contain multiple herbs and medications, it is difficult to separate out what is beneficial and why that is so.

Unani Medicine

Unani Medicine originated in Greece and claims to be based on teachings of Hippocrates and Galen. Now practiced mostly in India, it is based on balancing four temperaments or humors of bodily fluid—blood, phlegm, yellow bile, and black bile [68]. Unani practitioners believe that everything is made up of air, earth, water, and fire; illness results from imbalance of elements. Unani medical practitioners diagnose by assessing temperaments and use herbal remedies, dietary practices, and aromatic therapies to restore balance [67].

Unani stresses health promotion and disease prevention, but there is no strong research to support practices [69]. Although listed in Cochrane CAM, there do not appear to be any published Cochrane reviews of Unani Medicine. NCCIH does not include it in their list of Complementary and Alternative Medicines. The National Health Portal of India [70] describes Unani as a "comprehensive medical system, which meticulously deals with the various states of health and disease. It provides promotive, preventive, curative and rehabilitative healthcare."

Therapeutic Massage

Massage therapists manipulate soft tissues of the body to normalize those tissues. Massage has been reported to be effective for low-back pain [71], as a non-pharmacologic option for treating migraine [72], as a means to prevent sports injury [73] and to promote recovery from injury. No impact on muscle function post-massage was noted. In general, massage therapy is considered safe, although aggressive massage can injure tissues and cause pain and bruising.

Hypnotherapy

Hypnosis is a practice that induces an altered state of consciousness. Hypnotherapy has the potential to help relieve the symptoms of a wide variety of diseases and conditions [15]. It can be used independently or along with other treatments. Hypnotherapy is reported to be as effective as cognitive behavioral therapy in reducing depressive symptoms [74] and has been reportedly used for coping with stress and anxiety, for pain control and management of fatigue [75].

Reflexology

Reflexology is a type of massage that applies differing pressures to feet, hands, and ears. This can be done by oneself or by a trained therapist. It is based on a theory that body parts are connected to certain organs and body systems and appropriate pressure in one area improves function in the connected area and improves overall health. There is some thought that reflexology can improve depression, stress, and anxiety, manage nausea and fatigue from chemotherapy, and help generally with relaxation.

A Cochrane review of non-pharmacological interventions to manage fatigue in patients with rheumatoid arthritis mentions that reflexology was one physical activity intervention that seemed to demonstrate a small beneficial effect on fatigue [76]. Reflexology was reported to reduce pain anxiety levels and improve sleep quality and quantity in burn patients [77]. If performed incorrectly, reflexology can cause pain and bruises.

Energy Therapies

Practitioners of energy therapies describe energy fields that arise from within the body (biofields) or external to it (electromagnetic fields) [78]. When energy is flowing freely through the body, an individual has good emotional, physical, and spiritual health. Illness denotes blocked energy flow. Therapies are intended to improve the body's energy field either through direct touch (by placing the hands in or through an individual's biofields) or remotely (near or remote depending on the practitioner). Examples of energy therapy modalities include Reiki, Prana and Therapeutic Touch, and Qi gong.

Reiki is a Japanese form of energy therapy said to transfer life energy from a practitioner to a client through light touch or hands held a distance away from the client's body. Illness or stress are thought to indicate a low life force energy and Reiki therapy is used to transfer energy to and relax the client, reduce their pain, and assist with healing and general well-being. Several studies indicate some positive effect (better than placebo) of Reiki therapy in palliative care patients [79], particularly for managing anxiety and depression. However, a Cochrane CAM review found insufficient evidence to state that Reiki was useful for treating anxiety or depression [80].

Therapeutic touch was developed by Krieger and Kunz in the early 1970s based on the theory that mind, body, and emotions form a complex energy field [81]. Practitioners move their hands just above the body to identify and remove harmful energy that is causing blockages and replace it with their own healthy energy. Healing touch, which is similar to therapeutic touch, was established by Mentgen in the 1980s, and uses gentle touch on the body to help it heal its own energy fields. Therapeutic touch as reviewed by Cochrane CAM does not appear to have any published evidence of the effectiveness of therapeutic touch [82].

Qi gong is an ancient Chinese system of movement and meditation that is practiced to balance and cultivate life energy. It is usually slow, coordinated movement carried out calmly with rhythmic breathing and meditation. It is embraced by many as a form of exercise or martial arts training like Tai Chi. One review article supports Qi gong as a therapy for hypertension [83].

There is also bioelectromagnetic therapy which uses a wide variety of machines to produce an effect in the biological processes of the target organism [84]. For example, magnetic healing therapy uses magnets placed on different parts of the body, believed to help unblock the energy flow around the body.

Hydrotherapy

Hydrotherapy is used in CAM (particularly naturopathy), occupational therapy, and physiotherapy (including sports medicine and rehab) that involves the use of water for pain relief and treatment. The term encompasses a broad range of approaches and therapeutic methods that use physical properties of water to stimulate blood circulation and treat symptoms of certain diseases. Therapies include use of water jets, underwater massage, whirlpool baths, hot and cold (cryotherapy) temperatures, and mineral baths. Proponents assert that alternating temperatures result in improved blood flow for more rapid return of cellular breakdown by-products to the lymphatic system. Experimental evidence suggests that contrast hydrotherapy helps reduce injury in acute stages by stimulating blood flow and reducing swelling.

Balneotherapy is a water therapy distinct from hydrotherapy. As far back as 1700 BC, balneotherapy used mudpacks, douches, soaks, and wraps to treat pain and swelling, and for relaxation. It is still popular in Europe. Proponents of the therapy believe that mineral water boosts immune systems and relieves arthritis symptoms, although evidence of this is lacking to date [85].

Exercise or Movement Therapy

There are alternative therapies built around the principle that proper body movement and alignment lead to well-being. They include Feldenkrais, Rolfing, Alexander Technique, Yoga, Tai Chi, and Pilates among many others.

The Feldenkrais Method is a type of exercise therapy based on physics, biomechanics, and human development devised by Israeli Moshé Feldénkrais during the mid-twentieth century. The method is claimed to reorganize and repair connections between the motor cortex of the brain and the body to improve body movement and well-being. Feldenkrais practitioners evaluate how a patient moves, especially habitual movement patterns that could be inefficient or strained and attempt to teach new patterns (either passively led by a practitioner or actively performed by the recipient) using gentle, slow, repeated movements. Slow repetition is believed to be necessary to impart a new habit and allow it to feel normal. Feldenkrais method is promoted as a way to improve one's singing voice [86]. One study of visually impaired patients with nonspecific chronic neck and/or scapular pain reported that patients using the Feldenkrais method had significantly less pain than controls [87].

Dr. Ida P. Rolf developed Rolfing in the mid-1900s based on a believe that the body muscles, bones, nerves, and organs are a continuous tissue network with specific patterns or order, not separate structures. Rolfing is said to use deep tissue massage and patient education for improved posture and body alignment to reorganize the connective tissues throughout the body and restore balance. This is purported to reduce pain, improve flexibility, and increase energy. Diagnosis involves identifying asymmetries in the skeleton and fascia, identifying them as "areas of constriction". Deep tissue massage reorganizes fascia and collagen, allowing muscles to relax, reduce pain, and increase mobility. Research in this area appears to be very limited currently.

The Alexander Technique was developed in the 1890s by F. M. Alexander to correct posture and bring the body into natural alignment to help it function efficiently [88]. Its series of movements is reported to aid relaxation and improve breathing. Some practitioners claim benefits for asthmatics (although a Cochrane review indicated there was insufficient evidence to show a benefit for asthmatics by using the Alexander Technique) or for vocations like singing, athletics, and dancing that require good breath control. It is also said to be useful in treating repetitive stress injuries like carpal tunnel syndrome, backache, or stiff neck and shoulders, and to benefit patients with back pain, tension, or stress.

For some, Yoga is a religious practice but for many it is exercise. Yoga is part of Ayurvedic therapy that uses postures, breathing management, and meditation. NCCIH reports that Yoga helps manage lower back pain and neck pain, may help with weight loss and smoking cessation, and probably helps ease anxiety and depression. Cochrane reviews report no demonstrable improvement in pain management, but show benefits from Yoga in regard to asthma. Risks from yoga include strains and sprains particularly in older individuals.

Tai Chi is an ancient Chinese martial art that has gained popularity as a form of meditative exercise through repetition of controlled motions. It is said to improve muscle strength, flexibility, and balance and provide benefit in managing many chronic health conditions such as Parkinson disease, osteoarthritis, chronic obstructive pulmonary disease, and improving cognitive capacity [89].

Pilates is a form of exercise developed in the early twentieth century by Joseph Pilates to alleviate ill health. Although thought to be beneficial in improving fitness and balance, there is only limited research citing benefit of Pilates in treating Parkinson's disease [90] or as a preferred exercise plan for the elderly [91]. A Cochrane review of benefits for low back pain stated that although Pilates was better than no exercise [92], it was not demonstrably better than other forms of exercise.

Cochrane reviews of a variety of other exercise modalities report some positive change—slight pain reduction, improved physical function and fitness, less fatigue—but caution that evidence is of low quality [93, 94]. Although a variety of exercise styles were evaluated, none appeared significantly more beneficial than others.

Biofeedback

Biofeedback is a type of mind-body therapy that uses feedback from monitoring procedures and equipment to teach a patient relaxation techniques and mental exercises so the patient can control involuntary body responses, such as blood pressure, skin temperature, muscle tension, and heart rate. Patients work with a biofeedback therapist to learn relaxation techniques and mental exercises. In initial sessions, electrodes are attached to the skin to measure bodily states, but eventually the techniques can be practiced without a therapist or equipment. Biofeedback has been shown to be helpful for headache pain [95]. It may be helpful in stroke recovery and medical conditions including asthma, Raynaud's disease, irritable bowel syndrome, incontinence, headaches, cardiac arrhythmias, high blood pressure, and epilepsy.

A Cochrane systematic review of "mind and body therapy" found low level evidence to support effectiveness of a variety of therapies in improving pain, mood, or physical functioning [96].

Bach Flower Remedies

The Bach flower system was originated in the early 1900s by Dr. Edward Bach who believed that flowers can affect emotions positively. He believed that energy from different flowers had differing capacities to remove emotional pain and suffering, which over time harm health and impair healing. A systematic review of randomised clinical trials showed that there was no effect from use of flower remedies [97].

Anthroposophic Medicine

Anthroposophic medicine was founded in the early 1920s by Rudolf Steiner and Ita Wegman. It is described as an integrative multimodal treatment system based on a holistic understanding of man, nature, disease, and treatment that includes formative forces and a three-fold human constitution [98]. It employs medicines derived from plants, minerals, and animals, art therapy, eurythmy therapy, and rhythmical massage, counseling, psychotherapy, and specific nursing techniques such as external embrocation (a liquid rubbed on the body to relieve pain from sprains or strains). Anthroposophic practitioners claim that all acute and chronic diseases can be treated, with a focus on children's diseases, family medicine, and particularly chronic diseases. These claims are not borne out in peer-reviewed literature.

Neural Therapy

Neural therapy is described as a gentle, natural healing technique developed in the early 1900s, by Ferdinand and Walter Huneke in Germany [99], and is now also practiced in other countries in Europe and the United States. It involves injecting local anesthetics into autonomic nerve ganglia, peripheral nerves, scars, glands, acupuncture points, trigger points, and other tissues. Neural therapy is based on the theory that trauma, infection, or surgery can damage the autonomic nervous system and produce long-standing disturbances in electrochemical or electromagnetic functions of tissues. This results in dysfunction that can last indefinitely unless repaired. When the autonomic nervous system is injured or not functioning correctly, blood flow goes out of synch with demand, resulting in incomplete healing. Proponents report that there may be an instant reaction to therapy or repeated injections may be required to achieve resolution of illness or pain [100]. There appears to be little current research published on this topic and what is published relates to pain relief [101].

gSo-BA Rig-PA

gSo-BA Rig-PA, a traditional Bhutanese medicine, is one of the oldest surviving medical traditions in the world [102]. Systems such as Chinese medicine, Indian Ayurvedic medicine, Unani medicine, and Greco-Roman medicine influenced the way traditional gSo-BA Rig-PA evolved, but Buddhist philosophy is said to be the mainstream of this holistic medical system. gSo-BA Rig-PA's principles are based on the perception that the human body is composed of three main elements: rLung (Air), mKhris-pa (Bile), and Bad-kan (Phlegm). When these elements are balanced in the body, a person is said to be healthy. The pathophysiology is different from other medical systems and the close link to Buddhism is reflected in spiritual dimensions and a perception that all suffering is caused by ignorance. The treatment of diseases includes behavioral modification, physiotherapy, herbal medicines, minor surgery, and spiritual healing [103].

Siddha Medicine

Siddha medicine is an ancient medical system of India practiced by Tamils/Dravidians of peninsular South India [104]. The word Siddha means established truth. The mystic findings of Siddha medicine are contained in medicine, yoga, and astrology. Fundamental Principles of Siddha include theories of Five Elements (Aimpootham) and Three Forces/Faults (Mukkuttram). The Eight Methods of Examination (Envakai Thervukal) are used to determine diagnosis, etiology, treatment, and prognosis. Siddha is said to have safe herbal and herbo-mineral treatments for psoriasis, eczema, alopecia, diabetic ulcer, warts, vitiligo, pemphigus, pompholyx, leprosy, and many more very common and rare diseases. Lifestyle modifications including diet are important.

Meditation

Meditation is practiced in numerous religious traditions [15]. Early records of meditation (*dhyana*) are found in ancient Indian texts, the Vedas, and meditation is important in Hinduism and Buddhism. Muslims perform Salah which is a mandatory act of devotion that is akin to meditation. Meditation practices vary between traditions and within them. Typically, an individual focuses on a particular object or thought to achieve calm and mental clarity. In the last century, Asian meditative techniques have been adapted by other cultures in non-spiritual contexts such as business and health. Transcendental Meditation, a particular form of meditation, emerged in the 1940s under Maharishi Mahesh Yogi. Where mindfulness meditation is focused on the present, transcendental meditation focuses an individual on experiencing "being". It has been suggested that meditation may reduce stress, anxiety, depression, and pain, and enhance peace, perception, self-concept, and well-being.

Ozone Therapy

Ozone (O_3) gas has dangerous effects, but also has therapeutic effects [105]. Medical O_3 is used to disinfect and treat disease. Mechanism of actions is by inactivation of bacteria, viruses, fungi, yeast, and protozoa, stimulation of oxygen metabolism, and activation of the immune system. In treatment of external wounds, it is used as a transcutaneous O_3 gas bath in a closed system. Ozonized water is applied in dental medicine (a number of PubMed publications support treating with ozone) as a spray or compress.

A Cochrane CAM review of ozone used in treating diabetic foot ulcers was unable to draw firm conclusions due to limited evidence [106]. Other published reports include successful use of ozone in treating fibromyalgia [107] or low back pain [108].

Aromatherapy

Aromatherapy uses essential oils that contain concentrated extracts from roots, leaves, seeds, or blossoms of plants to promote healing when inhaled or applied topically. Like herbal therapy, aromatherapy can be traced back at least 5000 years. Some purported uses include treating inflammation or infections, promoting relaxation and calm, easing depression, nausea, and insomnia. A Cochrane systematic review, which looked at naturopathic therapies for surgery patients, noted that aromatherapy and music therapy seemed to reduce pain, stress, and anxiety [57]. Aromatherapy combined with massage was shown to improve sleep quality in burn patients [109], but it was also noted that massage alone had the same effect.

There is some reported risk with the use of essential oils especially for pregnant women, children, or pets. Essential (concentrated) oils should not be applied directly to skin and people should avoid prolonged exposure to aerosols without ventilation.

Summary

Consideration must be given to the beliefs held by both the patient/consumer and the health care provider when evaluating a patient and determining a plan for care. Communication and actively listening are very important for effective exchange of beliefs and information. Many complementary medicine users consider complementary therapies to be completely separate from and unrelated to mainstream healthcare. They may believe, unfortunately inaccurately, that "natural" means totally "safe" and cannot cause any harm. A practical problem with trying to integrate complementary and mainstream therapies is a lack of trust. A perception of mistrust by mainstream healthcare providers can result in reticence when patients seek mainstream health care solutions. Nearly 70% of adults reported not talking to their doctors about CAM treatments, either because of skepticism about how much they think their physicians know or because physicians don't ask about their use [110]. This can be problematic because of potential interactions or interference of one therapy with another.

These days, healthcare providers more frequently seek patient care solutions that include complementary therapies as chronic conditions continue to defy modern therapies. As reliable information becomes more readily available, the shift to include complementary therapies in mainstream health care will continue and, hopefully, contribute to a stronger body of research into what is effective care. Many people hold a strong belief in the benefit of complementary therapies, but there are still questions to be answered about whether and which alternative therapies are safe and effective. It can be difficult to "prove" alternative therapies as there can be a large (and real) spiritual component. The present-day surge in complementary therapy use and promotion makes it very important to study the efficiency and efficacy of complementary therapies, so consumers can make informed health care choices. In 2021, it is a telling sign that although there are many published complementary medicine research studies (279,000 on PubMed for "complementary medicine"), the number of research studies of complementary medicine is very low or nonexistent in mainstream specialty publications. Fortunately, increased government interest in regulation and standardization of complementary medicine should improve the quality of information available about complementary therapies and, in doing so, improve the accuracy of therapeutic claims and safer use of therapies.

In general, people should be wary of claims that are "too good to be true" as they likely are that. A guarantee of results should definitely be received cautiously. Simply because it has been published does not make research claims "true". Health care providers and patients should look for reliable and consistent sources of information about use of a particular therapy for a symptom or condition. Alternative therapies may have benefits which should be considered, especially if the benefits are supportive of and "complementary" to recommended mainstream therapies. However, limitations must be acknowledged and addressed.

Health care providers and consumers should seek current, reliable information before undertaking inclusion of complementary and alternative therapies into their health care regimens. There is a growing body of knowledge that will, over time, prove or refute health care claims. No health care therapy—whether mainstream or alternative—should be undertaken without a risk/benefit analysis.

References

1. Hollinghurst S, Shaw A, Thompson E. Capturing the value of complementary and alternative medicine: including patient preferences in economic evaluation. Complement Ther Med. 2008;16(1):47–51.
2. Coulter ID, Willis EM. The rise and rise of complementary and alternative medicine: a sociological perspective. Med J Aust. 2004;180(11):587–9.
3. Nahin R, Barnes P, Stussman B, Bloom B. Costs of complementary and alternative medicine (CAM) and frequency of visits to CAM practitioners. Natl Health Stat Report. 2009;30(18):1–14.
4. Americans Spent $30.2 Billion out-of-pocket on complementary health approaches: national center for complementary and integrative health; 2016. Available from: https://www.nccih.nih.gov/news/press-releases/americans-spent-302-billion-outofpocket-on-complementary-health-approaches.
5. Esmael N. Complementary and alternative medicine: use and public attitudes 1997, 2006, and 2016. The Fraser Institute 2017.
6. Posadzki P, Watson L, Alotaibi A, Ernst E. Prevalence of use of complementary and alternative medicine (CAM) by patients/consumers in the UK: systematic review of surveys. Clin Med (Lond). 2013;13(2):126–31.

7. Clarke TC, Barnes PM, Black LI, Stussman BJ, Nahin R. Use of Yoga, meditation, and chiropractors among U.S. adults aged 18 and over: National Center for Health Survey; 2018. Available from: https://www.cdc.gov/nchs/data/databriefs/db325-h.pdf.
8. Goertz C, Finch MD, Bray RM, Williams TV, Hourani LL, Hadden LS, Colleran HL, Jonas SB. Military report more complementary and alternative medicine use than civilians. J Altern Complement Med. 2013;19(6):509–17.
9. Who Global Report on Traditional and Complementary Medicine 2019. The World Health Organization; 2019. Report No.: ISBN 978-92-4-151543-6.
10. NG J. Insight into the characteristics of research published in traditional, complementary, alternative, and integrative medicine journals: a bibliometric analysis. BMC Complement Med Ther. 2021;21(1):185.
11. Jonas W. Hospitals creating optimal healing environments 2011. Available from: http://www.samueliinstitute.org/File%20Library/Our%20Research/OHE/CreatingOHEs.pdf.
12. Mission Statement for NCCIH: NCCIH National Center for Complementary and Integrative Health; [updated September 25 2019]. Available from: https://www.nih.gov/about-nih/what-we-do/nih-almanac/national-center-complementary-integrative-health-nccih.
13. Wieland L, Manheimer E, Berman B. Development and classification of an operational definition of complementary and alternative medicine for the Cochrane collaboration. Altern Ther Health Med. 2011;17(2):50–9.
14. Seaward B. Managing stress: principles and strategies for health and Well-being. 8th ed. Sudbury, MA: Jones and Bartlett Learning; 2013.
15. Tabish S. Complementary and alternative healthcare: is it evidence-based? Int J Health Sci (Qassim). 2008;2(1):V–IX.
16. Linde K, Allais G, Brinkhaus B, Fei Y, Mehring M, Shin B, et al. Acupuncture for the prevention of tension-type headache. Cochrane Database Syst Rev [Internet]. 2016; Available from: https://www.cochranelibrary.com/cdsr/doi/10.1002/14651858.CD007587.pub2/full
17. Dear JC, Zheng Z, Xue CCL, Liu JP, Shang J, Scott SW, et al. Acupuncture for Treating Fibromyalgia. 2013;5
18. Kober A, Scheck T, Schubert B, Strasser H, Gustorff B, Bertalanffy P, et al. Auricular acupressure as a treatment for anxiety in prehospital transport settings. Anesthesiology. 2003;98(6):1328.
19. Yb Y, Tse S. The effectiveness of relaxation acupoint stimulation and acupressure with aromatic lavender essential oil for non-specific low back pain in Hong Kong: a randomised controlled trial. Complement Ther Med. 2004;12(1):28–37.
20. Yip Y, Tse S. An experimental study on the effectiveness of acupressure with aromatic lavender essential oil for sub-acute, non-specific neck pain in Hong Kong. Complement Ther Clin Prac. 2006;12(1):18–26.
21. Kang HS, Sok SR, Kang J. Effects of Meridian acupressure for stroke patients in Korea. J Clin Nurs. 2009;18(15):2145–52.
22. Hu S, Stritzel R, Chandler A, Stern R. P6 acupressure reduces symptoms of vection-induced motion sickness. Aviat Space Environ Med. 1995;66(7):631–4.
23. Kim S, Lee SH, Kim MR, Kim EJ, Hwang DS, Lee J, et al. Is cupping therapy effective in patients with neck pain? A systematic review and meta-analysis. BMJ Open. 2018;8(11):e021070.
24. Dennehy CE, Tsourounis C. Dietary supplements and herbal medications. In: BG K, editor. Basic & clinical pharmacology. 15th ed. New York: McGraw Hill; 2021. p. 1179–94.
25. About Natural Health Product Regulation in Canada: Government of Canada; 2016 [updated 2016-08-11]. Available from: https://www.canada.ca/en/health-canada/services/drugs-health-products/natural-non-prescription/regulation.html
26. Government of Canada Pathway for Licensing Natural Health Products used as Traditional Medicines: Government of Canada; [updated 2012-12-20]. Available from: https://www.canada.ca/en/health-canada/services/drugs-health-products/natural-non-prescription/legislation-guidelines/guidance-documents/pathway-licensing-traditional-medicines.html#a1.1

27. FDA 101: Dietary Supplements: US Food and Drug Administration; 2015 [updated 07/15/2015]. Available from: https://www.fda.gov/consumers/consumer-updates/fda-101-dietary-supplements.
28. Bubela T, Koper M, Boon H, Caulfield T. Media portrayal of herbal remedies versus pharmaceutical clinical trials: impacts on decision. Med Law. 2007;26(2):363–73.
29. Barrett B, Kiefer D, Rabago D. Assessing the risks and benefits of herbal medicine: an overview of scientific evidence. Altern Ther Health Med. 1999;5(4):40.
30. McKay D, Jeffrey B, Blumberg J. A review of the bioactivity and potential health benefits of chamomile tea (Matricaria recutita L.). Phytother Res. 2006;20(7):519.
31. Karsch-Völk M, Barrett B, Kiefer D, Bauer R, Ardjomand-Woelkart K, Linde K. Echinacea for preventing and treating the common cold. Cochrane Database Syst Rev. 2014;2(2)
32. Block KI, Mead M. Immune system effects of echinacea, ginseng, and astragalus: a review. Integr Cancer Ther. 2003;2(3):247–67.
33. Matsutomo T. Potential benefits of garlic and other dietary supplements for the management of hypertension. Exp Ther Med. 2020;19(2):1479–84.
34. Berginc K, Albin KA. The effect of garlic supplements and phytochemicals on the ADMET properties of drugs. Expert Opin Drug Metab Toxicol. 2012;8(3):295–310.
35. Hilton M, Stuart E. Ginkgo biloba for tinnitus. Cochrane Database Syst Rev. 2004;2
36. Mei N, Guo X, Ren Z, Kobayashi D, Wada K, Guo L. Review of Ginkgo biloba-induced toxicity, from experimental studies to human case reports. J Environ Sci Health C Environ Carcinog Ecotoxicol Rev. 2017;35(1):1–28.
37. Alkhatib A, Tsang C, Tiss A, Bahorun T, Arefanian H, Barake R, et al. Functional foods and lifestyle approaches for diabetes prevention and management. Nutrients. 2017;9(12):1310.
38. Ng Q, Venkatanarayanan N, Ho C. Clinical use of Hypericum perforatum (St John's wort) in depression: a meta-analysis. J Affect Disord. 2017;1:211–21.
39. Soleymani S, Bahramsoltani R, Rahimi R, Abdollahi M. Clinical risks of St John's wort (Hypericum perforatum) co-administration. Expert Opin Drug Metab Toxicol. 2017;13(10):1047–62.
40. Carod-Artal F. Hallucinogenic drugs in pre-Columbian Mesoamerican cultures. Neurologia. 2015;30(1):42.
41. Krebs TS, Johansen P. Psychedelics and mental health: a population study. PLoS One. 2013;8(8):e63972.
42. Kyzar E, Nichols C, Gainetdinov R, Nichols D, Kalueff A. Review: psychedelic drugs in biomedicine. Trends Pharmacol Science. 2017;38(11):992.
43. Maduro R. Curanderismo and Latino views of disease and curing. West J Med. 1983;139:868–74.
44. Mothibe M, Sibanda M. African traditional medicine: South African perspective. African Traditional Medicine. 2019;
45. Kamaka ML, Paloma DSL, Maskarinec G. Recommendations for medical training: a native Hawaiian patient perspective. Hawaii Med J. 2011;70(11)
46. Periyakoil V. Traditional health beliefs: theories of illness: Stanford school of medicine; 2021. Available from: https://geriatrics.stanford.edu/ethnomed/hawaiian_pacific_islander/fund/health_beliefs.html#:~:text=Central%20to%20Native%20Hawaiian%20understanding,person%20are%20all%20in%20harmony.
47. Rapa Nui; The rebirth of ancestral medicine 2021. Available from: https://moevarua.com/en/the-rebirth-of-ancestral-medicine/.
48. Shaouli Shahid S, Finn L, Bessarab D, Thompson S. Understanding, beliefs and perspectives of aboriginal people in Western Australia about cancer and its impact on access to cancer services. BMC Health Serv Res. 2009;9(132)
49. Maher P. A review of 'Traditional' aboriginal health beliefs. Aust J Rural Health. 2002. Available from:;7:229. https://doi.org/10.1046/j.1440-1584.1999.00264.x.
50. Logan L. Creating space for indigenous healing practices in patient care plans. Can Med Educ J. 2020;11(1):e5–e15.

51. Blignault I, Hunter J, Mumford J. Integration of indigenous healing practices with western biomedicine in Australia, Canada, New Zealand and the United States of America: a scoping review protocol. JBI Database System Rev Implement Rep. 2018;16(6):1354–60.
52. Loudon I. A brief history of homeopathy. J R Soc Med. 2006;99(12):607–10.
53. McCarney RW, Lasserson TJ. Homeopathy for chronic asthma. Cochrane Database Syst Rev. 2004;26
54. Hawke K, van Driel ML, McGuire TM, King D. Homeopathic medicinal products for preventing and treating acute respiratory tract infections in children. Cochrane Database Syst Rev. 2018;4:CD005974.
55. Homeopathy: What you need to know: national center for complementary and integrative health; 2021. Available from: https://www.nccih.nih.gov/health/homeopathy.
56. Foxlee R, Wejfalk J, Dooley L, Del Mar CB. Topical analgesia for acute otitis media. Cochrane Database Syst Rev. 2006;2011:CD005657.
57. Lederer AK, Schmucker C, Kousoulas L, Fichtner-Feigl S, Huber R. Naturopathic treatment and Complementary medicine in surgical practice. Dtsch Arztebl Int. 2018;115(49):815–21.
58. Ernst E. Chiropractic: a critical evaluation. J Pain Symptom Manag. 2008;35(5):544–62.
59. Bryans R, Descarreaux M, Duranleau M, Marcoux H, Potter B, Ruegg R, Shaw L, Watkin R, White E. Evidence-based guidelines for the chiropractic treatment of adults with headache. J Manip Physiol Ther. 2011;34(5):274–89.
60. Blanchette MA, Da Silva RB, Boruff J, Harrison P, Bussières A. Effectiveness and economic evaluation of chiropractic care for the treatment of low Back pain: a systematic review of pragmatic studies. PLoS One. 2016;11(8):e0160037.
61. Iben A, Charlotte L. Chiropractic maintenance care–what's new? A systematic review of the literature. Chiropr Man Therap. 2019;27(63)
62. Difference between an Osteopath and a Chiropractor: UK Health Centre; 2019 [updated September 2021]. Available from: https://www.healthcentre.org.uk/osteopaths/osteopath-difference-chiropractor.html.
63. Dobson D, Vlieger AM, Prescott P, Lewith G. Manipulative therapies for infantile colic. Cochrane Database of Systematic Reviews Review–Intervention. 2012.
64. Lad V. Ayurveda: a brief introduction and guide 2016. Available from: https://www.ayurveda.com/resources/articles/ayurveda-a-brief-introduction-and-guide.
65. Sridharan K, Ramaratnam S, Panneerselvam D. Ayurvedic treatments for diabetes mellitus. Cochrane Database Syst Rev. 2011:CD008288.
66. Liu JP, Liu Y, Wei ML, Grimsgaard S. Herbal medicines for treatment of irritable bowel syndrome. Cochrane Database of Systematic Reviews. 2006.
67. Wong C. Health benefits of Ayurvedic herbs, 4 traditional herbal remedies used for healing 2021 [updated august 20, 2021]. Available from: https://www.verywellhealth.com/popular-ayurvedic-herbs-88822.
68. Alama A, Sofi G, Tarique BMD. Understanding hypothyroidism in Unani medicine. Journal of Integrative Medicine. 2019;17(6):387–91.
69. Itrat M. Methods of health promotion and disease prevention in Unani medicine. J Educ Health Promot. 2020;9(168):168.
70. Unani, The Science of Health and Healing: NHP CC DC; 2016 [updated Dec 24, 2016]. Validated by NHP Admin. Available from: https://www.nhp.gov.in/unani_mty.
71. Furlan AD, Baskwill A, Irvin E, Imamura M. Massage for low-back pain. Cochrane Database Syst Rev. 2015;9(CD001929)
72. Chaibi A, Russell MB. Manual therapies for migraine: a systematic review. J Headache Pain. 2011;12(2):127–33.
73. Weerapong P, Kolt S. The mechanisms of massage and effects on performance, muscle recovery and injury prevention. Sports Med. 2005;35(3):235–56.
74. Fuhr K, Broch A, Cyrny B, Hinkel J, Jaberg J, Petrasch M, Schweizer C, Stiegler A, Zeep C, Batra A. Efficacy of hypnotherapy compared to cognitive behavioral therapy for mild to moderate depression–results of a randomized controlled rater-blind clinical trial. J Affect Disord. 2021;286(1):166–73.

75. Michalopoulos M. Mind/body healing: hypnotherapy, functional/integrated medicine, epigenetics, cancer & the immune system. J Heart Centered Therapies. 2018;21(1)
76. Cramp F, Hewlett S, Almeida C, Kirwan JR, Choy EHS, Chalder T, et al. Non-pharmacological interventions for the management of patient-reported fatigue in rheumatoid arthritis 2013. Available from: https://www.cochrane.org/CD008322/MUSKEL_non-pharmacological-interventions-for-the-management-of-patient-reported-fatigue-in-rheumatoid-arthritis.
77. Alinia-najjara R, Bagheri-Nesami R, AfshinShorofi S, Nouraddin M, Kiarash S. The effect of foot reflexology massage on burn-specific pain anxiety and sleep quality and quantity of patients hospitalized in the burn intensive care unit (ICU). Burns. 2020;46(8):1942–51.
78. Rubik B, Muehsam D, Hammerschlag R, Jain S. Biofield science and healing: history, terminology, and concepts. Glob Adv Health Med. 2015;(Published online 2015 Nov 1):8–14.
79. Billot M, Daycard M, Wood C, Tchalla A. Reiki therapy for pain, anxiety and quality of life. BMJ Support Palliat Care. 2019;9(4):434–8.
80. Joyce J, Herbison G. Reiki for depression and anxiety 2015. Available from: https://doi.org/10.1002/14651858.CD006833.pub2.
81. Krieger D, Kunz D. The process of therapeutic touch 2017. Available from: http://therapeutictouch.org/.
82. Robinson J, Biley FC, Dolk H. Therapeutic touch for anxiety disorders. Cochrane Database Syst Rev. 2007:CD006240.
83. Wang XX, Li P, Xiaoke MD, Yuqing Z. Qigong for hypertension: a systematic review. 1 ed. J A, editor 2015.
84. Muehsam D, Chevalier G, Barsotti T, Gurfein B. An overview of biofield devices. Glob Adv Health Med. 2015;4:42–51.
85. Verhagen AP, Bierma-Zeinstra SMA, Boers M, Cardoso JR, Lambeck J, de Bie R, et al. Balneotherapy (or spa therapy) for rheumatoid arthritis 2015.
86. Nelson S, Blades-Zeller E. Singing with your whole self: the Feldenkrais method and voice. Lanham, MD: Scarecrow Press; 2002.
87. Lundqvist L, Zetterlund CO, Richter H. Effects of Feldenkrais method on chronic neck/scapular pain in people with visual impairment: a randomized controlled trial with one-year follow-up. Arch Phys Med Rehabil. 2014;95(9):1656–61.
88. Dennis JA, Cates C. Alexander technique for chronic asthma Cochrane. Syst Rev. 2012; Available from: https://www.cochrane.org/CD000995/AIRWAYS_alexander-technique-chronic-asthma
89. Huston P, McFarlane B. Health benefits of tai chi: what is the evidence? Can Fam Physician. 2016;2021:881–90.
90. Suárez-Iglesias D, Miller K, Seijo-Martínez M, Ayán C. Benefits of Pilates in Parkinson's disease: a systematic review and meta-analysis. Medicina (Kaunas). 2019;55(8):476.
91. Engers PB, Rombaldi AJ, Portella EG, da Silva M. The effects of the Pilates method in the elderly: a systematic review. Rev Bras Reumatol Engl Ed. 2016;56:352–65.
92. Yamato TP, Maher C, Saragiotto B, Hancock M, Ostelo R, Cabral C, et al. Pilates for low back pain: cochrane systematic reviews 2015. Available from: https://www.cochrane.org/CD010265/BACK_pilates-for-low-back-pain.
93. Bidonde J, Busch AJ, Schachter CL, Webber SC, Musselman KE, Overend TJ, et al. Mixed exercise programmes for adults with fibromyalgia 2019. Available from: https://www.cochrane.org/CD013340/MUSKEL_mixed-exercise-programmes-adults-fibromyalgia.
94. Kim SY, Busch AJ, Overend TJ, Schachter CL, van der Spuy I, Boden C, et al. Flexibility exercise training for adults with fibromyalgia. Cochrane Syst Rev. 2014; Available from: https://www.cochrane.org/CD013419/MUSKEL_flexibility-exercise-training-adults-fibromyalgia
95. Kondo K, Noonan KM, Freeman M, Ayers C, Morasco BJ, Kansagara D. Efficacy of biofeedback for medical conditions: an evidence map. J Gen Intern Med. 2019;34(12):2883–93.
96. Theadom A, Cropley M, Smith H, Feigin V, McPherson K. Interventions focusing on the link between the mind and body for adults with fibromyalgia. Cochrane Syst Rev. 2015; Available from: https://www.cochrane.org/CD001980/MUSKEL_interventions-focusing-link-between-mind-and-body-adults-fibromyalgia

97. Ernst E. Bach flower remedies: a systematic review of randomised clinical trials. Swiss Med Wkly. 2010;140:w13079.
98. Kienle GS, Albonico HU, Baars E. Anthroposophic medicine: an integrative medical system originating in Europe. Glob Adv Health Med. 2013;2(6):20–31.
99. Harris GR. Neural therapy and its role in the effective treatment of chronic pain. Practical Pain Management. 2011;9(6)
100. Huenke J. Neural therapy by Huneke 1999.
101. Frank B. Neural therapy. Phys Med Rehabil Clin N Am. 1999;10(3):573–82, viii.
102. Wangchuk P, Wangchuk D, Aagaard-Hansen J. Traditional Bhutanese medicine (gSo-BA rig-PA): an integrated part of the formal health care services. Southeast Asian J Trop Med Public Health. 2007;38(1):161–7.
103. Wangyal R, Tidwell T, Dhondrup W, Yungdrung T, Dhondrup G, He Q, et al. Dataset of materia medica in Sowa Rigpa: Tibetan medicine botanicals and Gawé Dorjé's classification system. Data Brief. 2020;33:106498.
104. Thas J. Siddha medicine–background and principles and the application for skin diseases. Clin Dermatol. 2008;26(1):62–78.
105. Elvis AM, Ekta JS. Ozone therapy: a clinical review. J Nat Sci Biol Med. 2011;2(1):66–70.
106. Jian Liu J, Zhang P, Tian J, Li L, Li J, Tian JH, et al. Ozone therapy for treating foot ulcers in people with diabetes. Cochrane Database Syst Rev. 2015;2015
107. Tirelli U, Cirrito C, Pavanello M, Piasentin C, Lleshi A, Taibi R. Ozone therapy in 65 patients with fibromyalgia: an effective therapy. Eur Rev Med Pharmacol Sci. 2019;23(4):1786–8.
108. de Andrade PR, de Oliveira-Neto OB, Barbosa LT, Santos IO, de Sousa-Rodrigues CF, Barbosa F. Effectiveness of ozone therapy compared to other therapies for low back pain: a systematic review with meta-analysis of randomized clinical trials. Rev Bras Anestesiol. 2019;69(5):493–501.
109. Rafii F, Ameri F, Haghani H, Ghobadi A. The effect of aromatherapy massage with lavender and chamomile oil on anxiety and sleep quality of patients with burns. Burns. 2020;46(1):164–71.
110. Crute S. The best medicine. AARP The Magazine. 2008:58–64.

Diets

23

Agnes Czibulka

Introduction

Many chronic conditions such as cardiovascular disease, neurodegenerative disease, cancer, and chronic infections have one thing in common: they all have low level chronic inflammation at their root. The standard Western diet contains foods high in saturated fatty acids, trans fatty acids, refined carbohydrates, sodium, and processed foods. The anti-inflammatory diet is associated with reduced chronic inflammation. It contains minimal processed foods, but is full of monounsaturated and omega-3 polyunsaturated fatty acids, nuts, vegetables, seeds, legumes, whole grains, and lean protein. The main components of an anti-inflammatory diet are Mediterranean, Dietary Approaches to Stop Hypertension (DASH), and Traditional Asian dietary patterns and contain a combination of foods that reduce chronic and systemic inflammation.

The Mediterranean diet is a plant-based diet with 3–9 servings of vegetables, 2 servings of fruits, and 1–3 servings of whole grains a day. Hallmark of this traditional diet is regular consumption of garlic and its relatively high fat content with one third of calories coming from fat. The majority of this fat is monounsaturated from olive oil, the rest is polyunsaturated from fish, nuts, and seeds.

Accumulating evidence indicates that the five most important adaptations induced by the Mediterranean dietary pattern are:

1. Lipid lowering effect.
2. Protection against oxidative stress, inflammation, and platelet aggregation.
3. Modification of hormones and growth factors involved in the pathogenesis of cancer.

A. Czibulka (✉)
Clinical Assistant Professor of Yale University Department of Surgery/Otolaryngology, New Haven, CT, USA

© The Author(s), under exclusive license to Springer Nature Switzerland AG 2023

B. W. Blakley, J. E. Blakley (eds.), *Functional Illness of the Head and Neck*,
https://doi.org/10.1007/978-3-031-12998-8_23

4. Inhibition of nutrient sensing pathways by specific amino acid restriction.
5. Gut microbiota-mediated production of metabolites influencing metabolic health [1].

Research investigating the association between diet and inflammatory markers has studied many components of the Mediterranean diet, finding a decrease of numerous inflammatory markers such as decreased CRP, IL-6, IL-1B and reduced LDL and TNF-alpha [2].

There is no single Asian diet, but generalizations can be made. Similar to the Mediterranean diet, Asian diets are composed of unprocessed, nutrient dense foods. A variety of seeds, nuts, soy, whole grains, vegetables, and lean proteins like fish are included. Whole soy products such as edamame, tofu, and tempeh are consumed daily providing a variety of nutrients and phytochemicals including vitamin C, magnesium, calcium, and potassium. Fermented vegetables such as kimchi enrich this diet with probiotic lactic acid bacteria. An inverse association was found between soy food consumption and interleukin-6, TNF-alpha, and soluble TNF receptors 1 and 2 [3]. Another staple of the Asian diet are mushrooms. They are rich in anti-inflammatory components, such as polysaccharides, phenolic and indolic compounds, mycosteroids, fatty acids, and vitamins [4]. Mushrooms act as prebiotics to foster the growth of healthy gut microbiota. Mushrooms are one of the few natural food sources of vitamin D which is important for vegetarians. Traditionally, shiitake mushrooms are used for diseases that involve depressed immune function such as environmental allergies, fungal infection, frequent flu and colds, bronchial inflammation, infectious diseases, heart disease, and hypertension. Antibiotic, anticarcinogenic, antiviral, and immunogenic compounds have been isolated both intracellularly and extracellularly. In a study after 4 weeks of shiitake mushrooms consumption, increased T-cell and NK-T cell proliferation and activity and increased IL-4, IL-10, and TNF-alpha were found. Increase in secretory IgA implied improved gut immunity [5].

Like the Mediterranean diet, the Dietary Approaches to Stop Hypertension (DASH) diet emphasize fruits, vegetables, and low-fat dairy. It also focuses on reducing sodium and assuring sufficient intake of potassium, calcium, magnesium, and fiber.

Overall, at the top of the list of undesirable foods is refined sugars. It is most commonly consumed as sucrose and high fructose corn syrup. Nearly 15% of the calories in a typical American diet are derived from added sugars. Excessive consumption of sucrose and high fructose corn syrup is an important contributing factor to many of the chronic health problems in a Western society. Refined sugar contains no vitamins, minerals, or micronutrients and it replaces the healthy micronutrients. Over the last few decades, a significant amount of the sucrose has been replaced by the high fructose syrup, which is more harmful than sucrose. It is not widely appreciated that high sugar intake is a major contributing factor to many symptoms and conditions including fatigue, anxiety, depression, migraine headaches, tension headaches, and candidiasis, beside the well-known effect on chronic diseases such as Type 2 diabetes, nonalcoholic fatty liver disease, and cardiovascular diseases.

The Human Microbiome

The term "microbiome" refers to the community of fungi, viruses, and bacteria in a location, the latter being the most prominent. Today, it is known that 50% of all cells within the human body are not of human origin and over 90% of microorganisms do not routinely cause disease. These microorganisms are understood to play essential roles in maintaining the health and normal physiological function of the human body. These microorganisms are found throughout the body, from the oral cavity to the stomach, lung, intestinal, and urogenital tracts. Each of these locations has its own unique set of microbes and is influenced by many factors including age, sex, genetics, environment, diet, and lifestyle.

The microbiota of the gastrointestinal tract is essential for the proper functioning of several physiological systems, including the immune, digestive, and nervous systems. The microflora participate in the digestive system by supporting the breakdown of complex carbohydrates and by producing vitamins and nutrients, including vitamin K and B12, niacin, pyridoxine, and others [6]. They also function as the first line of defense in the digestive tract and participate in training of the developing immune system. Microflora take part in detoxification and in the modulation of the nervous system through the gut-brain axis [7–10].

In 2008, the National Institute of Health funded the Human Microbiome Project (HMP) to analyze the human microbiome and determine its role in human health and disease. As a result, the taxonomic distribution, prevalence, and abundance of microbial taxa that inhabit a healthy human body sites were codified [11]. The project concluded that the microbiome begins at birth, whether via Cesarean section or vaginal delivery. Unlike the human genome, the human microbiome does not appear to be passed down through generations, but may be genetically influenced. There is no evidence for a core microbiome either within an individual or within a population. However, 40% of the microbiome genes are shared by 50% of the population. It changes as an individual ages, but stays remarkably constant from childhood through middle adulthood. Bacterial cells appear in a 1:1 ratio with human cells. There is a very close association between the human microbiome and the external environment, including lifestyle factors. There is evidence for a close association and interaction between the mucosal immune system and the human microbiome. Antibiotic usage greatly affects the human microbiome on a low term or permanent basis through selection of resistant organisms, horizontal gene transfer, and by long-term alteration of the microbiota.

The human intestines contain more than 100 trillion microorganisms that maintain a symbiotic relationship with the host. The upper portion of the digestive tract has low quantities of bacteria, most of which are aerobes, while the lower portion of the gastrointestinal system contains high densities of microbes most of which are anaerobes. The quality and quantity of microflora and their metabolites are constantly altered by host dietary choices, stress, and antibiotic exposure, to name only a few.

Probiotics are used for the prevention, and in some instances, the treatment of specific diseases because appropriate probiotic therapy can optimize systemic and local immune system activity. Data specific to respiratory tract infections are relatively sparse, but point to potential benefits on duration and severity of illness. Most studies do not support a role for probiotic therapy as a preventive measure against respiratory tract infections. Since antibiotic administration often alters the gut microflora balance, there can be an important role for a course of probiotic therapy to prevent antibiotic-associated diarrhea, and the alteration of the microbiome.

Recent research is expanding toward disease-specific use of probiotics. Intestinal bacteria have been shown to participate in the regulation of psychological processes. Two studies from 2016 showed the importance of Lactobacillus and Bifidobacterium families in depression and anxiety [7, 8]. Lactobacillus species are shown to prevent diarrhea associated with antibiotics.

Bifidobacterium infantis has been successfully used in the treatment of irritable bowel syndrome. Clostridium difficile colitis is treated with Saccharomyces boulardii. Transfer of intestinal flora through fecal bacterial therapy from one individual to another was first studied in 1958. The cure rate for chronic and recurrent Clostridium difficile is 90% with fecal bacterial therapy. Studies have shown that Lactobacillus reuteri can accelerate gastric emptying time and decrease regurgitation episodes in infants. Bifidobacterium lactis has been found to decrease whole gut transit time in a dose-dependent fashion and also decrease functional gastrointestinal symptoms, including vomiting, regurgitation, abdominal pain, nausea, and gurgling. The above studies support the efficacy of probiotics in maintaining healthy gut microbiota with potential beneficial effects on LPR [12–20].

Manufacturers differ in their recommendations on how best to take probiotic therapy, but most agree that in order to minimize exposure to gastric acid, probiotic should be taken on an empty stomach. Some brands pasteurize products, which kills the bacteria. This unfortunately nullifies their medicinal powers, so it is crucial to find brands that are labeled raw or unpasteurized. Daily dosage for infants is 1–10 billion CFU and 10–20 billion CFU for older children and adults. Caution should be used when considering probiotic therapy in immunocompromised patients and premature infants.

Regularly consuming foods that support diverse microorganisms can be simple. Prebiotic and probiotic foods are becoming more widely available in supermarkets. Prebiotics are indigestible food components (dietary fibers) that support the growth of beneficial gut microbiota in the colon. Foods rich in prebiotics are onions, garlic, leeks, bananas, artichokes, soy beans, asparagus, and whole wheat foods. Fermented foods rich in probiotics include sauerkraut, miso, kombucha, kimchi, pickled vegetables, tempeh, and cultured dairy foods that contain live bacteria such as bifidobacteria and lactobacilli.

One of the most interesting new areas of research is the interplay of our environment, diet, and genetics to modulate the risk of common diseases. Interesting new research shows that healthy fat intake with increased mono and polyunsaturated fat and decreased saturated fat over 2 years partially restores a healthy gut microbiome in obese patients with coronary heart disease, depending on the degree of metabolic dysfunction [21]. Studies also suggest that genetically susceptible individuals develop intolerance to dysregulated gut microflora and chronic inflammation develops as a result of environmental triggers, resulting in inflammatory bowel disease. Nutritional interventions such as the Specific Carbohydrate Diet (SCD), the low fermentable oligosaccharides, disaccharides, monosaccharides, polyol (FODMAP) diet, and the Mediterranean diet have shown strong anti-inflammatory properties and great promise for improving disease symptoms in inflammatory bowel disease.

We have begun to rethink how we view the trillions of microorganisms that inhabit the human body. Instead of invaders, one can view the microbiota as part of a very efficient mutualistic ecosystem.

ENT Diseases

Laryngopharyngeal Reflux

Gastroesophageal Reflux Disease GERD and laryngopharyngeal reflux (LPR) are largely driven by our western lifestyle. Poor diet, being overweight, and chronic stress are all contributing factors. Dietary advice and proton pump inhibitors (PPIs) are the mainstream treatment plan. Unfortunately, prolonged PPI therapy can result in poor absorption of essential nutrients, including calcium, iron, magnesium, and vitamins [22]. Long-term use is associated with multiple diseases. PPIs double the rates of Clostridium difficile colitis and bacterial colonization with resistant microbes in intensive care unit settings. Chronic acid inhibition may lead to bacterial overgrowth of the stomach and proximal small intestine. Research shows that patients treated with PPIs carry an increased load of intragastric bacteria [23]. PPIs reduce gastric acidity and in fact current use of PPIs is associated with an increased risk of bacterial gastroenteritis [24]. PPIs are also associated with an increased risk of community-acquired pneumonia [25]. PPIs are one of the most frequent causes of drug-induced acute interstitial nephritis [26].

Other means to treat LPR are lifestyle modifications, diet, weight loss, exercise, positional sleep, and alternative treatments with herbal therapies. Most of these data are based on studies done for GERD. Multiple small meals throughout the day are preferred. The evening meal should be 3–6 hours before planned nighttime sleep. Avoidance of late meals has shown decreased gastric and esophageal acidity [27]. Koufman and colleagues showed the advantage of a strict low acid diet in PPI-resistant LPR patients [28]. This temporary two week long diet avoids foods with pH below 4 as well as chocolate, caffeine, citrus, and spicy and acidic foods.

Botanicals to assist the diet are demulcent herbs containing mucilaginous materials to directly coat and soothe the lining of the GI tract. They are ingested before meals in order to coat and protect the mucosa. Commonly used demulcent plants include aloe vera, marshmallow root, slippery elm root, and licorice root. Licorice root has long been used for gastric inflammation because of its muco-protective effect. The deglycyrrhizinated form of licorice is recommended (DGL) for long-term use to avoid side effects from its mineralocorticoid properties. DGL is taken in a chewable tablet before meals and at bedtime, dosage ranging from 700 to 1200 mg, with a maximum daily dose of 5000 mg. Another herbal product is Iberogast, which contains the following herbs: lemon balm, licorice, peppermint, chamomile flower, milk thistle, caraway, celandine, candytuft, and angelica root. It is fast acting and effectively relieves stomach pain, bloating, gas, heartburn, and diarrhea. It also increases gastric motility [29].

Melatonin increases blood flow and protects the gastric mucosa from free radicals in stress-induced ulcers and from damage caused by NSAIDs. It has an inhibitory action on the secretion of HCl and Pepsin. It can be used alone or in combination with omeprazole, whose healing effect it accelerates [30]. Daily dosing is between 3 and 6 mg.

Ginger is a well-known promotility agent and can be helpful in the aging population to ameliorate the slowing of gastric emptying that occurs with age. It can be taken 30 minutes prior to meals with a maximum dose of 1200 mg 3 times a day.

Oral Leukoplakia

Oral leukoplakia is a term that refers to white or grayish patches of skin in the mouth or tongue. Cause is not always known, but includes tobacco, alcohol, or other regular irritants.

Vitamin A has been shown to be effective in treating leukoplakia in an acute topical format [31]. There is evidence of its recurrence after cessation of treatment. Therefore, topical treatment should be supplemented with oral Vit A in capsule form in the short term and reorganization of diet to include daily intake of foods high in Vitamin A in order to maintain levels in the long term. There is also substantial evidence and no contraindication for the regular inclusion of black tea and turmeric in the diet [32, 33].

Once lesions have healed and Vitamin A containing foods have been included in the diet daily, capsules can be phased out. Monitoring of Vitamin A levels should take place at 1 month, 6 month, and 1 year past discontinuation of supplementation. After that, yearly testing is recommended for the next 5 years to ascertain that dietary changes have become habitual.

To bolster Vitamin A levels in diet, include foods from the “Animal” and “Vegetable” categories at least once a day and as often as possible from the “Fruit” and “Extra” categories [34].

1. Animal sources: Liver, eggs, milk, cheese, yogurt, and oily fish such as herring, mackerel, and salmon.
2. Vegetable sources: sweet potatoes, spinach, pumpkin, red pepper, broccoli, tomatoes, carrots, and all other dark green, red, orange, and yellow vegetables.
3. Fruit sources: cantaloupe, mangoes, apricots, papayas, mandarins, guavas, and other orange fruits.
4. Extra sources: black tea, turmeric, spirulina, cod liver oil.

Vitamin A supplementation is controversial in patients who use tobacco or alcohol as it may combine with these substances in an adverse manner and increase the likelihood of cancer and hepatotoxicity. Along with checking Vitamin A levels, signs of these complications should be monitored [35].

Aphthous Ulcers

Aphthous ulcers are whitish painful ulcerative lesions of the oral mucosa. Pathogenesis is not well understood. Possible causes include trauma to the local mucosa due to a variety of reasons including dental treatments, friction due to a broken tooth, vigorous brushing, and caustic foods and food additives such as cinnamon, citric acid, and acetic acid. Nutritional deficiencies can result in decreased resilience of the oral mucosa. Food allergies are another possible implication and worth investigation through an elimination diet if removal of irritants and vitamin supplementation doesn't resolve lesions.

Assessing possible local irritants is a logical first step. Helping the patient think through what comes in regular contact with their oral mucosa during their daily routine will help identify possible culprits. Citric acid is a common food additive found in flavored drinks, candies, and medications. Acetic acid is included in many dressings and condiments. Physical trauma due to sharp edges on teeth, dentures, overly vigorous dental hygiene should also be considered.

If levels of Vitamin B 12, folic acid, iron, or zinc are low, supplementation with these nutrients has shown great success in healing mucosal ulcers [36–42]. Returning these levels of nutrients to normal levels should start with suppplemetation, but more importantly, patients should be educated about their natural occurence in foods. Once ulcers have healed and the patient is confident in including these nutrients in their daily diet, supplements can be phased out. Check nutrient levels at 1 month, 2 month, and 6 months to ensure successful maintenance of proper levels to prevent recurrence.

Food sources of the nutrients discussed:

Vitamin B 12: liver, clams, sardines, beef, tuna, trout, nutritional yeast, milk, yogurt, cheese, eggs.

Folic acid: liver, green leafy vegetables, Brussels sprouts, kidney beans, chickpeas, lentils, asparagus, beets, broccoli, citrus fruits, wheat germ, papaya, avocado.

Iron: live mussels, oysters, beef, sardines, eggs, turkey, chicken, tuna, mackerel, leafy greens, broccoli, beans, and lentils.

Zinc: meat, shellfish, legumes, hemp seeds, pumpkin seeds, sesame seeds, cashews, milk, cheese.

The addition of Omega-3 oil supplements to the diet has also been shown to improve outcome [43–45].

The debate over whether Sodium Lauryl Sulfate (SLS) containing toothpastes contributes to the problem has been ongoing with studies falling on both sides of the arguments. Some scientists argue that regular use of this detergent denatures the oral mucin layer. A meta-analysis in 2019 concluded that the use of SLS-free toothpastes reduced the number of ulcers, duration of ulcer, number of episodes, and ulcer pain [46].

Herpes Simplex

Herpes simplex virus 1 (HSV-1) causes the oral blisters that scab in a characteristic manner and are commonly known as "cold sores." The WHO estimates that 67% of the world's population are infected with HSV-1. The virus is acquired when oral mucosa comes in contact with the virus. Once an infection is established, the virus moves into the central nervous system and resides in the trigeminal ganglion. Blisters recur when the virus reactivates and travels down the trigeminal nerve. Triggers include fever, sunburns, stress, and local trauma.

A correlation has been observed between dietary lysine/arginine ratio and herpes outbreaks. One study demonstrated that a person's serum lysine concentration needs to exceed 165 nmol/ml in order to achieve a decreased rate of recurrence [47]. A different study found that 1200 mg a day of L-Lysine monochloride decreased recurrence [48]. Tissue culture analysis performed as part of a third study reported that viral replication was enhanced when amino acid ratio of arginine/lysine favored arginine.

A practical approach to putting these findings to use includes Lysine supplementation starting with 1200 mg/day. Measuring serum concentrations at regular intervals will inform the patients on whether they are successful at maintaining the desirable minimum level of 65 nmol/ml. In addition to lysine supplementation, patient should be provided with a list of foods high in arginine and begin to decrease their consumption. The patient will also need a list of foods that are high in lysine and begin to increase their consumption. Once symptoms have not recurred for three months and the patient has successfully shifted their dietary amino acid consumption to favor lysine over arginine, begin to wean lysine supplements while continuing to monitor blood serum levels. The goal is a permanent shift in diet that maintains this advantageous ratio.

Foods high in lysine and low in arginine: yogurt, cheese, cottage cheese, cream cheese, milk, cream, papaya, mango, apricot, apple, pear, fig, avocado, salmon, swordfish, tuna, halibut, cod, tomato, beet, avocado, and turnip.

Vitamin C, aka ascorbic acid, has been shown to be of help both as a preventive measure taken internally and topically during an acute outbreak. In one study, blisters were treated with an ascorbic acid containing solution just three times in one day and achieved significant healing improvements [49]. Vitamin C has also been shown to decrease recurrence when taken orally for prophylaxis at 1000 mg twice a day [50]. Here again the goal is to make this a regular part of the patient's diet. Starting out with Vitamin C capsules is a good place to begin, but it is preferable to shift the diet to include the foods which naturally provide this nutrient.

Foods high in Vitamin C: citrus fruits, peppers, strawberries, kale, kiwis, broccoli, persimmons, papayas, brussels sprouts, tomatoes, and peas. Acerola cherry and Camu powders mixed with water, juice, or yogurt are a great whole foods option to boost daily Vitamin C consumption.

When considering topical treatment for an acute outbreak of blisters, place Melissa Officinalis, aka Lemonbalm, on top of the list. Numerous articles have sung its praise in inhibiting virus replication and attachment to host cells [51].

Herpes Zoster

Herpes zoster and its sequelae, postherpetic neuralgia (PHN), cause significant discomfort for our population over 50. Thankfully, there are several easy and inexpensive approaches both for preventing outbreaks as well as managing the pain of acute flare-ups. When the varicella zoster virus living in the body is reactivated, it can cause painful blisters. When the pain lingers for long periods of time after the blisters have healed, it is termed postherpetic pain.

Recent research has demonstrated that inflammation can stimulate pain receptors and the reactive oxygen species (ROS), the free radical produced during this process, accumulate to produce further pain. Vitamin C has been shown to have an analgesic effect on this pain [52] and to successfully prevent PHN [53, 54]. Patients with HZ with low levels of Vitamin C can start by taking Vitamin C capsules to raise their levels into the normal range. The eventual goal is to include Vitamin C containing foods in the diet on a daily basis. Foods high in Vitamin C: citrus fruits, peppers, strawberries, kale, kiwis, broccoli, persimmons, papayas, brussels sprouts, tomatoes, and peas. Acerola cherry and Camu powders mixed with water, juice, or yogurt are a great whole foods option to boost daily Vitamin C consumption.

Vitamin D supplementation for preventing HZ reactivation is being examined, but has not been thoroughly substantiated. Two studies have shown that patients with low Vitamin D levels are more likely to experience reactivation of Herpes Zoster [55, 56]. Several other studies have examined the association between Vitamin D levels and HZ reactivation as well as the effect of Vitamin D supplementation on HZ, but the results are inconclusive at this point. Considering the importance of Vitamin D for many aspects of health, it is a worthwhile effort to check levels and bring them within the normal range. To raise Vitamin D levels, patients may start with capsules, but in the long term the best approach is to include high Vitamin D foods in their daily diet and regular sun exposure in small doses without sunburns. Foods that naturally contain high levels of Vitamin D are fatty fish such as salmon (wild caught is substantially better than farmed), sardines and herring, and egg yolks from chicken raised in the pasture. Cod liver oil is a traditional supplement that contains ample Vitamin D. Monitor levels monthly while the patient gets used to including these foods in their regular diet.

Xerostomia

Xerostomia is a medical term to describe the condition when the salivary glands do not produce enough saliva to keep the mouth properly moisturized. A bit of detective work will go a long way, as proper treatment will depend on identifying the root cause. Common causes range from medications' side effects and radiation therapy's side effects to mouth breathing and aging.

Zinc deficiency has been associated with xerostomia in several studies [57]. Zinc supplementation can relieve symptoms of xerostomia [58]. Zinc deficiency can be resolved by a regular intake of foods with significant zinc content. Foods with notable zinc content, with one serving covering at least 20% of daily intake, are: oysters, beef, crab, lobster, pork, baked beans, and pumpkin seeds. Beans and grains contain valuable amounts of zinc, but the phytic acid content makes their bioavailability low. Many traditional cultures soak and even sprout their grains and legumes prior to cooking. Modern studies have shown that these practices increase the bioavailability of micronutrients including zinc. Zinc nutritional status can be difficult to ascertain because laboratory tests measuring serum zinc levels do not reflect cellular zinc availability. If zinc deficiency is suspected based on clinical symptoms and a review of diet, it is a prudent choice to consider supplementation. If supplementation shows a positive response, then restructuring the diet to increase regular intake through food will provide a long-term resolution to the symptoms of xerostomia.

Mouth breathing is a common cause of xerostomia that can be resolved with some work on the patient's part. Mouth breathing is associated with a variety of health detriments including abnormal dental development, sleep disturbance, snoring, sleep apnea, tooth decay, halitosis, and cardiovascular disease [59]. Chronic mouth breathers are missing out on the many health benefits of nitric oxide (NO) produced in the sinuses, including improved arterial oxygenation and antiviral properties [60]. While most people naturally breathe through their nose while at rest, many do not realize that they breathe through their mouth while talking, exercising, and sleeping. The nitric oxide produced in the sinuses is brought down into the lungs during breathing and has a significant contribution to the levels of NO in the respiratory tract. Nasal breathing reduces respiratory tract infections by filtering the air before it travels further into the respiratory tract and also by treating it with NO which has antiviral properties [61]. Switching from mouth breathing to nasal breathing requires self-observation and dedication on part of the patient. Changing breathing habits during talking means slowing down and developing awareness of how one breathes between sentences.

At first, patients may feel out of breath when making the switch to nasal breathing and worry that they are not getting enough oxygen. Observing blood oxygen levels via a fingertip oximeter found in most pharmacies can help calm these concerns. Making the switch to nasal breathing during sleep can be a bit more challenging. There are many aids to help with this process on the market. Patients can find specially made tape and headbands designed to help the mouth stay closed while sleeping. Special tape and plugs are also available to help keep nostrils open and improve airflow while laying down.

Radiation therapy for head and neck cancers can cause mucositis as well as xerostomia. We cannot remove the cause of these symptoms, but we can ameliorate the side effects in several ways. Turmeric, aloe vera, ginger, and honey have all been shown to prevent and reduce the severity of radiation-induced mucositis [62–68].

Melatonin is commonly known for its effects on regulating circadian and seasonal rhythms. Scientists are discovering that its benefits are far wider reaching to include modulation of the immune system [69], radio protection, radio sensitization of cancer cells, and general anti-inflammatory [70, 71] and antioxidant properties [72]. Melatonin's radio protective effects have been thoroughly documented in animal models. For example, Fernandez-Gil et al. [70] demonstrated that melatonin protects the small intestines from toxic products formed during radiation of the oral mucosa. In their study they used a 3% melatonin gel applied to the oral cavity which protected the rat's small intestine from the significant oxidative damage that otherwise resulted from the oral radiation they received.

There isn't much research data in this area using human subjects. In 1998, Vijayalaxmi et al. published a study in which the radio protective effects of orally administered melatonin on human lymphocytes were documented. Subjects received 300 mg of melatonin orally and their blood was collected 1 and 2 hours later. The blood samples were exposed to 1Gy of gamma radiation and the lymphocytes were examined for DNA damage. The samples showed an increase in melatonin both 1 and 2 hours after supplementation as compared to the samples taken before supplementation and DNA damage was reduced in the samples taken after supplementation. In 2020, Jarosław et al. published a study in which patients undergoing radiation therapy for breast cancer were allocated to a melatonin emulsion or placebo group. The results showed that patients who received the melatonin emulsion experienced reduced radiation dermatitis compared to the placebo group. It is worth noting here that melatonin has also been shown to possess the ability to radiosensitize cancer cells while protecting healthy ones.

Melatonin is used for a variety of conditions and has a very good safety profile. A possible schedule for taking melatonin to protect oral mucosa during radiation could look like this: The night before radiation treatment take 5 milligrams. On the day of treatment take 5 mg 1 hour before radiation. For the two weeks following treatment take 10 milligrams each night. Always dissolve the contents of the capsule (or crush tablet) in 2 tablespoons of water. Swish around the mouth for 2 minutes, then gargle and swallow.

Vertigo and Meniere's Disease

Many practitioners have observed that vertigo is a common symptom of reactive hypoglycemia and insulin resistance is common in patients with Meniere's disease. Consumption of a diet designed to improve glucose metabolism and insulin sensitivity results in improvement of the symptoms.

Patients with Meniere's disease are typically advised to avoid caffeine, nicotine, and alcohol. Conventional treatment may include reduction of fluid levels in the body with a low sodium diet (1.5 g a day) and diuretics given for the same reason. Natural diuretics such as dandelion can also be used.

Both food and inhalant allergies are found to be an important factor or at least a contributing factor in some patients with vertigo. Food allergies are implicated more often than inhalants.

Nutritional supplementation with lipoflavinoids has been shown to decrease microvascular permeability; these flavonoids might therefore decrease excessive secretion of endolymph. Vitamin B6, Niacin, and Thiamine are frequently used as supplementation. Vitamin B6 works by increasing the secretion of gamma-aminobutyric acid. Niacin is believed to work by promoting the dilatation of labyrinthine blood vessels.

Otitis Media and Sinusitis

Infections (viral, bacterial, or fungal) and allergies are the most common causes of sinusitis and otitis media. Otitis media is one of the most common health problems in children. The cause of otitis media is unclear, but it is frequently associated with eustachian tube dysfunction. Similarly, sinusitis will develop when the normal drainage passageway of the sinuses is obstructed either by inflammation or by anatomical abnormalities.

Dietary factors in both cases are related to the consumption of large amounts of refined sugar and have been shown to impair immune function. Ingestion of 100 g of sucrose, fructose, or glucose caused a transient decrease in the ability of neutrophils to phagocytose bacteria [73].

Food and environmental allergies can both be contributing factors of sinusitis. The swelling of the nasal mucosa caused by the underlying allergy will obstruct the drainage pathway. As a result of inflammation and from the suppression of immune function driven by the allergic reaction, sinusitis will develop more often. Food allergy is a common factor in children who suffer from recurrent otitis media, but inhalational allergies can also contribute. Desensitization therapy has been successful in some children [74–76]. In a high proportion of cases, identification and avoidance of allergenic foods resulted in improvement and resolution of chronic middle ear fluid retention [77–79]. Elimination diet for food allergies is the first step and immunotherapy for the environmental allergies advised.

Nutritional supplements such as Vitamin C, D, and A should be considered; Vit D levels should be checked to guide dosing. Vitamin A is especially important as it plays a role in immune function and helps with the integrity of epithelial tissue including the mucous membrane of the respiratory tract. Another treatment option is Serratia peptidase, a proteolytic enzyme with fibrinolytic and anti-inflammatory activities, thus reducing the viscosity of exudates, facilitating drainage [80].

References

1. Tosti V, Bertozzi B, Fontana L. Health benefits of the Mediterranean diet: metabolic and molecular mechanisms. J Gerontol A Biol Sci Med Sci. 2018 Mar;73(3):318–26.
2. Mazzocchi A, Leone L, Agostoni C, Pali-Schöll I. The secrets of the Mediterranean diet. Does [only] olive oil matter? Nutrients. 2019;11(12):2941. https://doi.org/10.3390/nu11122941. https://www.ncbi.nlm.nih.gov/pmc/articles/PMC6949890/
3. Wu SH, Shu XO, Chow WH, Xiang YB, Zhang X, Li HL, et al. Soy food intake and circulating levels of inflammatory markers in Chinese women. J Acad Nutr Diet. 2012;112(7):996–1004.
4. Muszyńska B, Grzywacz-Kisielewska A, Kała K, Gdula-Argasińska J. Anti-inflammatory properties of edible mushrooms: a review. Food Chem. 2018;243:373–81.
5. Dai X, Stanilka JM, Rowe CA, Esteves EA, Nieves C, Spaiser SJ, et al. Consuming Lentinula edodes (Shiitake) mushrooms daily improves human immunity: a randomized dietary intervention in healthy young adults. J Am Coll Nutr. 2015;34(6):478–87. https://doi.org/10.1080/07315724.2014.950391. https://pubmed.ncbi.nlm.nih.gov/25866155/
6. LeBlanc JG, Milani C, de Giori GS, Sesma F, van Sinderen D, Ventura M. Bacteria as vitamin suppliers to their host: a gut microbiota perspective. Curr Opin Biotechnol. 2013;24(2):160–8. http://www.ncbi.nlm.nih.gov/pubmed/22940212

7. Sarkar A, Lehto SM, Harty S, Dinan TG, Cryan JF, Burnet PW. Psychobiotics and the manipulation of bacteria-gut-brain signals. Trends Neurosci. 2016;39(11):763–81. http://www.ncbi.nlm.nih.gov/pubmed/27793434
8. Sherwin E, Sandhu KV, Dinan TG, Cryan JF. May the force be with you: the light and dark sides of the microbiota-gut-brain axis in neuropsychiatry. CNS Drugs. 2016;30(11):1019–41. http://www.ncbi.nlm.nih.gov/pubmed/27417321
9. Rhee SH, Pothoulakis C, Mayer EA. Principles and clinical implications of the brain-gut-enteric microbiota axis. Nat Rev Gastroenterol Hepatol. 2009;6(5):306–14. http://www.ncbi.nlm.nih.gov/pubmed/19404271
10. Foster JA, McVey Neufeld K-A. Gut-brain axis: how the microbiome influences anxiety and depression. Trends Neurosci. 2013;36(5):305–12. http://www.ncbi.nlm.nih.gov/pubmed/23384445
11. Belizário JE, Napolitano M. Human microbiomes and their roles in dysbiosis, common diseases, and novel therapeutic approaches. Front Microbiol. 2015;6:1050. https://www.frontiersin.org/articles/10.3389/fmicb.2015.01050/full
12. Hempel S, Newberry SJ, Maher AR, Wang Z, Miles JN, et al. Probiotics for the prevention and treatment of antibiotic-associated diarrhea. JAMA. 2012;307(18):1959–69. http://www.ncbi.nlm.nih.gov/pubmed/22570464
13. Yuan F, Ni H, Asche CV, Kim M, Walayat S, Ren J. Efficacy of *Bifidobacterium infantis 35624* in patients with irritable bowel syndrome: a meta-analysis. Curr Med Res Opin. 2017;33(7):1191–7. http://www.ncbi.nlm.nih.gov/pubmed/28166427
14. Aroniadis OC, Brandt LJ, Greenberg A, Borody T, Kelly CR, Mellow M, et al. Long-term follow-up study of fecal microbiota transplantation for severe and/or complicated clostridium difficile infection. J Clin Gastroenterol. 2015;50(5):398–402. http://www.ncbi.nlm.nih.gov/pubmed/26125460
15. Francavilla R, Miniello V, Magista AM, De Canio A, Bucci N, Gagliardi F, et al. A randomized controlled trial of lactobacillus GG in children with functional abdominal pain. Pediatrics. 2010;126(6):e1445–52. http://www.ncbi.nlm.nih.gov/pubmed/21078735
16. Ait-Belgnaoui A, Durand H, Cartier C, Chaumaz G, Eutamene H, Ferrier L, et al. Prevention of gut leakiness by a probiotic treatment leads to attenuated HPA response to an acute psychological stress in rats. Psychoneuroendocrinology. 2012;37(11):1885–95. http://linkinghub.elsevier.com/retrieve/pii/S0306453012001291
17. Qin H-L, Shen T-Y, Gao Z-G, Fan X-B, Hang X-M, Jiang Y-Q, et al. Effect of lactobacillus on the gut microflora and barrier function of the rats with abdominal infection. World J Gastroenterol. 2005;11(17):2591–6. http://www.ncbi.nlm.nih.gov/pubmed/15849817
18. Indrio F, Riezzo G, Raimondi F, Bisceglia M, Filannino A, Cavallo L, et al. Lactobacillus reuteri accelerates gastric emptying and improves regurgitation in infants. Eur J Clin Invest. 2011;41(4):417–22. https://doi.org/10.1111/j.1365-2362.2010.02425.x.
19. Garofoli F, Civardi E, Indrio F, Mazzucchelli I, Angelini M, Tinelli C, et al. The early administration of lactobacillus reuteri DSM 17938 controls regurgitation episodes in full-term breastfed infants. Int J Food Sci Nutr. 2014;65(5):646–8. https://doi.org/10.3109/09637486.2014.898251.
20. Waller PA, Gopal PK, Leyer GJ, Ouwehand AC, Reifer C, Stewart ME, et al. Dose-response effect of Bifidobacterium lactis HN019 on whole gut transit time and functional gastrointestinal symptoms in adults. Scand J Gastroenterol. 2011;46(9):1057–64. https://doi.org/10.3109/00365521.2011.584895.
21. Haro C, García-Carpintero S, Rangel-Zúñiga OA, Alcalá-Díaz JF, Landa BB, Clemente JC, et al. Consumption of two healthy dietary patterns restores microbiota dysbiosis in obese patients with metabolic dysfunction. Mol Nutr Food Res. 2017;61(12):1700300.
22. Malfertheiner P, Megraud F, O'Morain C, Bazzoli F, El-Omar E, Graham D, Hunt R, Rokkas T, Vakil N, Kulpers EJ. Current concepts in the management of helicobacter pylori infection: the Maastricht III consensus report. Gut. 2007;56(6):772–81.
23. Gregor JC. Acid suppression and pneumonia: a clinical indication for rational prescribing. JAMA. 2004;292(16):2012–3.
24. Hassing RJ, Verbon A, de Visser H, Hofman A, Stricker BH. Proton pump inhibitors and gastroenteritis. Eur J Epidemiol. 2016;31(10):1057–63. https://www.ncbi.nlm.nih.gov/pmc/articles/PMC5065595/

25. Zedtwitz-Liebenstein K, Wenisch C, Patruta S, Parschalk B, Daxbock F, Graninger W. Omeprazole treatment diminishes intra- and extracellular neutrophil reactive oxygen production and bactericidal activity. Crit Care Med. 2002;30(5):1118–22.
26. Sierra F, Suarez M, Rey M, Vela MF. Systematic review: proton pump inhibitor-associated acute interstitial nephritis. Aliment Pharmacol Ther. 2007;26(4):545–53.
27. Duroux P, Bauerfeind P, Emde C, Koelz HR, Blum AL. Early dinner reduces nocturnal gastric acidity. Gut. 1989;30(8):1063–7.
28. Koufman JA. Low-acid diet for recalcitrant laryngopharyngeal reflux: therapeutic benefits and their implications. Ann Otol Rhinol Laryngol. 2011;120(5):281–7.
29. Pilichiewicz AN, Horowitz M, Russo A, Maddox AF, Jones KL, Schemann M, et al. Effects of Iberogast on proximal gastric volume, antropyloroduodenal motility and gastric emptying in healthy men. Am J Gastroenterol. 2007;102(6):1276–83. https://doi.org/10.1111/j.1572-0241.2007.01142.x.
30. Kandil TS, Mousa AA, El-Gendy AA, Abbas AM. The potential therapeutic effect of melatonin in gastro-esophageal reflux disease. BMC Gastroenterol. 2010;10(1):7. https://doi.org/10.1186/1471-230X-10-7.
31. Gorsky M, Epstein JB. The effect of retinoids on premalignant oral lesions: focus on topical therapy. Cancer. 2002;95(6):1258–64.
32. Halder A, Raychowdhury R, Ghosh A, De M. Black tea (Camellia sinensis) as a chemopreventive agent in oral precancerous lesions. J Environ Pathol Toxicol Oncol. 2005;24(2):141–4.
33. Rai B, Kaur J, Reinhilde J, Singh J. Possible action mechanism for curcumin in pre-cancerous lesions based on serum and salivary markers of oxidative stress. J Oral Sci. 2010;52(2):251–6. https://www.jstage.jst.go.jp/article/josnusd/52/2/52_2_251/_article
34. Winn DM. Diet and nutrition in the etiology of oral cancer. Am J Clin Nutr. 1995;61(2):437S–45S.
35. Leo MA, Lieber CS. Alcohol, vitamin A, and beta-carotene: adverse interactions, including hepatotoxicity and carcinogenicity. Am J Clin Nutr. 1999 Jun;69(6):1071–85.
36. Kozlak ST, Walsh SJ, Lalla RV. Reduced dietary intake of vitamin B12 and folate in patients with recurrent aphthous stomatitis. J Oral Pathol Med. 2010;39(5):420–3.
37. Volkov I, Rudoy I, Freud T, Sardal G, Naimer S, Peleg R, et al. Effectiveness of vitamin B12 in treating recurrent aphthous stomatitis: a randomized, double-blind, placebo-controlled trial. J Am Board Fam Med. 2009;22(1):9–16.
38. Sun A, Chen HM, Cheng SJ, Wang YP, Chang JY, Wu YC, Chiang CP. Significant association of deficiencies of hemoglobin, iron, vitamin B12, and folic acid and high homocysteine level with recurrent aphthous stomatitis. J Oral Pathol Med. 2015;44(4):300–5.
39. Yıldırımyan N, Özalp Ö, Şatır S, Altay MA, Sinder A. Recurrent aphthous stomatitis as a result of zinc deficiency. Oral Health Prev Dent. 2019;17(5):465–8.
40. Chiang CP, Chang JY, Wang YP, Wu YH, Wu YC, Sun A. Recurrent aphthous stomatitis–etiology, serum autoantibodies, anemia, hematinic deficiencies, and management. J Formos Med Assoc. 2019;118(9):1279–89.
41. Chen H, Sui Q, Chen Y, Ge L, Lin M. Impact of haematologic deficiencies on recurrent aphthous ulceration: a meta-analysis. Br Dent J. 2015;218(4):E8. https://doi.org/10.1038/sj.bdj.2015.100. https://www.nature.com/articles/sj.bdj.2015.100
42. Ozler GS. Zinc deficiency in patients with recurrent aphthous stomatitis: a pilot study. J Laryngol Otol. 2014;128(6):531–3. https://doi.org/10.1017/S0022215114001078. https://pubmed.ncbi.nlm.nih.gov/24849699/
43. Hadian Z, Moghadamnia AA, Kazemi S, Shirzad A. Effect of omega-3 on recurrent aphthous stomatitis and improvement quality of life. Int J Dent. 2021;2021:6617575. https://doi.org/10.1155/2021/6617575. https://pubmed.ncbi.nlm.nih.gov/33628246/
44. Nosratzehi T, Akar A. Efficacy of omega-3 in treatment of recurrent aphthous stomatitis; a randomised, double-blind, placebo-controlled study. Chin J Dent Res. 2016;19(3):159–64. https://doi.org/10.3290/j/cjdr.a36681. https://pubmed.ncbi.nlm.nih.gov/27622219/
45. El Khouli AM, El-Gendy EA. Efficacy of omega-3 in treatment of recurrent aphthous stomatitis and improvement of quality of life: a randomized, double-blind, placebo-controlled study.

Oral Surg Oral Med Oral Pathol Oral Radiol. 2013;117(2):191–6. https://doi.org/10.1016/j.oooo.2013.09.003. https://www.oooojournal.net/article/S2212-4403(13)00484-7/fulltext
46. Alli BY, Erinoso OA, Olawuyi AB. Effect of sodium lauryl sulfate on recurrent aphthous stomatitis: a systematic review. J Oral Pathol Med. 2019;48(5):358–64. https://doi.org/10.1111/jop.12845. https://pubmed.ncbi.nlm.nih.gov/30839136/
47. Thein DJ, Hurt WC. Lysine as a prophylactic agent in the treatment of recurrent herpes simplex labialis. Oral Surg Oral Med Oral Pathol. 1984;58(6):659–66.
48. McCune MA, Perry HO, Muller SA, O'Fallon WM. Treatment of recurrent herpes simplex infections with L-lysine monohydrochloride. Cutis. 1984 Oct;34(4):366–73.
49. Hovi T, Hirvimies A, Stenvik M, Vuola E, Pippuri R. Topical treatment of recurrent mucocutaneous herpes with ascorbic acid-containing solution. Antivir Res. 1995;27(3):263–70.
50. Kim GN, Yoo WS, Park MH, Chung JK, Han YS, Chung IY, et al. Clinical features of herpes simplex keratitis in a Korean tertiary referral center: Efficacy of oral antiviral and ascorbic acid on recurrence. Korean J Ophthalmol. 2018;32(5):353–60. https://doi.org/10.3341/kjo.2017.0131. https://pubmed.ncbi.nlm.nih.gov/30311457/
51. Schnitzler P, Schuhmacher A, Astani A, Reichling J. Melissa officinalis oil affects infectivity of enveloped herpesviruses. Phytomedicine. 2008;15(9):734–40. https://doi.org/10.1016/j.phymed.2008.04.018. https://pubmed.ncbi.nlm.nih.gov/18693101/
52. Carr AC, McCall C. The role of vitamin C in the treatment of pain: new insights. J Transl Med. 2017;15(1):77. https://doi.org/10.1186/s12967-017-1179-7. https://www.ncbi.nlm.nih.gov/pmc/articles/PMC5391567/
53. Chen JY, Chu CC, Lin YS, So EC, Shieh JP, Hu ML. Nutrient deficiencies as a risk factor in Taiwanese patients with postherpetic neuralgia. Br J Nutr. 2011;106(5):700–7. https://doi.org/10.1017/S0007114511000481. https://pubmed.ncbi.nlm.nih.gov/21473799/
54. Wang K, Jiang H, Li W, Qiang M, Dong T, Li H. Role of vitamin C in skin diseases. Front Physiol. 2018;9:819. https://doi.org/10.3389/fphys.2018.00819. https://pubmed.ncbi.nlm.nih.gov/30022952/
55. Chao CT, Lee SY, Yang WS, Yen CJ, Chiang CK, Huang JW, et al. Serum vitamin D levels are positively associated with varicella zoster immunity in chronic dialysis patients. Sci Rep. 2014;4:7371. https://doi.org/10.1038/srep07371. https://pubmed.ncbi.nlm.nih.gov/25487609/
56. Chao CT, Lai CF, Huang JW. Risk factors for herpes zoster reactivation in maintenance hemodialysis patients. Eur J Intern Med. 2012;23(8):711–5. https://doi.org/10.1016/j.ejim.2012.08.005. https://pubmed.ncbi.nlm.nih.gov/22958951/
57. Bao Z-X, Yang X-W, Shi J, Liu L-X. Serum zinc levels in 368 patients with oral mucosal diseases: a preliminary study. Med Oral Patol Oral Cir Bucal. 2016;21(3):335–40. https://doi.org/10.4317/medoral.21079. https://pubmed.ncbi.nlm.nih.gov/27031065/
58. Arbabi-Kalati F, Arbabi-Kalati F, Deghatipour M, Moghadam AA. Evaluation of the efficacy of zinc sulfate in the prevention of chemotherapy-induced mucositis: a double-blind randomized clinical trial. Arch Iran Med. 2012;15(7):413–7. https://pubmed.ncbi.nlm.nih.gov/22724877/
59. Jefferson Y. Mouth breathing: adverse effects on facial growth, health, academics, and behavior. Gen Dent. 2010;58(1):18–25.
60. Lundberg JO, Settergren G, Gelinder S, Lundberg JM, Alving K, Weitzberg E. Inhalation of nasally derived nitric oxide modulates pulmonary function in humans. Acta Physiol Scand. 1996;158(4):343–7.
61. Kukwa W, Guilleminault C, Tomaszewska M, Kukwa A, Krzeski A, Migacz E. Prevalence of upper respiratory tract infections in habitually snoring and mouth breathing children. Int J Pediatr Otorhinolaryngol. 2018;107:37–41. https://doi.org/10.1016/j.ijporl.2018.01.022. https://pubmed.ncbi.nlm.nih.gov/29501308/
62. Shah S, Rath H, Sharma G, Senapati SN, Mishra E. Effectiveness of curcumin mouthwash on radiation-induced oral mucositis among head and neck cancer patients: A triple-blind, pilot randomised controlled trial. Indian J Dent Res. 2020;31(5):718–27. https://doi.org/10.4103/ijdr.IJDR_822_18. https://pubmed.ncbi.nlm.nih.gov/33433509/

63. Arun P, Sagayaraj A, Mohiyuddin SM, Santosh D. Role of turmeric extract in minimising mucositis in patients receiving radiotherapy for head and neck squamous cell cancer: a randomised, placebo-controlled trial. J Laryngol Otol. 2020:1–6. https://doi.org/10.1017/S0022215120000316. https://pubmed.ncbi.nlm.nih.gov/32029014/
64. Sahebjamee M, Mansourian A, Hajimirzamohammad M, Zadeh MT, Bekhradi R, Kazemian A, Manifar S, Ashnagar S, Doroudgar K. Comparative efficacy of aloe vera and benzydamine mouthwashes on radiation-induced oral mucositis: a triple-blind, randomised, controlled clinical trial. Oral Health Prev Dent. 2015;13(4):309–15.
65. Nair GR, Naidu GS, Jain S, Nagi R, Makkad RS, Jha A. Clinical effectiveness of aloe vera in the management of oral mucosal diseases: a systematic review. J Clin Diagn Res. 2016;10(8):ZE01–7. https://doi.org/10.7860/JCDR/2016/18142.8222. https://pubmed.ncbi.nlm.nih.gov/27656587/
66. Szejk M, Kołodziejczyk-Czepas J, Żbikowska HM. Radioprotectors in radiotherapy-advances in the potential application of phytochemicals. Postepy Hig Med Dosw. 2016;70(0):722–34. https://doi.org/10.5604/17322693.1208039. https://pubmed.ncbi.nlm.nih.gov/27356603/
67. Jayalekshmi JL, Lakshmi R, Mukerji A. Honey on oral mucositis: a randomized controlled trial. Gulf J Oncolog. 2016;1(20):30–7.
68. Khanal B, Baliga M, Uppal N. Effect of topical honey on limitation of radiation-induced oral mucositis: an intervention study. Int J Oral Maxillofac Surg. 2010;39(12):1181–5.
69. Morteazee K, Potes Y, Mirtavoos-Mahyari H, Motevaseli E, Shabeeb D, Musa AE, et al. Boosting immune system against cancer by melatonin: a mechanistic viewpoint. Life Sci. 2019;238:116960. https://doi.org/10.1016/j.lfs.2019.116960. https://pubmed.ncbi.nlm.nih.gov/31629760/
70. Carrascal L, Nunez-Abades P, Ayala A, Cano M. Role of melatonin in the inflammatory process and its therapeutic potential. Curr Pharm Des. 2018;24(14):1563–88.
71. Hardeland R. Aging, melatonin, and the pro- and anti-inflammatory networks. Int J Mol Sci. 2019;20(5):1223. https://doi.org/10.3390/ijms20051223. https://www.ncbi.nlm.nih.gov/pmc/articles/PMC6429360/
72. Zhang HM, Zhang Y. Melatonin: a well-documented antioxidant with conditional pro-oxidant actions. J Pineal Res. 2014;57(2):131–46.
73. Sanchez A, Reeser JL, Lau HS, Yahiku PY, Willard RE, McMillan PJ, et al. Role of sugars in human neutrophilic phagocytosis. Am J Clin Nutr. 1973;26(11):1180–4.
74. Viscomi GJ. Allergic secretory otitis media: an approach to management. Laryngoscope. 1975;85(4):751–8.
75. McMahan JT, Calenoff E, Croft DJ, Barenholtz L, Weber LD. Chronic otitis media with effusion and allergy: modified RAST analysis of 119 cases. Otolaryngol Head Neck Surg. 1981;89(3):427–31.
76. Whitcomb NJ. Allergy therapy in serous otitis media associated with allergic rhinitis. Ann Allergy. 1965;23:232–6.
77. Noun LJ. Chronic otorrhea due to food sensitivity. J Allergy. 1942;14:82–6.
78. Ruokonen J, Paganus A, Lehti H. Elimination diets in the treatment of secretory otitis media. Int J Pediatr Otorhinolaryngol. 1982;4(1):39–46.
79. Nsouli TM, Nsouli SM, Linde RE, O'Mara F, Scanlon RT, Bellanti JA, et al. Role of food allergy in serous otitis media. Ann Allergy. 1994;73(3):215–9.
80. Mazzone A, Catalani M, Costanzo M, Drusian A, Mandoli A, Russo S, Guarini E, Vesperini G. Evaluation of Serratia peptidase in acute or chronic inflammation of otorhinolaryngology pathology: a multicentre, double-blind, randomized trial versus placebo. J Int Med Res. 1990;18(5):379–88.

Functional Medicine in the Pediatric Otolaryngology Patient

24

Steven Engebretsen, Dustin Jones, and Nathan J. Gonik

Introduction

Pediatric otolaryngology complaints are common among visits to pediatricians. Overall, ear nose, and throat-related concerns account for up to 50% of outpatient visits in children [1]. The symptoms are often significant and can range from acute infection or feeding disruptions to respiratory difficulty. Parental concerns often reach beyond the acute presentation to questions focused on long-term outcomes. Will my child develop normal speech? Is my child going to stop breathing one night? Do we need hearing aids? Will my child need to be on antibiotics forever? As Otolaryngologists taking care of children, we are charged with caring for several vital organ systems that can impact a child's well-being and impact their long-term development.

Traditionally, we have focused on treating symptoms as they present. Our guidelines are designed to guide the care of our management of presenting symptoms with definitive management. If a child has sinusitis symptoms for more than 10 days or has worsening symptoms—treat with antibiotics [2, 3]. A child that has more

S. Engebretsen (✉)
Michigan State University College of Osteopathic Medicine, East Lansing, MI, USA

Detroit Medical Center Department of Otolaryngology, Detroit, MI, USA
e-mail: Sengebre@dmc.org

D. Jones
Michigan State University College of Osteopathic Medicine, East Lansing, MI, USA

Miami Valley Hospital Department of Otolaryngology, Dayton, Ohio, USA

N. J. Gonik
Department Otolaryngology Head and Neck Surgery, Wayne State University School of Medicine, Detroit, MI, USA

Children's Hospital of Michigan, Detroit, MI, USA

© The Author(s), under exclusive license to Springer Nature Switzerland AG 2023

B. W. Blakley, J. E. Blakley (eds.), *Functional Illness of the Head and Neck*,
https://doi.org/10.1007/978-3-031-12998-8_24

than seven tonsil infections in a year should undergo tonsillectomy [4]. Conventional medicine trains us to look for a morphological change [5]. And that is necessary. However, more often than not, presentations fall between the focus of guideline action statements. Or, after treating a disease process a child returns with recurrent symptoms. We acknowledge predisposing factors in our histories and our literature but rarely address them. Daycare attendance, pacifier use, tobacco exposure, allergies, nutritional deficiencies, socioeconomic status, and many other factors are often considered but rarely focus our clinical attention.

A functional medicine approach requires the clinician to look beyond a single diagnosis and address the factors that lead to disease. While this may seem like a new age approach, it is rooted in the bedrock of the vocation of medicine. Dr. William Osler in his lectures on the history of medicine attributed the following to Hippocrates: "Each disease has its own nature, and that no one arises without a natural cause" [6]. Understanding the nature and cause of a disease is the key to preventing progression and inviting resolution.

Functional Medicine Pediatric Otolaryngology

Functional medicine (FM) is a moniker often commingled with other terms like Complementary and Alternative Medicine. While FM practitioners will often utilize complementary treatment options, like acupuncture, osteopathic manipulation, or homeopathy, those interventions along with standard allopathic care are simply methods of addressing bodily dysfunction. As described by the Institute of Functional Medicine, FM starts with the standard of care and adds new strategies and tools, from evidence-based medicine, to find the root cause of conditions [7].

As a field, pediatric otolaryngology requires this type of approach. There is an interplay between the most common pediatric head and neck ailments. Gastroesophageal reflux (GER) generally coexists with laryngomalacia and swallowing disorders. Otitis media is often associated with GER disease (GERD) and in some cases may be triggered by allergy. Further, it is well established that treating adenotonsillar hypertrophy may improve other conditions varying from asthma to sleep apnea or eustachian tube dysfunction [3]. Searching for the common risk factors and addressing underlying predispositions allow the clinician to treat multiple disease processes at once and blunt the progression of chronic disease states. At the core of the FM approach is a focus on genetic, environmental, and lifestyle factors that increase susceptibility to disease. It is helpful to think in terms of the Functional Medicine Tree [7]. While the otolaryngologist is often included in one of the distal branches, the best outcomes are achieved when we look down towards the roots and address the antecedents, mediators, and triggers that predated symptoms. The rest of this chapter will focus on evidence-based approaches and current trends in our field that incorporate these philosophies.

Multidisciplinary Care of Pediatric Patients

A widespread trend within the field of Pediatric Otolaryngology that embraces aspects of FM is the multidisciplinary team. The concept of a medical home for children with complicated medical histories was pioneered in the management of hemophilia, sickle cell disease, and cystic fibrosis [8–10]. Rather than seeing individual specialists, the patient sees multiple specialists on a regular basis and improves outcomes by reducing hospitalizations and preventing complications. This more holistic approach takes physicians out of their silos and encourages the use of preventative interventions and collaboration in care. Similarly, the concept of aerodigestive teams allows the pediatric otolaryngologist to better assess the source of airway complaints to achieve improved outcomes in children with airway anomalies [11, 12]. Boesch et al. used a Delphi approach to define an Aerodigestive patient. They note, "a pediatric aerodigestive patient is a child with a combination of multiple and interrelated congenital and/or acquired conditions affecting airway, breathing, feeding, swallowing, or growth that require a coordinated interdisciplinary diagnostic and therapeutic approach to achieve optimal outcomes." [13] Essential aerodigestive team members include Otolaryngology, Pulmonology, Gastroeneterology, Speech Pathology, and Nutrition. Frequent collaborators include Allergy/Immunology, Genetics, Social work, Psychology, and other specialists. Offering patients complimentary interventions like aroma therapy, mind–body therapies, and acupuncture are intriguing additions that are not universally employed. The acknowledgment by all practitioners involved that there is an interplay between the successful functioning of each organ system is key to success. Further coordinating care between specialists reduces the burdens on family including missed work, costs of care, and stress of coordination further improving the quality of life for the entire family unit.

A Functional Approach to Common Pediatric Otorhinolaryngologic Conditions

As a specialty, the unified airway theory has been universally adopted among Otolaryngologists. The physical continuity of the esophagus, lower airway, and the upper airway extends to the middle ear via the eustachian tube. These areas demonstrate shared histology with pseudostratified respiratory epithelium and similar susceptibilities to inflammatory mediators. The Rhino-Bronchial Syndrome describes the spread of inflammation from the nose to the bronchi. Through natural drainage pathways, infected material descends from the osteomeatal complex, the spheno-ethmoidal recess, and the rhino-pharynx leading to inflammation of the lower airways [14, 15]. This is also the location of the adenoid tissue and the entrance of Waldeyer's ring that can harbor biofilm or viral replication which can easily pass through the eustachian tube [16–18]. It is proposed that these anatomic communications may be the first step in an inflammatory cascade affecting the entire airway [19]. Consequently, any process that leads to inflammation in one area of the aerodigestive tree may have an impact on the entire system.

Pediatric Gastroesophageal Reflux

Perhaps the most striking example of incorporating aspects of Functional Medicine into the treatment of a common pediatric condition is in the management of pediatric GERD. In 2018, the North American Society for Pediatric Gastroenterology Hepatology and Nutrition (NASPGHAN) released updated guidelines on treating GERD in infants and older children [20]. The authors highlight the following changes from previous recommendations: " [1] It focuses on reducing acid suppression whenever possible with short empiric trials of 4–8 weeks recommended for GERD symptoms; [2] it shifts away from attributing respiratory and laryngeal symptoms to GERD; [3] it adds an algorithm for typical symptoms to incorporate reflux testing to further characterize patients to differentiate patients with reflux based diagnoses versus functional diagnoses and [4] it adds a recommendation for change of formula to a protein hydrolysate or amino acid-based formula before acid suppression in infants," see Fig. 24.1.

Recent evidence suggests that treating infants with proton pump inhibitors (PPIs) is ineffective and may increase the risk of respiratory infections [20]. Further, multiple studies have demonstrated a lack of association between the acidity and volume of refluxate and symptoms of gastrointestinal (GI) distress in infants [20–23]. Interestingly, these guidelines are a concerted attempt, from a large organizing body, to look beyond treating a primary complaint and addressing its antecedents, systematically. Assessing a child's diet and determining whether there is a better nutritional alternative supersedes medication administration. These recommendations come on the back of mounting evidence that intolerance of milk, soy, and other protein sources and allergic or eosinophilic responses to the contents of breast milk or formula are frequently associated with GI symptoms.

The guidelines address other functional interventions for pediatric reflux and acknowledge evidence of potential benefits from probiotic administration but could not make a recommendation based on the quality and generalizability of the studies. Similarly, the authors mention but do not feel there is enough evidence to advocate for, homeopathy, chiropractic, and other alternative treatment modalities.

Sadly, there are few studies investigating alternative therapies for reflux in children. Extrapolating adult data is potentially risky and may suggest efficacy in interventions that are not clinically relevant. For instance, magnesium alginate use has been shown to reduce symptoms of reflux and dyspepsia in children and adults [24, 25]. However, preparations with aluminum must be used with caution in young children that are more prone to toxicity and overdose [26].

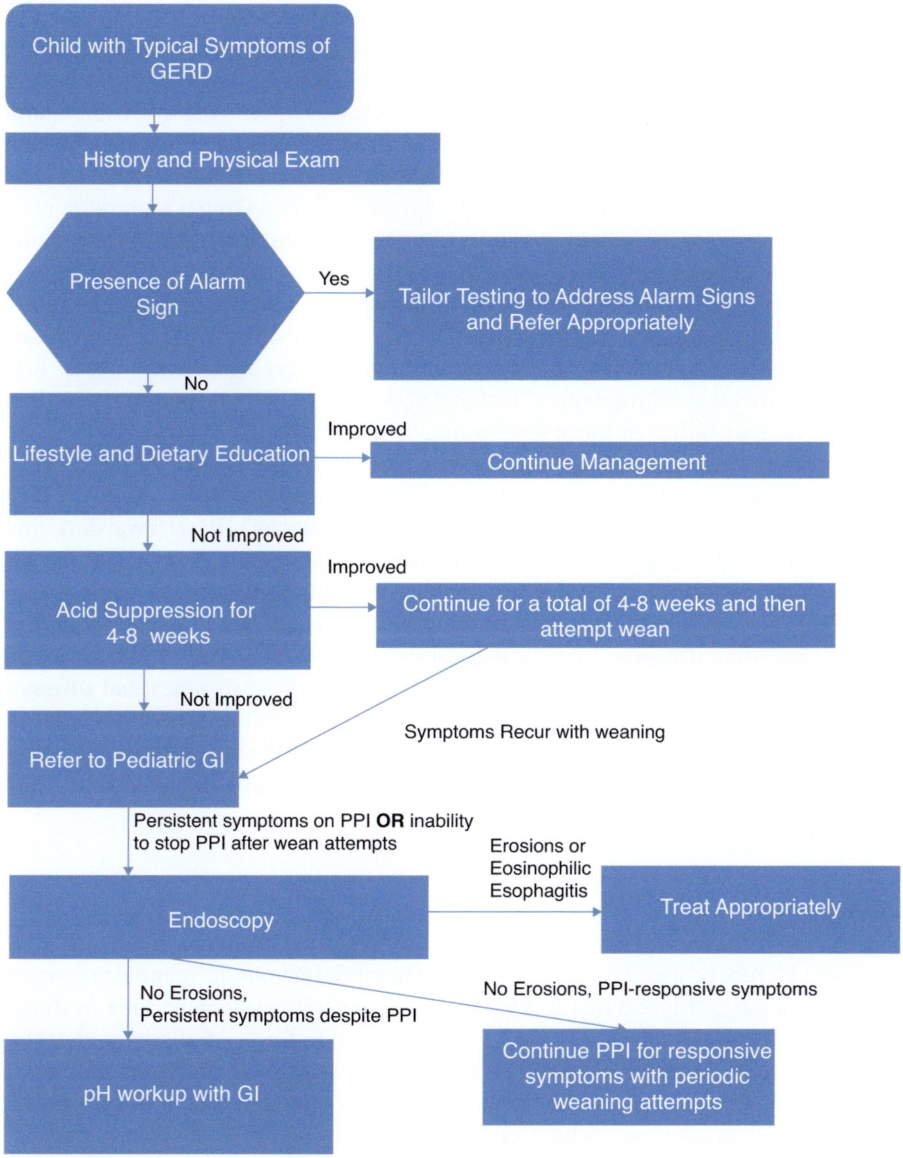

Fig. 24.1 Algorithm for treatment of children with GERD (*GERD* Gastroesophageal Reflux Disease; *PPI*=Proton Pump Inhibitor)

Iberogast, a combination of 9 herbal supplements (bitter candy tuft, lemon balm leaf, chamomile flower, caraway fruit, licorice root, angelica root, milk thistle fruit, peppermint leaf, and greater celandine herb) has been studied in vitro as well as in adults. It is thought to improve inflammatory mediators by increasing prostaglandin E and reducing leukotrienes. There are no published studies in children. Although often effective in adults, with a low incidence of adverse reactions, its use in children is unstudied and must be considered with caution [27]. Ginger root, often used as a kitchen spice or ingredient in many cultures, has been demonstrated to provide a pro-kinetic, cholinergic effect that can improve gastric emptying and gastrointestinal motility [28]. While ginger has not been studied in children, it has been safely used as an antiemetic during pregnancy. The most common side effects are related to gastrointestinal symptoms of dyspepsia and discomfort with higher doses. It is known to have an antithrombotic effect and should be used with caution in children with bleeding disorders or those undergoing surgery [29].

Acupuncture has been studied in both children and adults in treating nausea, vomiting, and reflux [30]. PC6 (neiguan), ST36 (zusanli), ST43 (xiangu), CV12 (zhongwan), ST25 (tianshu), SP4 (gongsun), LV3 (taicong), BL21 (weishu), and LI4 (hegu) have been targeted individually and in combination. A review of the literature demonstrated the safety of acupuncture and similar therapies even in young children [31]. It is important to realize that reflux, irritable bowel and dyspepsia in children are often triggered by emotional stressors. The mind-body-gut connection will often lead to somaticized symptoms manifesting in gastrointestinal distress. Several trials espouse the benefits of hypnotherapy, mindfulness, and biofeedback among other methods of promoting relaxation [30]. With the age-appropriate application, there is minimal risk and the potential to significantly alleviate short- and long-term symptoms.

Allergy

In 1998, Derebery and Berliner reviewed the otolaryngologic manifestations of allergic disease and found that in 151 adult patients with eustachian tube dysfunction and evidence of allergy/atopy, 92% were positive for food allergy and 100% were positive for inhalant allergy [32]. The prevalence of food allergy in children is between 3% and 7%. The vast majority of these allergies are related to cow's milk proteins, chicken eggs, soy, wheat, peanut, tree nuts, and shellfish. The majority of these are non-IgE or a mix of IgE and non-IgE mediated reactions [33, 34]. Inflammatory cascades from food allergy can have more systemic impacts on absorption, especially for micronutrients. The most common deficiencies are in vitamin D, followed by iron, zinc, fatty acids, and B vitamins. Subsequently, it is important not to overlook the possible feeding difficulties in a child if there is a food allergy suspected. As seen in many pediatric aerodigestive clinics, this can have an impact on the entire aerodigestive management [33].

Cow's milk protein allergy (CMPA) has shown the strongest correlation with nasal congestion and rhinitis as may be encountered by the otolaryngologist. It has been suggested that cow's milk protein allergy leads to more severe otolaryngologic diseases. One study comparing children with and without CMPA noted that 76% of the CMPA group required otolaryngologic surgery compared with only 8.6% of the control group. The CMPA group was also uniformly maximally treated for GERD at the time of surgery [35].

Food allergies have dramatic effects on the quality of life of affected children and families [36–38]. The younger the child, the worse they tend to score in each quality-of-life domain, and children with food allergies often score worse than those with sickle cell or intestinal failure. This poor scoring is thought to be due both to daily symptoms and the fear of IgE-mediated, life-threatening, anaphylactic reactions [34].

The relationship between allergies and inflammation of the aerodigestive system is well defined in the condition of eosinophilic esophagitis (EoE). EoE is a disorder characterized by dense esophageal eosinophilia occurring in association with upper gastrointestinal symptoms that, oftentimes, do not respond to acid suppression therapy [39]. This disease process can affect both adults and children and has a male predilection. The definitive diagnosis is made with esophagoscopy and biopsy of the esophageal mucosa showing greater than 15 eosinophils per high-power field. A suggestive endoscopic finding includes "trachealization" of the esophageal mucosa in which the mucosa appears to have a series of tracheal rings. In patients with EoE, about 70% of children and 40% of adults have tested positive for food allergies. Additionally, patients with EoE have a higher degree of atopic disease including allergic rhinoconjunctivitis, asthma, and atopic dermatitis and subsequent improvement of symptoms with the treatment of their allergies. EoE has also been associated with otolaryngologic processes including recurrent croup and otitis media with effusion [40]. Food avoidance or allergy desensitization is effective in improving both histopathologic inflammation and end organ symptomatology [41]. However, systematic elimination diets can be difficult to maintain, and their application must be weighed against the severity of symptoms and the likelihood of adherence.

Environmental allergies impact pediatric otolaryngology conditions both directly and indirectly. The correlation between allergy and otitis media is well described. The "shock organ theory" proposes that antigen activation causes inflammation in middle ear mucosa leading to a secretory response and the creation of otitis media and effusions [42]. The "eustachian tube dysfunction theory" proposes that allergy causes edema and inflammation of the nasal mucosa, which in turn leads to mucociliary impairment. Both of these theories have been supported in clinical and animal studies and it is likely a combination of the two results in reduced middle ear ventilation and chronic otitis [43, 44] Still another theory proposes that the chronic allergy-mediated inflammation of lymphoid tissues results in retrograde aspiration of nasopharyngeal secretions into the middle ear [45]. Inflammatory markers including IL-4, IL-5, T-lymphocytes, and eosinophils, common in allergic presentations are often sampled in middle ear effusions [45].

Rhinosinusitis describes an inflammatory condition affecting the nasal and paranasal sinus mucosa. Pediatric rhinosinusitis affects 1–9% of the pediatric population in the United States each year and accounts for more than 1.8 billion dollars in indirect healthcare expenditures and more than 20 million prescriptions each year. Risk factors are similar to those of otitis media and asthma and include exposure to smoke, industrialized upbringing, short duration of breastfeeding, late exposure to allergens, and early exposure to certain viruses including respiratory syncytial virus [46]. The "hygiene hypothesis" suggests that our typical lifestyles and sanitation reduce exposure to pathogens at a young age resulting in poorly developed immune systems. Studies in Amish children demonstrate higher exposure to bacterial endotoxin and reduced prevalence of allergic sensitization and asthma [47]. Regarding early exposure to allergens, there seems to be conflicting evidence. The LEAP study in 2015 demonstrated improvements in peanut sensitization in infants given doses of peanut before 6 months old. The American Association of Pediatricians now recommends the introduction of peanuts to high-risk children between 4 and 6 months of age [23]. Conversely, the Urban Environment and Childhood Asthma study determined that higher environmental allergen exposure in the home resulted in a higher risk of subsequent asthma development in young children [48]. On the same note, elevated levels of traffic-related air pollution (TRAP) in young children are known to predispose them to atopic conditions. There appears to be an interesting interplay between early exposure to inflammatory triggers. While some exposures reduce later inflammatory conditions and build a stronger immune system, others predispose to heightened and pathologic immune responses. This is an area of ongoing research.

There are numerous alternative treatment options for acute and chronic upper airway inflammation. As hyaluronic acid, resveratrol, cucurbitacin extract, enoxolone, probiotics, and bacteriotherapy are under investigation, it is hard to draw conclusions about their individual or combined effectiveness. Each complementary medicine approach has early studies showing promise but requires further investigation and as such we will not make recommendations for or against their use [19].

Nutrition

The nutritional status of any pediatric patient greatly influences their growth and development. When considering the otolaryngology patient, there are important influences from the macronutrient and micronutrient components of the diet that impact the microbiome and the immune system. On gross physical examination, children who are malnourished or obese draw attention to well-established acute and chronic health concerns. Even for those that appear healthy to the eye, micronutrient deficiency or imbalance can result in the breakdown of bodily barriers and impair our innate protection. When there is a considerable concern, and in patients that are failing to thrive, it is important to involve the care of qualified dieticians, gastroenterologists, allergists, or social workers to collaboratively optimize diet and health.

A Finnish cross-sectional study from Tapiainen et al. compared the prevalence of acute otitis media (AOM) in daycare children with their consumption of sweets [49]. Their analysis noted an increased risk of acute otitis media events in those that often consumed sweet pastries and jams and a protective effect against Staph Aureus carriage and the development of AOM in those that consumed fruits and berries. It is notable that only 20% of participants in the study indicated regular intake of fresh fruits. These findings identify a potentially modifiable risk factor for AOM in the general diet of the child. Importantly, reports have noted that the diet of children tends to decline after the first year of life when the child partakes in family meals and the consumption of fresh vegetables, fruits, and healthy fats often decreases [50, 51].

Xylitol is a sugar alcohol that has been promoted to potentially reduce ear infections and ear aches in children [49]. Xylitol use has been best described as reducing dental carries when used in chewing gum. It is a sugar alternative that is absorbed more slowly than glucose and is metabolized independent of insulin, resulting in less of an effect on blood sugars. It may also have an independent immune modulation aspect that could contribute to a reduction in respiratory infections [52]. A recent Cochrane review found moderate evidence that prophylactic administration of xylitol among daycare centers can reduce the incidence of AOM. However, as with most research on micronutrients, the data are ultimately mixed among other subpopulations such as patients with recurrent otitis media or in the treatment of patients with an acute respiratory illness [53]. It is an interesting option that is often found in chewing gum and lozenge formulations.

Acid

We have already discussed many of the dietary changes that may be necessary to avoid food allergies and eosinophilic esophagitis that may coexist with and contribute to GERD. Jamie Koufman, MD a pediatric otolaryngologist, has published several patient or parent-targeted books on the effects of the western diet, in particular acid consumption, on acid reflux disease and other otolaryngology-related disorders. She coined the term "respiratory reflux" to describe the effects of increased exposure to acid on the rest of the aerodigestive tract. In a book she published alongside two other prominent pediatric otolaryngologists, *Acid Reflux in Children*, the authors describe the various ways that acid is introduced in everyday foods [54]. Pepsin produced in digestive juices is activated at a lower pH. If present, when acidic foods are consumed, they will become activated causing symptoms long after the initial reflux event. Congress enacted the Low-Acid Canned Food Regulation (CFR) in 1973, charging the Food and Drug Administration (FDA) with ensuring that preserved canned foods maintain a pH of 4.6 or less. Many carbonated beverages may contain a pH as low as 2.6, similar to lemons or limes. Even baby foods that are shelf-stable may contain concerning levels of acid to reduce the risk of bacterial contamination. A pH-balanced diet is recommended in patients with a variety of head and neck complaints and may play a role in reducing the burden of disease.

Micronutrients

Vitamin D

Micronutrients are part of the complex process of disease and health. Vitamin D is the most studied micronutrient impacting the upper aerodigestive tract. In the last 10 years, there have been 41,000 peer-reviewed studies on vitamin D [55]. Many findings have been established which are too broad to discuss in this text. However, in otolaryngic conditions, supplementation has been presented as both a potential prevention and treatment strategy [56, 57].

The pathophysiologic mechanism of Vitamin D on immunity is multifaceted. Data exists to support the improved defense of the immune system against viral and bacterial infections with supplementation [58]. Other studies suggest that hypovitaminosis D may be involved in the initial stages of inflammation. Vitamin D has documented antimicrobial effects, decreases inflammation, promotes antimicrobial factors within the host and influences the microbiome. Vitamin D suppresses the pro-inflammatory cytokines IL-10 and TNF alpha and also suppresses the NFκB pathway [59–62]. Animal models have noted 47–50% thicker mucosa in vitamin D deficient rats which correlates with NF-κB suppression and increased mucin production [63]. This may also be due to a decrease in bactericidal nitric oxide in the supplemented subject or increased squamous metaplasia in the deficient patient. Vitamin D has also been shown to up-regulate the peptide cathelicidin in some subjects, which is an endogenous antimicrobial with activity against *Haemophilus influenzae*, *Streptococcus pneumoniae*, and *Moraxella catarrhalis* [64, 65]. Considering these concepts together, theoretically, vitamin D could very well impact both allergic rhinitis and otitis media directly and synergistically.

Many studies have evaluated vitamin D use in clinical settings; however, most are of low to moderate quality. Low vitamin D has been associated with otitis media, but it is important to note that hypovitaminosis D and otitis media share risk factors such as winter months and younger age [57]. One randomized clinical trial in Italy noted a higher incidence of otitis media in the control group (65.5%) compared to those receiving a supplement (44.8%) [66]. A 2016 meta-analysis and systematic review concluded that low levels of vitamin D were not associated with otitis media in general [67]. In a sub-analysis of the same study, they noted that AOM was associated with vitamin D levels. The discrepancy in these findings may be due to the weighting and methodology of the meta-analysis and the low-quality studies that were included. Since that review was published, other studies and reviews have been published with similarly mixed results [57, 58].

Another well-designed randomized controlled trial compared pediatric supplementation at a standard dose of vitamin D at 400 IU/day to a high dose at 2000 IU/day. The study reported no difference in upper respiratory illness between the groups [68]. Secondary outcomes, such as the frequency of outpatient visits, emergency department visits, and antibiotic prescriptions also did not improve with higher doses. The researchers concluded that vitamin D may exhibit a threshold effect and that daily low-dose vitamin D supplementation, as recommended by the

American Academy of Pediatrics to prevent rickets, could be sufficient for upper respiratory infection prophylaxis [69]. Perhaps, at the time of this publication the best conclusion to draw from the available evidence may be that Vitamin D is not a cure, but a component of the overall treatment paradigm and prevention of OM subtypes.

Studies assessing pharyngotonsillitis and vitamin D levels have had similarly mixed results [70–72]. While the studies are more limited, the evidence in pediatric rhinosinusitis suggests a more definitive correlation. Zisi et al. noted that children with chronic rhinosinusitis with nasal polyposis or acute fungal rhinosinusitis were more likely to be vitamin D deficient than those with rhinosinusitis without polyps [58, 73]. In another study, hypovitaminosis D was found to be a risk factor for complications of acute rhinosinusitis [74]. Vitamin D supplementation has been associated with lower rates of allergic rhinitis and atopy and improved rhinosinusitis symptoms in general [58, 75, 76]. There are few studies focusing specifically on children and many studies are not of high enough quality to establish generalizable guidelines. At this time, vitamin D proponents suggest that it may be an inexpensive and effective prophylactic measure with other health benefits and a minimum side effect profile [77]. Considerations of skin type, geographic location, sun exposure, and economic impact are important in counseling regarding supplementation.

Vitamin C

Vitamin C is well known in the general public and medical literature as a prophylactic and treatment for upper respiratory tract infections. Commercials on the television and radio espouse the benefits of mega-dose treatment at the first cold symptoms. L-Ascorbic acid acts as an antioxidant purported to protect host cells. Supplementation is supposed to augment the already high L-ascorbic acid levels found in phagocytes. Vitamin C was used heavily in decades past due to positive early clinical trials, however, use later declined as results were not replicated. Vitamin C has somewhat returned to favor of late, at least partially due to some favorable studies. A systematic review in 2019 failed to demonstrate the efficacy of vitamin C in preventing URTIs, but a decrease in the duration of infections by about 1.6 days was found compared to placebo. Interestingly, the reviewers found it more effective in children under 6-year-old and those with vigorous exercise programs [78]. Well-designed studies regarding Vitamin C and otolaryngology conditions are currently lacking. Vitamin C is water soluble and excreted in the urine. Even in large doses side effects are exceedingly rare.

Vitamin A/E

Vitamin A (retinol and retinoic acid) and vitamin E (tocopherol) are fat-soluble vitamins with antioxidant properties. No specific studies regarding the aerodigestive tract have been published to date. One study evaluating markers of allergy and inflammation after tonsillectomy identified less self-reported viral symptoms in those with higher Vitamin A levels and less allergy symptoms in those with higher vitamin E levels [75]. No other studies were found that show more direct clinical correlation and the results of these findings warrant further investigation. Supplementation with fat-soluble vitamins requires more supervision as overdosing or misuse can result in birth defects, hepatic injury, or other complications.

Other Micronutrients and Supplements

Iron is critical in normal cognitive and motor development. Iron is known to be involved in anti-inflammatory processes and there is evidence that it plays an important role in the DNA replication pathways of immunoprogenitor cells [79]. One study did identify higher rates of iron deficiency anemia in patients with otitis media and effusions compared to those with normal ear examinations. These findings are somewhat anecdotal and there is no clear causative association or recommendation for therapy, especially in children who are not anemic [80].

Zinc supplementation for adults and children has been a topic of interest for decades. Zinc is another essential nutrient involved in immune function. Despite acting as a vital micronutrient for both growth and immunity, there are no body stores of zinc, and it must be consumed regularly to maintain normal levels. The average diet contains high zinc sources found in animal proteins, nuts, beans, and seeds [81]. Studies have also shown pneumonia prevention and decreased mortality of up to 15% in previously deficient and subsequently supplemented populations and a protective effect, specifically in children, from acquiring pneumonia [82–84].

At the onset of the ongoing SARS-CoV-2 pandemic, consumers rushed to buy supplements in an attempt to bolster immunity in the face of the spreading disease. Within days, all vitamins with Zinc were bought and shelves were bare. Zinc continues to be one of the sought-after supplements for the prevention of viral illnesses despite evidence of only a marginal impact on symptoms in those that are not significantly deficient [85–87]. Treatment at the onset of symptoms may reduce upper respiratory infection duration [81, 87, 88]. In studies investigating otitis media, there were few true adverse events with commercially available doses of zinc and some studies suggested it conferred some additional protection.

Selenium is also worth mentioning in this context as it is often regarded as an immune modulator [86, 89]. Although early studies suggest there could be a deficiency of both zinc and selenium in patients requiring tympanostomy tube placement, there is little evidence demonstrating improvement with supplementation [89]. Similarly, it is suggested that patients with chronic otitis media may have lower selenium levels. There is still a lack of data describing benefits in otolaryngology-related diseases with selenium supplementation [90].

It is clear that a healthy, well-rounded diet is key to maintaining excellent health. It is also clear that those with deficiencies in a particular micronutrient will benefit from supplementation. Mega-dose vitamin treatments should garner concern. There is little evidence to suggest benefits beyond recommended dietary intake. In patients

Table 24.1 Role of micronutrients in immunity

Micronutrient impact on immunity		
Micronutrient	Innate immunity	Adaptive immunity
Vitamin E	Decreases PEG, COX, NO, IL-12, CD11+; decreases dendritic cell migration; increases NK activity and phagocytosis	Increases antibody production, IgM, IgE, plasma cell production, IL-2, T-cell proliferation, induced cell death; decreases T-cell activation
Vitamin D	Increases phagocytosis, killing antigens, cathelicidins, IL-10, TNF α, mannose receptor, NK activity, phagocytosis; decreases MHC-II, IL-23, IL-12	Increases apoptosis, IL-10, IL-4; decreases antibody production, IgM, IgE, plasma cell production, IL-17, Il-21, inflammation
Vitamin C	Increases phagocytosis, killing antigens, NK activity, phagocytosis, oxidant production	Increases antibody production, IgM, IgG, IgA, plasma cell production, IL-2, cytotoxic activity; polarizes T-helper cells
Folate	Increases production of NK cells	Increases expression of antigen-presenting cells, antibody-mediated immune response, and antibody production; assists T-helper cell response
Iron	Regulates production of cytokines, improves phagocytosis	Increases T-cell proliferation and cytotoxic T-cell function
Zinc	Protects against oxidants, aids in maintaining skin and mucosal cell membrane integrity	Promotes cytokine release, assists T-helper 1 cells, activates T cells
Copper	Aids neutrophil phagocytosis, increases IL-2 production	Increases T-cell proliferation and antibody production; improves cellular immunity by activating cytokines and chemokines
Selenium	Aids selenium-dependent enzymes resist oxidant production; supports NK cell function and leukocytes	Increases antibody production; promotes T-cell proliferation and differentiation

Table adapted from Akhtar et al. (*PEG* polyethylene glycol; *COX* cyclooxygenase; *Ig* immunoglobulin; *IL* interleukin; *MHC* major histocompatibility complex; *NK* Natural killer; *NO* nitric oxide; *TNF* tumor necrosis factor) [86]

with frequent or severe head and neck concerns, a review of their diet and symptoms may identify targets for directed supplementation to improve their response to infection and inflammatory cascade. A summary of the immune influences of various micronutrients is found in Table 24.1.

Socioeconomic Factors

In the functional medicine model, there are three main foci of socio-cultural factors—social determinants of health, social needs of health, and implicit bias of the practitioner. These three components are viewed as antecedents of health, mediators of health, and triggers, respectively [7, 91, 92].

The social determinants of health were developed by the world health organization and represent a list of critical antecedents to a person's health status [93]. The socioeconomic and socio-cultural factors of which the child is a part, play a role in decision making as a practitioner. Many of the factors considered above are highly dependent on the education level within the family. Supplementation and implementation of alternative therapies are more common in patients with higher socioeconomic status [49]. Interestingly, rates of obesity and malnourishment are highest in those with less access to healthcare [94]. Pediatric cochlear implantation results exemplify the contributions of social determinants of health. To achieve maximum benefit, and reach the best speech and reception outcomes, the child ideally will be supported by regular access to rehabilitation programs, therapy, education, and supportive modes of communication including spoken and sign languages [95, 96]. Yet, it is often seen that access and compliance with these programs are limited due to socioeconomic status, education level, and geography. Additionally, families with lower socioeconomic status may be at risk for poorer access to cochlear implantation and audiologic services in general. Due to this reality, social workers are critical in identifying and mitigating risk factors for complications and poor outcomes prior to surgical consideration [97–99].

As an antecedent of health, the socio-cultural factors are not traditionally viewed as an aspect that can be easily modified by the individual practitioner. These underlying differences may require broader public health interventions and support. However, the individual practitioner can help the patient by understanding the challenges they face and the resources available. As discussed in a review by Bergmark et al., the socioeconomic factors impacting patients often greatly impact the treatment modalities provided—sometimes impacting their length of life [100]. Addressing these concerns may require ancillary staff support in complex conditions such as described above with cochlear implantation. However, in the general ENT evaluation, the otolaryngologist should take an active role. Many regions have programs for childhood obesity which can complement treatment for obstructive sleep apnea or GERD. The American Academy of Otolaryngology—Head and Neck Surgery has recommended counseling of families regarding persistent obstructive sleep apnea in children, especially in the setting of obesity [4]. These regional programs are becoming more widely available in urban and rural areas. Many show benefits in both improved physical health in addition to the quality of life improvements and can be a referral site for otolaryngologists [101, 102].

Otolaryngologists have been championing some mediators of health in pediatric patients for many years. For example, known risk factors for otitis media include lack of breastfeeding, daycare attendance, older siblings, tobacco smoke exposure, and pacifier or push-and-pull plastic bottle caps [103]. Visits for AOM and rhinosinusitis are excellent times to discuss the recommendations and precautions families can take to improve the health of their children.

The impacts of socioeconomic disparities are also realized through the implicit bias of the practitioner and patient. As discussed above, a goal of the Functional Medicine approach is to share responsibility with the patient for their health. Several of the factors discussed above may become part of the conversation when counseling patients. Physicians may not be aware when they cross boundaries or make families uncomfortable. Multiple studies have shown through patient surveys that much of the perception of having received quality care depends on their engagement in care choices. Similarly, engaging patients does lead to better outcomes and satisfaction. Providing patients and families with the most personally appropriate information at each stage of their care is paramount [104]. It is imperative for providers to constantly assess their personal prejudices and interactions to continue to improve their communication with patients.

Conclusion

Even simple presentations may be mired by pre-existing antecedents and predilection for disease. Children may fall under the radar due to their age and lack of known comorbid conditions. The observant otolaryngologist will attempt to identify the antecedents, mediators, and triggers that led the pediatric patient to their current state. This does require a holistic approach and understanding of the interplay between diet, inflammation, allergy, and infection. Aside from treating the symptoms, addressing predispositions through multidisciplinary care and embracing other specialties and modes of treatment are key to achieving the best results. The application of evidence-based guidelines, proper diagnosis, and consideration of less traditionally taught interventions as discussed in this text will aid the otolaryngologist to alter the disease course of their patients.

References

1. Mace AD, Narula AA. Survey of current undergraduate otolaryngology training in the United Kingdom. J Laryngol Otol. 2004;118:217–20. https://pubmed.ncbi.nlm.nih.gov/15068520/
2. Wald ER, Applegate KE, Bordley C, Darrow DH, Glode MP, Marcy SM, et al. Clinical practice guideline for the diagnosis and management of acute bacterial sinusitis in children aged 1 to 18 years. Pediatrics Pediatrics. 2013;132. https://pubmed.ncbi.nlm.nih.gov/23796742/
3. Brietzke SE, Shin JJ, Choi S, Lee JT, Parikh SR, Pena M, et al. Clinical consensus statement: Pediatric chronic rhinosinusitis. Otolaryngol-Head Neck Surg. 2014;151(4):542–53. https://pubmed.ncbi.nlm.nih.gov/25274375/
4. Mitchell RB, Archer SM, Ishman SL, Rosenfeld RM, Coles S, Finestone SA, et al. Clinical practice guideline: tonsillectomy in children (update). Otolaryngol–Head Neck Surg. 2019;160(1_suppl):S1–42.
5. Helmut W, Schimmel VP. Functional medicine: the origin and treatment of chronic diseases. 2nd ed. Thieme; 1997.
6. Osler W. The evolution of modern medicine. 1913 [cited 2021 Mar 20]. https://www.gutenberg.org/files/1566/1566-h/1566-h.htm
7. Medicine TI of F. The institute for functional medicine. [cited 2021 Mar 20]. https://www.ifm.org/
8. Soucie JM, Nuss R, Evatt B, Abdelhak A, Cowan L, Hill H, et al. Mortality among males with hemophilia: relations with source of medical care. Blood. 2000 Jul 15;96(2):437–42.
9. Bhaumik U, Norris K, Charron G, Walker SP, Sommer SJ, Chan E, et al. A cost analysis for a community-based case management intervention program for pediatric Asthma. J Asthma. 2013;50(3):310–7. https://pubmed.ncbi.nlm.nih.gov/23311526/

10. Yang YM, Shah AK, Watson M, Mankad VN. Comparison of costs to the health sector of comprehensive and episodic health care for sickle cell disease patients. Public Health Rep. 1995;110(1):80–6. /pmc/articles/PMC1382078/?report=abstract
11. Rotsides JM, Krakovsky GM, Pillai DK, Sehgal S, Collins ME, Noelke CE, et al. Is a multidisciplinary aerodigestive clinic more effective at treating recalcitrant aerodigestive complaints than a single specialist? Ann Otol Rhinol Laryngol. 2017;126(7):537–43. https://pubmed.ncbi.nlm.nih.gov/28474959/
12. Collaco JM, Aherrera AD, Au Yeung KJ, Lefton-Greif MA, Hoch J, Skinner ML. Interdisciplinary pediatric aerodigestive care and reduction in health care costs and burden. JAMA Otolaryngol-Head Neck Surg. 2015;141(2):101–5. https://pubmed.ncbi.nlm.nih.gov/25473812/
13. Boesch RP, Balakrishnan K, Acra S, Benscoter DT, Cofer SA, Collaco JM, et al. Structure and functions of pediatric aerodigestive programs: a consensus statement. Pediatrics. 2018;141(3). https://pubmed.ncbi.nlm.nih.gov/29437862/
14. Wigand ME, Steiner W, Jaumann MP. Endonasale Nebenhöhlenchirurgie unter endoskopischer Kontrolle: Von der Radikaloperation zur Schleimhautrehabilitation. Endoscopy. 1978;10(4):255–60. https://pubmed.ncbi.nlm.nih.gov/738221/
15. Dykewicz MS. Rhinitis and sinusitis. J Allergy Clin Immunol. 2003;111. Available from: https://pubmed.ncbi.nlm.nih.gov/12592298/
16. Ciprandi G, Caimmi D, del Giudice MM, La Rosa M, Salpietro C, Marseglia GL. Recent developments in United Airways disease. Allergy Asthma Immunol Res. 2012;4:171–7. https://pubmed.ncbi.nlm.nih.gov/22754709/
17. Watkins DN, Lewis RH, Basclain KA, Fisher PH, Peroni DJ, Garlepp MJ, et al. Expression and localization of the inducible isoform of nitric oxide synthase in nasal polyp epithelium. Clin Exp Allergy. 1998;28(2):211–9. https://pubmed.ncbi.nlm.nih.gov/9515595/
18. Djupesland PG, Chatkin JM, Qian W, Haight JSJ. Nitric oxide in the nasal airway: a new dimension in otorhinolaryngology. Am J Otolaryngol–Head Neck Med Surg. 2001;22(1):19–32. https://pubmed.ncbi.nlm.nih.gov/11172211/
19. Varricchio A, La Mantia I, Brunese FP, Ciprandi G. Inflammation, infection, and allergy of upper airways: new insights from national and real-world studies. Italian J Pediatrics BioMed Central Ltd. 2020;46. /pmc/articles/PMC7008537/?report=abstract
20. Rosen R, Vandenplas Y, Singendonk M, Cabana M, Dilorenzo C, Gottrand F, et al. Pediatric gastroesophageal reflux clinical practice guidelines: joint recommendations of the North American society for pediatric gastroenterology, hepatology, and nutrition and the european society for pediatric gastroenterology, hepatology, and nutrition. J Pediatric Gastroenterol Nutrit. 2018;66:516–54. https://pubmed.ncbi.nlm.nih.gov/29470322/
21. Sultan N, Nazareno J, Gregor J. Association between proton pump inhibitors and respiratory infections: a systematic review and meta-analysis of clinical trials. Canadian Journal of Gastroenterology. 2008;22:761–6. https://pubmed.ncbi.nlm.nih.gov/18818790/
22. Leung AKC, Hon KL. Gastroesophageal reflux in children: an updated review. Drugs in Context. 2019;8. https://pubmed.ncbi.nlm.nih.gov/31258618/
23. Du Toit G, Roberts G, Sayre PH, Bahnson HT, Radulovic S, Santos AF, et al. Randomized trial of peanut consumption in infants at risk for peanut allergy. N Engl J Med. 2015;372(9):803–13. https://pubmed.ncbi.nlm.nih.gov/25705822/
24. Baldassarre ME, Di Mauro A, Pignatelli MC, Fanelli M, Salvatore S, Di Nardo G, et al. Magnesium alginate in gastro-esophageal reflux: a randomized multicenter cross-over study in infants. Int J Environ Res Public Health. 2020;17(1). https://pubmed.ncbi.nlm.nih.gov/31861951/
25. Leiman DA, Riff BP, Morgan S, Metz DC, Falk GW, French B, et al. Alginate therapy is effective treatment for GERD symptoms: a systematic review and meta-analysis. Dis Esophagus. 2017;30(5):1–9. https://pubmed.ncbi.nlm.nih.gov/28375448/
26. Tighe M, Afzal NA, Bevan A, Hayen A, Munro A, Beattie RM. Pharmacological treatment of children with gastro-oesophageal reflux, Cochrane Database of Systematic Reviews. 2014;2014. https://pubmed.ncbi.nlm.nih.gov/25419906/

27. Ottillinger B, Storr M, Malfertheiner P, Allescher HD. STW 5 (Iberogast®)-a safe and effective standard in the treatment of functional gastrointestinal disorders. Wiener Medizinische Wochenschrift. 2013;163(3–4):65–72. https://pubmed.ncbi.nlm.nih.gov/23263639/
28. Thomson M, Corbin R, Leung L. Effects of ginger for nausea and vomiting in early pregnancy: a meta-analysis. J Am Board Fam Med. 2014;27(1):115–22. https://pubmed.ncbi.nlm.nih.gov/24390893/
29. Thomson M, Al-Qattan KK, Al-Sawan SM, Alnaqeeb MA, Khan I, Ali M. The use of ginger (Zingiber officinale Rosc.) as a potential anti-inflammatory and antithrombotic agent. Prostaglandins Leukot Essent Fat Acids. 2002;67(6):475–8. https://pubmed.ncbi.nlm.nih.gov/12468270/
30. Yeh A, Golianu B. Integrative treatment of reflux and functional dyspepsia in children. Children. 2014;1(2):119–33. /pmc/articles/PMC4928719/
31. Jindal V, Ge A, Mansky PJ. Safety and efficacy of acupuncture in children: a review of the evidence. J Pediatr Hematol Oncol. 2008;30(6):431–42. https://pubmed.ncbi.nlm.nih.gov/18525459/
32. Derebery MJ, Berliner KI. Allergy for the otologist: external canal to inner ear. Otolaryngol Clin North Am. 1998;31(1):157–73. https://pubmed.ncbi.nlm.nih.gov/9530684/
33. Meyer R. Nutritional disorders resulting from food allergy in children. Pediatr Allergy Immunol. 2018;29(7):689–704.
34. Meyer R, Godwin H, Dziubak R, Panepinto JA, Foong RXM, Bryon M, et al. The impact on quality of life on families of children on an elimination diet for non-immunoglobulin e mediated gastrointestinal food allergies. World Allergy Organ J. 2017;10(1). /pmc/articles/PMC5320765/?report=abstract
35. Paddack A, Gibbons T, Smith C, Patil S, Richter GT. Food hypersensitivity and otolaryngologic conditions in young children. Otolaryngol–Head Neck Surg (United States). 2012;147(2):215–20.
36. Salvilla SA, Dubois AEJ, Flokstra-De Blok BMJ, Panesar SS, Worth A, Patel S, et al. Disease-specific health-related quality of life instruments for IgE-mediated food allergy. Allergy: European Journal of Allergy and Clinical Immunology. 2014;69:834–44. https://pubmed.ncbi.nlm.nih.gov/24836207/
37. King RM, Knibb RC, Hourihane JOB. Impact of peanut allergy on quality of life, stress and anxiety in the family. Allergy Eur J Allergy Clin Immunol. 2009;64(3):461–8. https://pubmed.ncbi.nlm.nih.gov/19076542/
38. Valentine AZ, Knibb RC. Exploring quality of life in families of children living with and without a severe food allergy. Appetite. 2011;57(2):467–74. https://pubmed.ncbi.nlm.nih.gov/21708202/
39. Lucendo AJ, Arias Á, Molina-Infante J. Efficacy of proton pump inhibitor drugs for inducing clinical and histologic remission in patients with symptomatic esophageal eosinophilia: a systematic review and meta-analysis. Clinical Gastroenterology and Hepatology. 2016;14:13–22.e1. https://pubmed.ncbi.nlm.nih.gov/26247167/
40. Kelly EA, Linn D, Keppel KL, Noel RJ, Chun RH. Otolaryngologic surgeries are frequent in children with eosinophilic esophagitis. Ann Otol Rhinol Laryngol. 2015;124(5):355–60. https://pubmed.ncbi.nlm.nih.gov/25385840/
41. Reed CC, Dellon ES. Eosinophilic Esophagitis. Medical clinics of North America. 2019;103:29–42. /pmc/articles/PMC6260964/
42. Bluestone CD. Eustachian tube function: physiology, pathophysiology, and role of allergy in pathogenesis of otitis media. J Allergy Clin Immunol. 1983;72(3):242–51. https://pubmed.ncbi.nlm.nih.gov/6886258/
43. Downs BW, Butehorn HF, Prazma J, Rose AS, Stamat JC, Pillsbury HC. Action of histamine on eustachian tube function. Otolaryngol–Head Neck Surg. 2001;124(4):414–20. https://pubmed.ncbi.nlm.nih.gov/11283499/
44. Hardy SM, Heavner SB, White DR, Mcqueen CT, Prazma J, Pillsbury HC. Late-phase allergy and eustachian tube dysfunction. Otolaryngol–Head Neck Surg. 2001;125(4):339–45. https://pubmed.ncbi.nlm.nih.gov/11593168/

45. Corso Eugenio D, Elena C, Jacopo G, Veronica S, Daniela L, Cesare Tiziana D, et al. Otitis media in children: which phenotypes are most linked to allergy? a systematic review.
46. Boolchandani H, Horwitz R, Soffer G. An integrative medicine review of primary prevention of allergy in pediatrics. Complementary Therapies in Medicine. 2021;58. https://pubmed.ncbi.nlm.nih.gov/33636296/
47. Stein MM, Hrusch CL, Gozdz J, Igartua C, Pivniouk V, Murray SE, et al. Innate immunity and asthma risk in amish and hutterite farm children. N Engl J Med. 2016;375(5):411–21. https://pubmed.ncbi.nlm.nih.gov/27518660/
48. Lynch SV, Wood RA, Boushey H, Bacharier LB, Bloomberg GR, Kattan M, et al. Effects of early-life exposure to allergens and bacteria on recurrent wheeze and atopy in urban children. J Allergy Clin Immunol. 2014;134(3). https://pubmed.ncbi.nlm.nih.gov/24908147/
49. Tapiainen T, Paalanne N, Arkkola T, Renko M, Pokka T, Kaijalainen T, et al. Diet as a risk factor for pneumococcal carriage and otitis media: a cross-sectional study among children in day care centers. PLoS One. 2014;9(3). /pmc/articles/PMC3944052/?report=abstract
50. Erkkola M, Kronberg-Kippilä C, Kyttälä P, Lehtisalo J, Reinivuo H, Tapanainen H, et al. Sucrose in the diet of 3-year-old Finnish children: Sources, determinants and impact on food and nutrient intake. Br J Nutr. 2009;101(8):1209–17. https://pubmed.ncbi.nlm.nih.gov/18755050/
51. Grimes CA, Riddell LJ, Campbell KJ, Nowson CA. Dietary salt intake, sugar-sweetened beverage consumption, and obesity risk. Pediatrics. 2013;131(1):14–21. https://pubmed.ncbi.nlm.nih.gov/23230077/
52. Salli K, Lehtinen MJ, Tiihonen K, Ouwehand AC. Xylitol's health benefits beyond dental health: a comprehensive review. Nutrients. 2019;11. /pmc/articles/PMC6723878/
53. Azarpazhooh A, Lawrence HP, Shah PS. Xylitol for preventing acute otitis media in children up to 12 years of age. Cochrane Database of Systematic Reviews. 2016;2016
54. Koufman MD, Jamie W, Zur JL, Karen G. Acid reflux in children: how healthy eating can fix your Child's asthma, allergies, obesity, nasal congestion, Cough & Croup. Katalitix.
55. Matsui MS, Vitamin D. Update. Current Dermatology Reports. 2020;9:323–30. /pmc/articles/PMC7556559/?report=abstract
56. Rosenfeld RM, Shin JJ, Schwartz SR, Coggins R, Gagnon L, Hackell JM, et al. Clinical practice guideline. Otolaryngol–Head Neck Surg (United States). 2016;154(1 Suppl):S1–41. https://pubmed.ncbi.nlm.nih.gov/26832942/
57. Walker RE, Bartley J, Camargo CA, Mitchell EA. Vitamin D and otitis media. Curr Allergy Asthma Rep. 2019;19(7):33.
58. Zisi D, Challa A, Makis A. The association between vitamin D status and infectious diseases of the respiratory system in infancy and childhood. Hormones. 2019;18:353–63. /pmc/articles/PMC7092025/?report=abstract
59. Hansdottir S, Monick MM, Lovan N, Powers L, Gerke A, Hunninghake GW. Vitamin D decreases respiratory syncytial virus induction of NF-κb–linked chemokines and cytokines in airway epithelium while maintaining the antiviral state. J Immunol. 2010;184(2):965–74. https://pubmed.ncbi.nlm.nih.gov/20008294/
60. Zhang Y, Leung DYM, Richers BN, Liu Y, Remigio LK, Riches DW, et al. Vitamin D Inhibits Monocyte/Macrophage Proinflammatory Cytokine Production by Targeting MAPK Phosphatase-1. J Immunol. 2012;188(5):2127–35. https://pubmed.ncbi.nlm.nih.gov/22301548/
61. Zhu Y, Mahon BD, Froicu M, Cantorna MT. Calcium and 1α, 25-dihydroxyvitamin D3 target the TNF-α pathway to suppress experimental inflammatory bowel disease. Eur J Immunol. 2005;35(1):217–24. https://pubmed.ncbi.nlm.nih.gov/15593122/
62. Coussens AK, Wilkinson RJ, Hanifa Y, Nikolayevskyy V, Elkington PT, Islam K, et al. Vitamin D accelerates resolution of inflammatory responses during tuberculosis treatment. Proc Natl Acad Sci U S A. 2012;109(38):15449–54. https://pubmed.ncbi.nlm.nih.gov/22949664/
63. Kim HB, Lim SH, Cho CG, Choi HS. Influence of vitamin D deficiency on progression of experimental otitis media in rats. Endocrinol Metab. 2018;33(2):296–304. https://pubmed.ncbi.nlm.nih.gov/29947185/

64. Bhan I, Camargo CA, Wenger J, Ricciardi C, Ye J, Borregaard N, et al. Circulating levels of 25-hydroxyvitamin D and human cathelicidin in healthy adults. J Allergy Clin Immunol. 2011;127(5):1302–1304.e1. https://pubmed.ncbi.nlm.nih.gov/21310475/
65. McGillivary G, Ray WC, Bevins CL, Munson RS, Bakaletz LO. A member of the cathelicidin family of antimicrobial peptides is produced in the upper airway of the chinchilla and its mRNA expression is altered by common viral and bacterial co-pathogens of otitis media. Mol Immunol. 2007;44(9):2446–58. https://pubmed.ncbi.nlm.nih.gov/17113647/
66. Martineau AR, Jolliffe DA, Hooper RL, Greenberg L, Aloia JF, Bergman P, et al. Vitamin D supplementation to prevent acute respiratory tract infections: systematic review and meta-analysis of individual participant data. BMJ. 2017;356. https://pubmed.ncbi.nlm.nih.gov/28202713/
67. Li HB, Tai XH, Sang YH, Jia JP, Xu ZM, Cui XF, et al. Association between vitamin D and development of otitis media: a PRISMA-compliant meta-analysis and systematic review. Medicine (United States). 2016, 95. https://pubmed.ncbi.nlm.nih.gov/27749530/
68. Aglipay M, Birken CS, Parkin PC, Loeb MB, Thorpe K, Chen Y, et al. Effect of high-dose vs standard-dose wintertime Vitamin D supplementation on viral upper respiratory tract infections in young healthy children. JAMA–J Am Med Assoc. 2017;318(3):245–54. /pmc/articles/PMC5817430/?report=abstract
69. Hueniken K, Aglipay M, Birken CS, Parkin PC, Loeb MB, Thorpe KE, et al. Effect of high-dose Vitamin D supplementation on upper respiratory tract infection symptom severity in healthy children. Pediatr Infect Dis J. 2019;38(6):569–76.
70. Shin JH, Kim BG, Kim BY, Kim SW, Kim SW, Kim H. Is there an association between vitamin D deficiency and adenotonsillar hypertrophy in children with sleep-disordered breathing? BMC Pediatr. 2018;18(1). https://pubmed.ncbi.nlm.nih.gov/29921246/
71. Yildiz I, Unuvar E, Zeybek U, Toptas B, Cacina C, Toprak S, et al. The role of vitamin D in children with recurrent Tonsillopharyngitis. Ital J Pediatr. 2012;38(1):25. /pmc/articles/PMC3453523/?report=abstract
72. Aydin S, Aslan I, Yildiz I, Aĝaçhan B, Toptaş B, Toprak S, et al. Vitamin D levels in children with recurrent tonsillitis. Int J Pediatr Otorhinolaryngol. 2011;75(3):364–7. https://pubmed.ncbi.nlm.nih.gov/21215466/
73. Mulligan JK, White DR, Wang EW, Sansoni SR, Moses H, Yawn RJ, et al. Vitamin D3 deficiency increases sinus mucosa dendritic cells in pediatric chronic rhinosinusitis with nasal polyps. Otolaryngol-Head Neck Surg (United States). 2012;147(4):773–81. https://pubmed.ncbi.nlm.nih.gov/22627120/
74. Elbistanlı MS, Koçak HE, Güneş S, Acıpayam H, Şimşek BM, Canpolat S, et al. Vit D deficiency is a possible risk factor in ARS. Eur Arch Oto-Rhino-Laryngology. 2017;274(9):3391–5. https://pubmed.ncbi.nlm.nih.gov/28608241/
75. Elenius V, Palomares O, Waris M, Turunen R, Puhakka T, Rückert B, et al. The relationship of serum vitamins A, D, e and LL-37 levels with allergic status, tonsillar virus detection and immune response. PLoS One. 2017;12(2). /pmc/articles/PMC5325266/?report=abstract
76. San T, Muluk NB, Cingi C. 1,25(OH)2D3 and specific IgE levels in children with recurrent tonsillitis, and allergic rhinitis. Int J Pediatr Otorhinolaryngol. 2013;77(9):1506–11. https://doi.org/10.1016/j.ijporl.2013.06.019.
77. Esposito S, Bianchini S, Bosis S, Tagliabue C, Coro I, Argentiero A, et al. A randomized, placebo-controlled, double-blinded, single-Centre, phase IV trial to assess the efficacy and safety of OM-85 in children suffering from recurrent respiratory tract infections. J Transl Med. 2019;17(1). /pmc/articles/PMC6708164/?report=abstract
78. Vorilhon P, Arpajou B, Vaillant Roussel H, Merlin É, Pereira B, Cabaillot A. Efficacy of vitamin C for the prevention and treatment of upper respiratory tract infection. A meta-analysis in children. Eur J Clin Pharmacol. 2019;75(3):303–11.
79. Muñoz C, Rios E, Olivos J, Brunser O, Olivares M. Iron, copper and immunocompetence. Br J Nutr. 2007;98(Suppl. 1):24–8.
80. Akcan FA, Dündar Y, Akcan HB, Cebeci D, Sungur MA, Ünlü İ. The association between iron deficiency and otitis media with effusion. J Int Adv Otol. 2019;15(1):18–21. /pmc/articles/PMC6483434/?report=abstract

81. Gulani A, Sachdev HS. Zinc supplements for preventing otitis media, vol. 2014. Cochrane Database of Systematic Reviews; 2014.
82. Lassi ZS, Moin A, Bhutta ZA. Zinc supplementation for the prevention of pneumonia in children aged 2 months to 59 months. Cochrane Database of Systematic Reviews. 2016;2016. https://pubmed.ncbi.nlm.nih.gov/27915460/
83. Yakoob MY, Theodoratou E, Jabeen A, Imdad A, Eisele TP, Ferguson J, et al. Preventive zinc supplementation in developing countries: impact on mortality and morbidity due to diarrhea, pneumonia and malaria. BMC Public Health. 2011;11. https://pubmed.ncbi.nlm.nih.gov/21501441/
84. Bhutta ZA, Black RE, Brown KH, Meeks Gardner J, Gore S, Hidayat A, et al. Prevention of diarrhea and pneumonia by zinc supplementation in children in developing countries: Pooled analysis of randomized controlled trials. J Pediatr. 1999;135(6):689–97. https://pubmed.ncbi.nlm.nih.gov/10586170/
85. Abioye AI, Bromage S, Fawzi W. Effect of micronutrient supplements on influenza and other respiratory tract infections among adults: a systematic review and meta-analysis. BMJ Global Health. 2021;6. https://pubmed.ncbi.nlm.nih.gov/33472840/
86. Akhtar S, Das JK, Ismail T, Wahid M, Saeed W, Bhutta ZA. Nutritional perspectives for the prevention and mitigation of COVID-19. Nutr Rev. 2021;79(3):289–300. /pmc/articles/PMC7454773/
87. Wang MX, Win SS, Pang J. Zinc supplementation reduces common cold duration among healthy adults: A systematic review of randomized controlled trials with micronutrients supplementation. Am J Trop Med Hyg. 2020;103(1):86–99. /pmc/articles/PMC7356429/
88. Singh M, Das RR. Zinc for the common cold. Cochrane Database of Systematic Reviews; 2015; 2015. https://pubmed.ncbi.nlm.nih.gov/25924708/
89. Linday LA, Dolitsky JN, Shindledecker RD. Nutritional supplements as adjunctive therapy for children with chronic/recurrent sinusitis: pilot research. Int J Pediatr Otorhinolaryngol. 2004;68:785–93.
90. Arikan TA, Kelles M. Plasma selenium and cadmium levels in patients with chronic otitis media in a Turkish population and their relation to inflammation markers. 2011; https://doi.org/10.1007/s12011-018-1520-x
91. Nölke L, Mensing M, Krämer A, Hornberg C. Sociodemographic and health-(care-)related characteristics of online health information seekers: a cross-sectional German study. BMC Public Health. 15(1):31. http://www.pubmedcentral.nih.gov/articlerender.fcgi?artid=4312446&tool=pmcentrez&rendertype=abstract
92. Andermann A. Taking action on the social determinants of health in clinical practice: a framework for health professionals. CMAJ. Canadian Medical Association. 2016;188:E474–83. /pmc/articles/PMC5135524/
93. World Health Organization. Social determinants of health–Global. In [cited 2021 Mar 20]. https://www.who.int/teams/social-determinants-of-health
94. Shifler Bowers K, Francis E, Kraschnewski JL. The dual burden of malnutrition in the United States and the role of non-profit organizations. Preventive Medicine Reports. 2018;12:294–7. https://pubmed.ncbi.nlm.nih.gov/30406007/
95. Geers AE, Mitchell CM, Warner-Czyz A, Wang NY, Eisenberg LS. Early sign language exposure and cochlear implantation benefits. Pediatrics. 2017;140(1):20163489. www.aappublications.org/news
96. Hyde M, Punch R. The modes of communication used by children with cochlear implants and the role of sign in their lives. Am Ann Deaf. 2011;155(5):535–49. https://muse.jhu.edu/article/425310
97. Lazaridis E, Therres MK, Marsh RR. How is the Children's implant profile used in the Cochlear implant candidacy process? Int J Pediatr Otorhinolaryngol. 2010;74(4):412–5. https://doi.org/10.1016/j.ijporl.2010.01.022.
98. Sharma SD, Cushing SL, Papsin BC, Gordon KA. Hearing and speech benefits of cochlear implantation in children: a review of the literature. Int J Pediatr Otorhinolaryngol. 2020;133(2019):109984.

99. Quittner AL, Cruz I, Barker DH, Tobey E, Eisenberg LS, Niparko JK, et al. Effects of maternal sensitivity and cognitive and linguistic stimulation on cochlear implant users' language development over four years. J Pediatr. 2013;162(2):343–8.e3. http://www.ncbi.nlm.nih.gov/pubmed/22985723
100. Bergmark RW, Sedaghat AR. Disparities in health in the United States: an overview of the social determinants of health for otolaryngologists. Laryngoscope Investig Otolaryngol. 2017;2(4):187–93.
101. Engebretsen S, Sorrells R, Yi-Frazier JP, Early KB. Longitudinal quality of life improvement in underserved rural youth with obesity. Obes Sci Pract. 2016;2(4):444–55.
102. Al-Khudairy L, Loveman E, Colquitt JL, Mead E, Johnson RE, Fraser H, et al. Diet, physical activity and behavioural interventions for the treatment of overweight or obese adolescents aged 12 to 17 years. Cochrane Database Syst Rev. 2017;2017(6)
103. Zernotti ME, Pawankar R, Ansotegui I, Badellino H, Croce JS, Hossny E, et al. Otitis media with effusion and atopy: is there a causal relationship? World Allergy Organization Journal. 2017;10. /pmc/articles/PMC5684754/?report=abstract
104. Espinel AG, Shah RK, McCormick ME, Krakovitz PR, Boss EF. Patient satisfaction in pediatric surgical care: a systematic review. Otolaryngol–Head Neck Surg (United States). 2014;150(5):739–49.

Glossary

5-HHT	5-hydroxytryptamine transporter, also known as SERT—serotonin transporter. 5-HHT is a protein that transports serotonin from the synaptic cleft back to the pre-synaptic neuron, removing the serotonin effect on the post-synaptic neuron. 5-HHT is thought to play a role in some psychiatric disorders including anxiety, depression, alcoholism, and suicidal ideation. Inhibition of 5-HHT is the basis for the action of serotonin reuptake inhibitors.
5-HT-1A and 5-HT-2A	Serotonin receptors.
ABRS	Acute bacterial rhinosinusitis, an acute bacterial infection of the paranasal sinuses.
ACR	American College of Rheumatology. ACR has created criteria for fibromyalgia.
ACT	Acceptance and commitment therapy—a psychological treatment approach involving awareness and acceptance of present experience, in the service of being engaged in valued life activities.
ACTH	Adrenocorticotropic hormone. ACTH is made in the pituitary gland and controls the production of cortisol.
ACTTION	Addiction Clinical Trial Translations Innovations Opportunities and Networks. A public-private partnership with the US Food and Drug Administration involved in fibromyalgia, pain and addictions research.
AED	Antiepileptic drugs.
AIP	Adaptive processing model. Under AIP memories are activated from memory and lead to the resolution of stressful events.
AP	Antipsychotic.
AR	Allergic rhinitis.
ARS	Acute rhinosinusitis, a true infection of the sinuses associated with constant, often unilateral facial pain for less than 12 weeks, and rhinorrhea. See Table 14.2.
BoNT-A	Botulinum neurotoxin A.

© Editors 2023

B. W. Blakley, J. E. Blakley (eds.), *Functional Illness of the Head and Neck*,
https://doi.org/10.1007/978-3-031-12998-8

BZD Benzodiazepine.

CBD Cannabidiol. One of the active ingredients in cannabis thought to modulate seizures, inflammation and other actions.

CBT Cognitive behavioral therapy. CBT is a psychological approach to dealing with bothersome issues wherein the therapist tries to alter the patient's attitude about bothersome symptoms. Mindfulness-based cognitive therapy (MBCT) is a third-wave form of CBT.

CFS Chronic fatigue syndrome. A disorder that features significant fatigue, myalgia and cognitive difficulties.

CGRP Calcitonin gene-related peptide. A peptide that interacts with a transmembrane receptor for pain sensations involved in migraine and other chronic pain syndromes.

CK Creating kinase. CK is an enzyme derived from muscle, often used to assess muscle damage.

COMT Catechol-*O*-methyltransferase an enzyme that adds a methyl group to terminate the action of catecholamines such as epinephrine and norepinephrine. TMD may also relate to COMT dysfunction.

COX Cyclooxygenase. COX enzymes oxygenate arachidonic acid resulting in prostanoids (prostaglandins, prostacyclin and thromboxane). COX-1 generate prostanoids for functions such as GI tract protection whereas COX-2 generates prostanoids important in cancer and inflammation. Early NSAIDs inhibited both COX-1 and COX-2 but more COX-2 "selective" drugs have been developed including celecoxib, diclofenac meloxicam, rofecoxib and others.

CRH Corticotropin releasing hormone. CRH is involved in stress response and the immune system. CRH is synthesized in the hypothalamus, transported to the anterior pituitary and causes release of adrenocorticotropic hormone.

CRP C-reactive protein, a non-specific marker of inflammation.

CRPS Complex regional pain syndrome. CRPS, is a poorly understood chronic disorder consisting of pain, swelling, and skin changes. Type I CRPS is also called "reflex sympathetic dystrophy" (RSD) without causative lesions such as surgery or trauma and type II called causalgia, which has some evidence of nerve damage so is neuropathic pain.

CRS Chronic rhinosinusitis. See Table 14.2.

CT Computed tomography.

DASH Dietary Approaches to Stop Hypertension. DASH diets emphasize fruits, vegetables and low-fat dairy foods.

DGL Deglycyrrhizinated form of licorice. DGL avoids the mineralocorticoid effects of licorice.

DHI Dizziness Handicap Inventory. A standardized tool used to assess the severity of dizziness.

DSM-5 Diagnostic and Statistical Manual of Mental Disorders version 5.0. The DSM-5 is the standard classification and definition for mental disorders developed by the American Psychiatric Association.

EBM	Evidence-based medicine. EBM is the application of the best evidence available in decision-making for individual patients. Notes should be made that EBM (1) does not always require randomized clinical trial evidence, (2) decisions are made for individual patients in their unique set of circumstances and (3) is not a constant "cook-book" recipe to apply always.
EMDR	Eye Movement Desensitization and Reprocessing. A psychological treatment focusing simultaneously on images, thoughts, emotions and/or bodily sensations associated with a traumatic event with stimulation such as lateral eye movements across the visual field.
ESR	Erythrocyte sedimentation rate—non-specific marker of inflammation.
ESS	Endoscopic sinus surgery.
EULAR	European League Against Rheumatism.
EvestG	A technique for analysis of large datasets of neural events recorded from the ear canals, possibly useful in quantitatively assessing a variety of neurological disorders.
FDA	Food and Drug Administration.
FM	Fibromyalgia. A poorly understood disorder that features generalized muscle pain and significant fatigue.
FODMAP	A diet low in fermentable oligosaccharides, disaccharides, monosaccharides and polyols. These are short-chain carbohydrates that the small bowel may have difficulty absorbing. FODMAP diet is recommended for irritable bowel and other disorders.
FSS	Functional somatic syndrome. A description of categories of body symptoms frequently encountered in many areas of medical practice that have no well-defined structural organic pathology including some types of pain, dizziness, heart palpitations, gastrointestinal distress, weakness, and generalized fatigue.
GABA	Gamma-amino butyric acid. GABA is the major inhibitory neurotransmitter. Low levels of GABA are associated with anxiety, mood disorders and chronic pain. It is structurally similar to gabapentin. Pregabalin is a related drug but neither gabapentin nor pregabalin bind to GABA receptors. GABA-ergic refers to drugs or substances that increase the effect of GABA such as benzodiazepines, as well as gabapentin and pregabalin.
GAD	Generalized anxiety disorder.
GERD	Gastro-esophageal reflux disease. GERD results when stomach acid passes back into the esophagus and may underly many problems in the throat and perhaps the ears, sinuses.
GRBAS	Grade, roughness, breathiness, asthenia and strain scale.
HAs	Hearing aids.
HEPA	High efficiency particulate air. HEPA filters remove ultra-fine particles from the air and are often used minimize allergy symptoms.

HPA	Hypothalamic-pituitary-adrenal axis. HPA relates to stress, energy metabolism, neuropsychiatric and endocrine function. The HPA is neuroendocrine relationship among the hypothalamus, pituitary and adrenal glands. The HPA is the central regulator of several hormones including cortisol. Disruption of the HPA is important in stress responses. Some authors report that increased sensitivity of the glucocorticoid receptor is thought to cause post-traumatic stress syndrome controlled by the hypothalamic paraventricular nucleus (PVN).
ICAR	International Consensus Allergy and Rhinosinusitis.
ICHD-3	International Classification of Headache Disorders, 3rd edition.
Ig	Immunoglobulin. Immunglobulin subclasses include IgE, IgA, IgG, IgD and IgM.
IL	Interleukin. Interleukins are a type of cytokine that consist of signaling proteins involved in the inflammatory response and some tumor responses via the endogenous immune system, originally thought to arise only from white blood cells. IL is often followed by a number indicating its specific IL. For example "IL-6" is interleukin-6.
INCS	Intranasal corticosteroids. Typical examples include fluticasone, mometasone, and budesonide.
JFIQ	Fibromyalgia Impact Questionnaire.
LDL	Low density lipoproteins. LDLs are "bad" lipoproteins that are associated with atherosclerosis.
LDN	Low dose naltrexone.
Limbic system	The area of the brain involved in emotions and memory. The limbic system affects autonomic nervous system, endocrine system, feeding and basic instincts. Anatomically the limbic system consists of (1) the limbic lobe, which consist of the cingulate gyrus and parahippocampal gyrus on the medial aspect of the cerebral cortex, (2) hippocampus, (3) amygdala and (4) hypothalamus. The limbic system is responsible for anger, instinct, impulsive, and primitive actions and is typically inhibited by the frontal lobe in normal humans but less so in animals. The hippocampus, amygdala, and prefrontal cortex are sometimes called the "emotional triad."
MAO	Monoamine oxidase is an enzyme that terminates the function of serotonin and dopamine. MAO inhibitors are antidepressants with relatively high incidence of side-effects such as hypertension, particularly if dietary precautions such as avoidance of aged cheeses, sauerkraut, cured meats, draft beer and fermented soy products are not followed.
MBCT	Mindfulness-based cognitive therapy—a psychological approach that uses mindfulness meditation to encourage acceptance of the present moment without trying to change it, push the experience away or cling to it in combination with CBT principles such as noticing thought distortions, used to treat tinnitus and other problems.

MBSR Mindfulness-based stress reduction. MBSR is one emerging psychological treatment for chronic pain and other functional disorders that uses mindfulness mediation and yoga exercises to encourage acceptance of the present moment without trying to change it, push the experience away, or cling to it.

MDD Major depressive disorder. MDD requires at least 2 weeks of symptoms of depression plus one of: (1) Depressed mood: For children and adolescents, this can also be an irritable mood, (2) Diminished interest or loss of pleasure in almost all activities, (3) Significant weight change or appetite disturbance, (4) Sleep disturbance (insomnia or hypersomnia), (5) Psychomotor agitation or retardation, (6) Fatigue; loss of energy, (7) Feelings of worthlessness, (8) Diminished ability to think or concentrate; indecisiveness, (9) Recurrent thoughts of death, recurrent suicidal ideation without a specific plan, a suicide attempt, or a specific plan for committing suicide.

ME Myalgic encephalitis—an older term for chronic fatigue syndrome.

MHC Major histocompatibility complex, also called Human leukocyte antigen (HLA). MHC genes on chromosome 6 that code cell surface proteins important in tissue compatibility and inflammation, usually using T-cell mediated immunity, and tissue typing.

MTD Muscle tension dysphonia—a voice disorder characterized by tension in the laryngeal and paralaryngeal muscles.

NAR Non-allergic rhinitis.

NK Natural killer. Natural killer cells are a subset of T-lymphocytes, particularly important in the inflammatory response to some viral infections.

NK-T Natural killer T-lymphocyte cells. NKT cells are a sub-type of natural killer (NK) cells. NK cells are not antigen-specific whereas NKT cells are.

NMDA *N*-methyl-d-aspartate.

NMS Neuroleptic malignant syndrome.

NO Nitric oxide. NO has vasodilator, neurotransmitter and other physiologic properties such as possible antiviral activity. Nitric oxide is free radical with many physiologic purposes such as vasodilator, antithrombotic, anti-atherogenic, and complex effects on the central nervous system effects and inflammation.

NSAIDs Non-steroidal anti-inflammatory drugs. NSAIDS, which include aspirin, inhibit the cyclo-oxygenase enzymes I and II (COX-I and COX-II). NSAIDs are commonly used to treat pain but can have adverse reactions on GI mucosa, renal function, as well as platelet dysfunction in spite of the observation that NSAIDs, except for aspirin, may be associated with myocardial infarction. NSAIDs specific for COX-II inhibition, such as celecoxib, have fewer GI and platelet side effects than NSAIDs that inhibit both forms of COX. Rofecoxib is a selective COX-II inhibitor that was taken off the market in 2004 due to an increased incidence of myocardial events.

OSA Obstructive sleep apnea.

PAMP Pattern-associated molecular patterns. PAMPs are patterns of molecules, conserved within a family of microbes, that are sensed by the innate immune system to trigger a response. PAMPs may be glycans and are recognized by toll-like receptors (TLRs) and pattern recognition receptors (PRRs).

PNES Psychogenic nonepileptic seizures. An older term is "pseudo-seizures".

PPI Proton pump inhibitor. PPIs are a family of drugs that reduce stomach acid production by H^+/K^+ ATPase in the parietal cells of the stomach. Typical examples are omeprazole, pantoprazole, esomeprazole but there are many others.

PPPD Persistent postural-perceptual dizziness. PPPD is a form of dizziness recognized by some medical societies as a specific disease.

PRRs Pattern recognition receptors. PRRs are sensors of peptides foreign to the body that are found outside of bacterial or other foreign cells used by the innate immune system to trigger an immune response.

PTA Pure tone average. Generally defined as the average auditory threshold of 500, 1000 and 2000 Hz.

PTSD Post traumatic stress disorder.

PVCD Paradoxical vocal cord dysfunction.

PVN Hypothalamic paraventricular nucleus. PVN is a major regulator of the Hypothalamic-Pituitary-Adrenal axis (HPA).

RCT Randomized controlled trial. RCTs are accepted techniques for valid research studies. Some are placebo-controlled and/or doubleblinded as well.

REDOX Oxidation/reduction. REDOX chemistry involves the exchange of electrons between chemical species and is a central consideration in many forms of pathology.

RF Reticular formation, which is an important center in the brain in the center of the midbrain, pons and medulla that regulates sensory and motor information and level of arousal and consciousness.

RLS Restless legs syndrome.

rTMS Repetitive transcranial magnetic stimulation. rTMS involves application of electromagnetic pulses to the surface of the skull in induce changes in nerve function deep to the skull. rTMS has been used mainly to treat depression, but other psychological problems and tinnitus applications have also been reported.

SCD Specific Carbohydrate Diet. SCD is basically a gluten-*free, grain-free, lactose-free, and refined sugar-free diet intended to eliminate certain long-chain carbohydrates that may support unhealthy bacteria from the microbiome. SCD is often used to treat Crohn's disease, ulcerative colitis and other G.I. disorders.*

SNOOP Systemic, Neurologic, Onset, Older, Positional, Prior, Papilledema, Precipitated by—a mnemonic for red flags for headache features.

SNRIs Serotonin and norepinephrine reuptake inhibitors. SNRIs are a family of antidepressants but are useful in many forms of functional illness. Examples include duloxetine, milnacipran and venlafaxine.

SSCD Superior semicircular canal dehiscence.

SSRIs Selective serotonin reuptake inhibitors. SSRIs are a family of antidepressant drugs, but are also used for many forms of functional illness. Examples include citalopram, fluoxetine, fluvoxamine, sertraline and paroxetine.

SSS Symptom severity scale. One of two scales used to confirm the diagnosis of fibromyalgia. The other scale is the widespread pain index (WPI).

TACs Trigeminal autonomic cephalalgias. TACs include cluster, paroxysmal hemicrania and others associate with autonomic features such as epiphora, lacrimation, conjunctival injection, or rhinits.

TCA Tricyclic antidepressants. TCAs are older than SSRIs or SNRIs and are as effective for treatment of depression but have more side effects. The most common TCAs are amitriptyline and nortriptyline.

tDCS Transcranial direct current stimulation. tDCS is one of the electromagnetic therapies, mainly applied for depression but its use in other disorders is under investigation. tDCS has some similarities to rTMS but uses direct current applied to the surface of the skull rather than magnetic pulses.

TENS Transcutaneous electrical stimulation. Tens involves application of electric current to surface electrodes.

TFI Tinnitus functional index, a questionnaire recommended to assess the severity of tinnitus.

TH-1 T-helper-1 lymphocytes. TH-1 cells are important in autoimmune disease and relate to the microbiotia.

TH-2 T-helper-2 lymphocytes. TH-2 cells are important in allergy and helminth infections and should be in "balance" with TH-1 cells.

THC 9-tetrahydrocannabinol, one of the active ingredients in cannabis that is thought to be responsible for the "high" feeling of marijuana as well as other effects.

THI Tinnitus Handicap Inventory. A standard research tool to assess the *severity* of tinnitus.

TLRs Toll-like receptors. TLRs are proteins, often derived from microbes, *that are important initiators of the innate immune system.*

TM Tympanic membrane.

TMD Temporomandibular joint dysfunction.

TMJ Temporomandibular joint.

TN Trigeminal neuralgia.

TNF Tumor necrosis factor, tumor necrosis factor alpha (TNF-α), cachexin, or cachectin. TNF-α is a cytokine protein important in acute phase inflammation.

TRP Transient receptor potential. Phosphorylation of TRP receptor proteins, notably TRPV1 (transient receptor potential vanilloid 1) involved in sensation of unpleasant stimuli such as pain. TRPV1 is also the capsaicin receptor responsible for the hot sensation in foods such as chilli peppers.

TSH Thyroid stimulating hormone. TSH levels are commonly used to screen for thyroid diasease.

VAS Visual analog scale.

VHI-10 Voice Handicap Index.

VVM Visual vestibular mismatch. A type of dizziness arising from visual inmput, thought to arise from difficulty of the vestibular system to compensate for eye movements, similar to PPPD.

WPI Widespread Pain Index. One of two scales used to confirm the diagnosis of fibromyalgia. The other scale is the symptom severity scale (SSS).

WRS Word recognition score, an audiological measure of the percent of words that a subject is able to accurately repeat when delivered at an appropriate intensity.

YLDs Years lived with disability.

Index

© Editors 2023

B. W. Blakley, J. E. Blakley (eds.), *Functional Illness of the Head and Neck*,
https://doi.org/10.1007/978-3-031-12998-8

MIX
Papier aus verantwortungsvollen Quellen
Paper from responsible sources
FSC® C105338

If you have any concerns about our products,
you can contact us on
ProductSafety@springernature.com

In case Publisher is established outside the EU,
the EU authorized representative is:
Springer Nature Customer Service Center GmbH
Europaplatz 3, 69115 Heidelberg, Germany

Printed by Libri Plureos GmbH
in Hamburg, Germany